Internal vs. External Events	Emphasis on Group Factors Cohesion	Developmental Stages	Levels of Intervention		
			Individual	Interpersonal	Group
Emphasis on events within the group. Relational patterns inside and outside the group may be linked.	Strong emphasis: Cohesion is a condition facilitating the operation of other factors and a therapeutic factor in its own regard.	The therapist supports the group to achieving the level of maturity required for the establishment of group cohesiveness.	Assists members in identifying with other members.	The most essential interventions occur at this level to foster interpersonal learning.	Mass group commentaries are used to remove group-level resistances.
Both internal and external events explored.	Group cohesion, a necessary property for the group's work, is expected to fluctuate within and between stages.	The stages invite the reemergence and reworking of the conflicts that arise in individual development.	Interpretive comments linking past and present may occur.	Through feedback, members learn about the effects of their organizing schemas on their interpersonal worlds.	Used to build cohesiveness, identify conflicts at the group-level, and restore the group frame.
Affects and cognitions emerging within the moment are emphasized along with the external situations activating them.	In some groups, commonalities in members' automatic thoughts, etc. may be used to strengthen cohesion.	Stages may make certain schema more available for exploration.	Assists members in identifying automatic thoughts, conditional beliefs, and schemas.	Members receive feedback from others in the process of testing conditional beliefs and in role plays.	Didactic comments made to the entire group.
Problems emerging both inside and outside the group are solved.	Minimal emphasis; close-ended structure and well-defined goals and processes are likely to promote cohesion.	Stages may affect the problems members identify, the alternatives they generate, and the solutions they select.	Assists members in individual problem identification.	Members receive feedback both to help them identify problems and to role play solutions.	Didactic comments made to the entire group.

Introduction to
Group Therapy

Introduction to
Group Therapy

Virginia Brabender

JOHN WILEY & SONS, INC.

ISBN 0-471-37889-5

Printed in the United States of America.

10 9 8 7 6 5 4 3 2 1

To my kind, wise, and beautiful daughter,
Gabrielle Mercedes

This text is the product of 20 years of teaching group therapy. This time has been divided between the clinic and the classroom. In the first decade I worked as a senior staff psychologist at Friends Hospital, where I was involved in training psychology interns. I had the great pleasure of doing cotherapy with them and leading a group therapy seminar for them. Many of these interns came into their internship year with little or no academic preparation in group therapy. My task, then, was to help them master the essentials well enough to be able to function effectively as cotherapists in the inpatient groups. I am grateful to those 30 or so interns who gave me the opportunity to make concepts clear to them and to myself. I also had the responsibility of chairing the Group Psychotherapy Task Force, which oversaw all group therapy activities at the hospital and attempted to build a climate within the institution that was receptive to group therapy. As in most psychiatric hospitals, the range of psychological problems was great and the time available for their treatment increasingly small. My position required me to help the members of the task force think about how to effect a match between the needs and resources of the potential member, the time frame, and the format of the group. This theme of matching is one that is developed throughout this text.

In the second decade of my professional life (and through the present) I have served on the faculty of the doctor of psychology program of Widener University. For 6 years I was director of internship training in the doctoral program. I was responsible for the placement of 60 or so students in various mental health sites in the Philadelphia area each year. I also monitored their clinical experiences at these placements. These administrative activities have influenced my writing on group therapy. By visiting students in their placements, I had the privilege of seeing the types of groups in which they were involved. Field supervisors routinely gave me feedback on what knowledge base and skills best equipped students to function effectively in therapy groups. I also have had the responsibility of teaching Introduction to Group Psychotherapy. Students' comments and questions have played an important role in guiding this text. Some topics have received relatively great emphasis because students have told me that an extensive coverage of them was helpful. For example, detailed discussion of issues pertaining to payment for group therapy was based upon my students' expression of appreciation when this often anxiety-arousing topic was handled in-depth in class.

From both my classroom and administrative experience, I have observed that students are called upon to use a variety of approaches at their work at different sites. Some of the sites were strongly cognitive-behavioral, others, psychodynamic, and so on. My realization was that any adequate course and text must capture the richness of group therapy as it is practiced today. Otherwise, students receive the erroneous impression that there is one truth about the practice of group therapy. Accordingly, I wanted to create a text in which diverse approaches are presented. In the first part of this text I describe potential goals of a therapy group, the potential resources within the group to foster positive change, and the therapist interventions by which these resources can be accessed. Examples from different theoretical orientations are provided. However, my treatment of certain topics may tap one orientation more fully than others because within that orientation, a more articulated view of the topic has been achieved. For example, my presentation of therapist reactions relies heavily on psychodynamic concepts because relative to the other approaches, psychodynamic thinkers have, in my perception, made greater headway in this area. In talking about feedback, an interpersonal view is summoned for the same reason. Group therapy across theoretical orientations involves a set of special ethical and legal considerations, and these are described in Chapter 9.

In the second part of the book, four theoretical approaches to group therapy are featured. This set represents only a sample of the theoretical frameworks present in the contemporary landscape. In deciding which four approaches to use, I had two criteria. I wanted approaches that contrasted with one another along a variety of dimensions. For example, the models are different in terms of goals, therapist activities, resources of the group deployed, and time frame. I wanted to show the reader that despite the variation, certain factors unique to the therapy group relative to other modalities could be used in all approaches. In this way the reader could see the red thread across approaches, a thread that helps to identify what group therapy is. The other criterion is idiosyncratic. I wanted to write about models I have had the opportunity to use. During my tenure at Friends Hospital I was fortunate to have used cognitive-behavioral, interpersonal, and problem-solving approaches. I had distinguished colleagues such as Ronald Coleman with whom to discuss the nuances of the cognitive-behavioral approach. My psychology intern, John Ficken, collaborated in the development of a cognitive-behavioral eight-session model for the treatment of inpatients with anxiety and depression. The late Erich Coche was a great resource to me in my effort to learn about the problem-solving approach to groups. It was Erich who showed me the great potential of weaving psychodynamic concepts into the problem-solving approach, and this theme was developed further by my colleague at Hahnemann University and later at Widener University, George Spivack. In my own long-term outpatient work, I have found object-relations and interpersonal approaches extremely helpful. The decision to include approaches ranging from the highly structured to the relatively unstructured was based upon my perception that certain factors must be summoned to enable any group approach to be maximally effective. By presenting these approaches together, I hoped to encourage the student to attend to these factors in whatever approach he or she may use in clinical settings.

When I begin to teach Introduction to Group Therapy each year, my hope is that by the semester's end each student will be more enticed to obtain the field experiences, supervision, and advanced courses to be a full-fledged group therapist. My hope for the reader of this text is the same.

VIRGINIA BRABENDER

A book is a group event and this book is no less so than others. Throughout the two and a half years of its development, many have contributed to the project by reading chapters, raising questions, offering references, and most importantly, providing encouragement. To all of you, I express my gratitude.

For giving me the opportunity to write this text, I wish to thank Dr. Florence Kaslow who first raised the idea with me. I wish to thank the editorial staff at John Wiley. I am grateful to Jennifer Simon, Associate Publisher, who immeasurably contributed to this text as a pedagogical tool by urging me (albeit ever so gently) always to keep the student in mind. Isabel Pratt, Editorial Program Assistant, also provided careful reading of the text and offered wonderful suggestions. Thank you to Carol Herrington at Publications Development Company of Texas for so competently seeing the manuscript through the production process.

In pursuing this project, I was blessed with a large number of readers each one of whom brought a unique perspective to my work that enriched it enormously. My thanks go to Drs. Patricia Bricklin, Francine Deutsch, Amiram Elwork, Rachel Ginzberg, Howard Roback, and Bruce Zahn, and also to my terrific graduate assistants, Nicole Greenspan and Amy Gulino. Students in my third-Year Introduction to Group Psychotherapy course contributed inestimably by responding to the vignettes included in this book. Their excellent questions enabled me to know where I needed to write with greater clarity or extend my ideas further. My colleague, April Fallon, was always available to discuss the fine points of conducting group psychotherapy.

My group members over many years of practice have taught me a great deal about psychotherapy groups. They, too, are contributors to this text.

I would like to thank Carol Bricklin for her amazingly able assistance with the administrative aspects of this project (particularly on the day when six chapters were inadvertently erased) and Kim D'Elletto for her competently and cheerfully rendered secretarial help.

My good fortune is to work in a setting supportive of scholarship. I would like to thank the administration of Widener University and most specifically, Dean of the School of Human Service Professions, Stephen C. Wilhite, for supporting me in this project. I would like to thank my colleagues in the Institute for Graduate Clinical Psychology for providing me with the kind of intellectually stimulating environment that fosters creativity.

Thanks to my children, Jacob and Gabrielle, who in fact were not at all patient as I wrote (and I am glad that they weren't) and to my husband Arthur whose love, and confidence sustains me daily.

V.B.

Section Two
Change Processes

Chapter 3
Development of the Group

Chapter 4
Mechanisms of Change

Chapter 12

The Cognitive-Behavioral Approach   365

Chapter 13

Interpersonal Problem Solving   401

GROUP THERAPY

Introduction

Renata was rather surprised when her therapist suggested that she join a therapy group. The therapist noted, "I just think that in the long run, you will make more rapid progress if you have an opportunity to get some feedback from some other people." She initially put off making a decision. She told the therapist she was having financial problems. However, the truth was she was frightened. But the recommendation of her therapist was difficult to dismiss, particularly given the painful struggles she had with others in her life. Eventually, when Renata said she would "try" a group, her therapist referred her to a mixed-gender group in which members remained an average of 2¹/₂ years.

Renata went through a number of preparatory sessions with the group therapist and began to have a glimmering of enthusiasm about the group. However, this positive feeling was dashed during her first session. The group began with members asking Renata about herself. Several members noted that they did not want Renata to feel "pressured" during her first session. Renata made a few vague comments and was relieved when the group shifted to another topic. One member, Maureen, accused two other members of talking about her in her absence. Maureen claimed she sensed she "got on their nerves" during the previous session. When she went to her car afterwards, she saw the two members standing together. They lowered their voices as she passed. The members were adamant in their denial, and Maureen seemed mollified. However, a lengthy discussion was launched about the dangers and benefits of parking lot discussion. Renata, who had learned something about avoiding topics from her time in individual therapy, silently concluded that the other members of the group must be avoiding their difficulties by absorbing themselves with this parking lot chatter. She was therefore incredulous when the therapist said the group had hit upon an important issue. Feeling that the group occupied itself with too many trivialities, she thought about leaving but remembered she had promised her individual therapist she would give it a "fair shake."

In the next few weeks, Renata observed other members closely. Another relatively new member, Oscar, articulated his suspicion that his coworkers were trying to sabotage him by reporting minor mistakes of his to the boss. He didn't know what was provoking this mean-spiritedness. Renata felt she knew exactly what his co-workers found so provoking about him, for she had been irritated with his patronizing way of describing his position on a topic several times as if members couldn't understand him the first time. Moreover, she noticed that when he understood or agreed with something another member said, he acted as though what that person said was obvious. When he could not comprehend another's points, he acted as if the person were speaking nonsense. She decided to express these observations to him, and she did so with all the sensitivity she could muster. Oscar tried to interrupt her several times, but the other members told him he must give himself a chance to be helped. She summed up her comments by saying, "Oscar, the way you treat others makes them feel stupid, and no one likes that."

When she completed her comment, another member, Emma, who had been in the group for several years, said that when she joined the group, she related to others in much the same way Oscar did. She added that she came to realize that her haughty manner was just a manifestation of her certainty that she could not hold her own with others on a genuine level. She had to use means like Oscar's to avoid that moment when she would feel weak and inferior and be seen that way, too. Other members talked about similar behaviors they used to bolster themselves but that sometimes backfired. Oscar did not directly respond to Emma's comments or those of the other members, but he listened intently. He seemed, at least to Renata, to derive something from their input.

As the months went by, Renata felt positively about her group involvement. She didn't talk as much as many of the other members, but she knew that when she did speak, members valued what she said. Often, she would make an observation and other members would then chime in. Because she liked herself in the group, she looked forward to sessions greatly.

In one session, two members had been talking about their difficulties with one another. Cathy had said that she felt that Maureen was overbearing in her demeanor toward her and the other members. She further stated that she resented the blunt and intrusive way Maureen questioned her about sensitive matters. Maureen defended herself, saying that she was merely doing her job as a group member. Renata had always felt herself to be very aligned with Cathy, so she decided to speak up. "But I bet you have a lot of the same difficulties with people out there. Sure, we're expected to ask questions and pursue . . . things. But it's the way you do it. Did you ever hear the expression 'bull in a china shop'?"

Maureen looked at her with astonishment. ". . . A bull?" she exclaimed. Renata responded, "Well, I didn't literally mean . . . you just come on so strong." Maureen responded, "You want me to be like you? I can't be like you. I can't be prim and watch everything I say. Your comments come out like these . . . perfect little packages. I feel I have no idea who you really are or what you think about anything."

Tom broke in, "It may be true Renata is ultracareful, but that doesn't mean Maureen couldn't benefit from—"

Renata interrupted. "What do you mean by 'ultracareful'?"

Tom hesitated, "Well, I've been really grateful for some of your comments about me. Yet, in a way, I think Maureen hit the nail on the head when she talked about your weighing everything and not saying anything until you can say it with exactly the right words. You're never just . . . spontaneous in here, and if you're the same way out there, it's hard to picture you having any relationships that are more than just surface." Renata began to tear. The therapist asked Renata how she felt about Tom's and Maureen's comments. Renata said somewhat tremulously, "Well, I'm sort of shaken. . . . I just didn't expect it tonight." Tom said gently, "I didn't mean to upset you. It's just that I see you as . . . a bud that is almost, well, too delicate to open."

Cathy quickly interrupted, "That's okay, we're a bouquet of closed buds." The other members, including Renata, laughed.

Renata then said, "Tom, what do you think my being careful has to do with my relationships? You are right: My relationships never seem to amount to too much . . . so maybe it's good we're talking about this."

In the months that followed, Renata engaged in considerable work looking at her interpersonal style and how certain of her behaviors interfered with her ability to achieve an intimate relationship. She also came to understand some of the fears about closeness that underpinned these behaviors. For example, she discovered her own hidden expectation that in the context of an intimate relationship, she would discover hidden parts of herself that would elicit shame. In fact, over the course of her group participation, she learned about much within herself that might have evoked shame. However, because other members were talking about the same feelings and urges, her discoveries were almost tolerable.

There are many different approaches to group therapy, four of which will be discussed in this text in some detail. Many of the dominant approaches use certain resources for psychological growth that are potentially abundant in groups and less available in other modalities. The vignette that opens this chapter showcases some of these resources.

Renata's individual therapist identified one major resource present in group treatment: *feedback* (or the offering of reactions) from the other group members. Over time, Renata was able to learn from the other group members how they saw her and how they reacted affectively to their perceptions. A powerful feature of the group is the presence of a number of viewpoints. The reader may have noticed how Renata was presented with a particularly powerful stimulus when Tom joined with Maureen. She could have easily dismissed Maureen's input as defensiveness on Maureen's part. A component of it was defensive in that Maureen was fending off the narcissistic hurt of Renata's observation. However, when it was paired with Tom's comments, it became more of a force to reckon with.

Another resource highlighted by this example is the type of relationships available for exploration. A major dimension of group work is the availability of both peer relationships and relationships with authority. Furthermore, the diversity of personality characteristics of different members provides a range of stimuli to which each member may respond. In that way, a group provides something of the richness of the world outside the group and the environment achieves ecological validity (Brunswick, 1956). Because of their inherent heterogeneity, groups provide a context where members can exhibit and address the difficulties that may have motivated their desire for treatment.

The reader may have noticed in the vignette that the members of the group did not merely comment on others but identified with them. That is, they considered how behaviors, or a feeling or impulse giving rise to a behavior, could be found in their own person. Through this discovery of common ground, members are able to move toward a higher degree of acceptance of aspects of themselves. For example, Emma helped Oscar to accept both the fact of his insensitive social behaviors ("haughty," in her words) and the motive sustaining the behavior, self-protection. This knowledge that he was not unique in possessing these qualities made the recognition of these qualities far less of a challenge to his self-regard. In fact, by acknowledging their presence, he had the potential comfort, if not the downright pleasure, of joining with another person.

Another example is Cathy's use of Tom's closed bud metaphor. Through the development of a common set of images (Ettin, 1994), members are able to construct a net in which disturbing experiences can be both contained and further explored. This element of sharing is far less present in individual therapy. Because the therapist has a caretaking role, acknowledging commonalities with patients may be more disturbing than reassuring to them.

The reader may have noticed that the therapist made only a single comment. Members proceeded through lengthy exchanges that the therapist neither initiated nor sustained. The therapist's lack of evident activity does not mean that the therapist's role is unimportant. In fact, much of this text will be devoted to the activities of the therapist in the group and how they differ across models. Nonetheless, in many contemporary approaches, much of the work that is done is member centered. Because this group has undergone considerable development (see Chapter 3), it has acquired a mode of operation that enables members to be helpful to one another. The potential in any group of constructive member-to-member interaction is a feature that is unique to group therapy.

This vignette and the analysis following it are offered to give the reader a glimmering of the distinctiveness of this modality and a sense of why Renata's individual therapist might have believed that the group could make a special contribution to her realization of her therapeutic goals. The vignette serves as a foundation for our exploration of this modality because it generates such critical questions as: How can the special features of group therapy be amplified? What kinds of patients would be particularly able to benefit from the special features of this modality? Questions such as these will be addressed throughout this text.

Effectiveness of Group Therapy

The special features of group therapy are of interest only if they can be shown to produce positive change in group members. The effectiveness of therapy groups relative to no treatment at all, to a placebo condition, or to another modality—most typically, individual therapy—has been examined in a variety of studies. Fuhriman and Burlinghame (1994), in a survey of the outcome literature on group therapy, noted that it was not until the 1970s that such studies had sufficient methodological rigor to yield valid and reliable results. For example, samples had been assigned to groups not randomly but on the basis of convenience.

By the 1970s, an awareness of the importance of methodology led to the design of sounder studies. Gradually, a pattern emerged showing the effectiveness of group therapy. For example, Toseland and Siporin (1986) reviewed all of the studies to date that used group treatment with a symptomatically heterogeneous group of patients and met a set of methodological criteria. All of the studies had to have random assignment of subjects to the groups being compared, a control group, and independent and dependent variables measured by one or more standardized instruments.

The investigators found that out of the 32 studies that met these criteria, 24 (or 75 percent) showed that group therapy and individual therapy did not have differential effectiveness (although both were superior to no treatment or minimal treatment). In eight studies, group treatment was superior to no treatment or individual treatment. The investigators also found that in studies for which attendance data was available, the rate of premature termination was lower for group patients than for individual patients.

Additional light is shed on the effectiveness of group therapy from reviews based upon the meta-analytic method (Smith, Glass, & Miller, 1980). The meta-analytic method is based upon a standard quantitative index or *effect size* that represents each measure of an outcome study. The effect sizes are then averaged across measures and studies and compared to those of a control condition. In this way, the effect of a given modality such as group therapy can be compared to that of other modalities or no treatment. Existing reviews based on meta-analyses include investigations in which group and individual treatments were directly compared and those in which they were not, for example, studies in which only individual treatment was administered.

As Fuhriman and Burlingame note, out of seven meta-analytic studies, five found no difference between individual and group therapy (Miller & Berman, 1983; Robinson, Berman, & Neimeyer, 1990; Shapiro & Shapiro, 1982; Smith et al., 1980; Tillitski, 1990). (Shapiro and Shapiro report a slight superiority of individual therapy over group therapy. However, this is a statistically nonsignificant finding. Both individual and group treatments substantially exceeded couple/family therapy.) However, two meta-analytic studies showed a superiority of individual over group treatment. Fuhriman and Burlingame wondered what set apart the two studies in which groups fared more poorly than the others. By reviewing the specific studies included in the two meta-analytic investigations, they found that in the majority of studies representing the group modality, group therapy was used specifically because of its convenience. They write, "no attempt was made to incorporate or capitalize upon unique properties deemed therapeutic to the group format. . . . [The studies] can best be described as individual treatment in the presence of others" (p. 16).

What this pattern of findings among meta-analytic studies suggests is that group therapy has its own special elements that should be deployed in order to maximize its benefits. Furthermore, when these elements are activated, group treatment is effective on a variety of outcome measures relative to no treatment or minimal treatment. It also is at least of comparable effectiveness to other modalities such as individual therapy. The reader had an opportunity to see some of the unique properties of group therapy in the description of Renata's group experience, for example, feedback from peers and the discovery of shared experiences. These properties will be described more comprehensively and formally in subsequent chapters.

Efficiency of Group Therapy

From its earliest days, group therapy has been appreciated for its efficiency. One of the earliest group therapists, Edward Lazell at St. Elizabeth's Hospital, Washington, D.C., saw in group therapy a way of treating schizophrenic patients, who were so large in numbers that they could not possibly be seen individually. He convened large groups of patients to hear lectures he would deliver on psychoanalytic concepts and organized participants into discussion groups. After World War II, group therapy became a celebrated modality again because of its efficiency. Scheidlinger (1993) wrote, "Faced with many psychiatric casualties, a few military psychiatrists were forced to use group treatment methods through sheer necessity" (p. 3).

Today, the efficiency of group therapy continues to be one of its appealing attributes. We practice in an era in which treatment is limited by time. Time is restricted by third-party payers such as managed health care organizations that often reimburse only for a limited number of sessions. The length of treatment is also curtailed by patients themselves in search of quick relief. MacKenzie reviewed utilization patterns of mental health services and found that the majority of individuals receive fewer than eight sessions. Moreover, fewer than 15 percent are still in treatment beyond 6 months. One implication of this finding is that to be serviceable to the vast majority of mental health recipients, any modality must be able to produce positive effects within a very brief period of time. In the prior section in which the efficacy of group therapy was established, a number of reviews were cited. These reviews are based primarily on group therapy interventions that are either brief or short-term in nature. These studies overwhelmingly show that therapy groups can produce positive position changes in a relatively brief period.

The other respect in which group therapy is efficient is in its capacity to treat multiple patients simultaneously. Group therapy places less demand on staff resources relative to individual therapy. MacKenzie (1995) estimated that in a given health care system, 15 percent of the patients in the system will require long-term therapy (approximately 50 sessions). If these patients receive individual therapy, they will utilize 37 percent of staff resources. If these same patients are treated in group therapy, the percentage drops to 25, freeing up staff time for the much larger group of patients who require crisis intervention (approximately 8 sessions). Roller (1997) noted, "A group therapist can treat from two to three times as many patients in one-half to one-third of the time" (p. xiii). Because of the savings in staff time, some managed care companies may be willing to increase the number of sessions, enabling the accomplishment of more ambitious goals.

Because in group therapy multiple clients are seen at one time, fees for group therapy are almost always substantially lower than they are for individual therapy. Thus, one consequence of group therapy's efficiency is that it is more affordable for poorer persons.

Value of Group Therapy: Perceived and Actual

Given the findings in the research literature—findings that have been available for nearly two decades—it may seem paradoxical that in many environments, particularly outpatient treatment, group therapy is not perceived as the treatment of choice. If a given treatment is as effective as another and is more efficient (both in terms of the tenure of the person in treatment as well as the number of persons treated by a given therapist in an interval), then why should it not be used in preference to individual therapy? Why should not the training of mental health professionals in group therapy skills occur as early and as extensively as they do in individual therapy skills? The answer is that there is a disparity between the actual and perceived value of group therapy (MacKenzie, 1994; Steenbarger & Budman, 1996), a disparity for which there are at least several causes.

First, for many years, the uniqueness of group therapy in relation to other modalities was not fully appreciated, in many cases even by group therapists themselves let alone the community of mental health practitioners or, more broadly still, the public. The problem was the false assumption that the mechanism of change was the same in the two modalities. If the change-producing elements in both individual therapy and group therapy are identical, then the latter would seem to provide group members with a more diluted exposure to these elements than would individual therapy. Consider these two examples. Suppose a psychodynamic therapist identifies insight as the change-producing factor in any treatment. In individual therapy, it might seem that the patient, being the therapist's exclusive focus, would have greater opportunity to be the recipient of the kinds of interpretive comments that lead to insight. Furthermore, the therapist's more ample exposure to the historical and contemporary details of the patient's life outside of therapy would provide the basis for more finely hewn interpretations.

Another example is a therapist providing cognitive behavioral treatment. If the most critical element of the treatment is the identification of individual cognitions, then individual therapy would give the therapist a greater fund of material to formulate more precisely what these cognitions are relative to group therapy, where the time is divided among members.

In fact, when the processes in group therapy that are emphasized are the same processes available in individual therapy, the former is a weaker form of treatment relative to its potential. Individual therapy conducted in a group *is* less potent individual therapy. It is only when the interactional processes of group therapy are given center stage that this modality realizes its potential. As the contrasts among the meta-analytic studies show, when these interactional processes are the focus of therapists and members, group therapy is at least as effective as individual therapy. However, as long as mental health professionals do not fully appreciate the distinctiveness of the processes of group therapy, the disparity will exist between the perceived and actual value of this modality.

Another factor is cultural. Culture may account for why group therapy has failed to be understood in its particularity. Western culture, especially Western Anglo-Saxon culture and particularly since the Enlightenment, has placed high value upon the individual beyond that of the group, and upon individual fulfillment rather than the commonweal (Skolnick, 2000). In this culture, individual therapy is highly valued specifically because it centers upon the individual. That is, it has primacy because it focuses upon the primary social unit of the culture. This is very different from other cultures that place highest priority upon the group. For example, in Eastern culture, the group is highly valued and the individual is understood in terms of his or her connection with, and contribution to, the group.

The cost of the Western cultural perspective can be seen in the array of social problems that beset the United States and other Western countries. School violence is an example par excellence. While many aspects of this phenomenon are unknown, one common pattern is that a youth or subgroup of youths are scapegoated by their peers. The scapegoated persons respond to this psychological aggression with acts of physical violence. This problem is one of group dynamics. Although certainly the youths who take such action bring difficulties to school, the interactions they have with their peers in school are central to the violence that emerges. As the reader will see, scapegoating is one solution that groups readily use to solve their problems, and one task in a group's development is to acquire more mature, constructive means of problem solving.

Rutan and Stone (1993) identify another example of the cost of this cultural emphasis upon the individual to the neglect of larger social units such as the couple, the family, and the community. An emphasis upon the individual, and in particular, individual gratification, has led to the erosion of intimate, stable relationships:

> There has been a strong trend in modern society to value happiness now at the expense of deepened relationship and firm foundations (Lasch, 1979; Marin, 1975). "Doing your own thing" is no longer countercultural ethos. It has become part of the value system in all sectors and strata of society. The ready option today is to change the relationship rather than resolve the

conflicts. This tendency has become both the cause and the effect of the dramatic instability of modern marriages and family life (at present the risk of a marriage ending in divorce in the United States is approaching one in two). (Rutan & Stone, 1993, p. 6)

As every practitioner knows, one of the most common presenting complaints of individuals entering therapy is the sense of emptiness and meaninglessness that the failure to sustain relationships of substance produces.

While the cultural emphasis on individualism may hinder a full appreciation of the value of group therapy, it is also true that group therapy is ideally suited to treating the relationship afflictions that are so prevalent today. Within this modality, the individual is always in focus. However, in focus, too, is the individual's relationship to each other member and to the group as a whole. As individuals grow in the group, relationships grow, and the community grows.

Summary

In this chapter, a vignette highlighted many of the special features of group therapy. These features distinguish group therapy from individual therapy and to some extent from modalities such as couple and family therapy. These features include the giving and receiving of feedback about one's interpersonal style based upon immediate experiences with other members of the group. Other benefits include the multiplicity of perspectives on oneself, the availability of both peer and authority relationships for exploration, and members' identifications with one another's experience. This list is a partial one, which will be expanded throughout the course of the text.

The success of group therapy in effecting positive change in members has been investigated in many studies. Generally, these studies show that group therapy is as effective as individual therapy and in some cases more so. However, an examination of patterns of results across different meta-analytic studies suggests that group therapy is most likely to produce positive results when the features that distinguish it from other modalities are emphasized within the treatment.

The efficiency of group therapy is inherent given that one or two therapists can simultaneously treat multiple clients. This feature generally makes group therapy more affordable. However, another aspect of its efficiency is that positive outcomes can occur after relatively brief intervals. Of course, longer-term involvements provide the opportunity for additional benefits. The efficiency of group therapy makes it compatible with the emphasis within contemporary health-care delivery systems on cost containment.

There is a disparity between the perceived and actual value of group therapy in the eyes of the public and the mental health community. While the comparable if not superior effectiveness of group therapy in relation to individual therapy has been well established, group therapy continues to be seen as a less desirable alternative. Reasons for this disparity include a failure of the professional mental health community to realize the distinctive processes that are activated in the therapy group, and the emphasis in Western culture upon individualism. Despite this disparity, group therapy is highly tailored to contemporary societal and personal needs.

Goals of Group Therapy

Group therapy is a tool for effecting change. To employ this tool to its fullest advantage, a professional must know what types of changes it can effect. Consider the following three situations in which such knowledge about what groups can do would be necessary for good clinical decision making:

Situation 1

The director of a residential treatment center for persons with depressive disorders considers introducing a group therapy program to help individuals deal more effectively with depressive symptoms. However, the director is not a specialist on groups and is uncertain about what groups can do for depressed people.

Situation 2

An intake worker in a community mental health center interviews a 35-year-old man who complains of having difficulty maintaining employment. After inquiry about his success in different types of relationships, she forms a hypothesis that this person has conflictual feelings toward authority figures that give rise to hostile behaviors toward supervisors at work. She wonders whether this man could better resolve this conflict in a therapy group.

Situation 3

Two psychology interns were asked to run a therapy group in a crisis unit of a psychiatric hospital. While there had been various activity therapy groups, the unit had not had a therapy group in operation previously. The average group member was likely to remain in the group for four sessions, but some could be present for only a single session. The interns could not imagine that in such limited time, goals such as symptom reduction, conflict resolution, or skill acquisition would be realistic possibilities. They asked their supervisor whether in such a short interval, there was anything that a group could do for its members.

The professionals in all these situations are called upon to make a clinical decision based on their knowledge of what a group can do. As these examples suggest, it is not only the group therapist who must possess this knowledge. Essentially, any mental health administrator or clinician can make decisions more effectively by an awareness of the full scope of this modality.

In this chapter, we will discuss four areas of change that can be instigated by group therapy participation. Knowledge of these areas of change will help practitioners in several ways. First, therapists will be aided in selecting specific goals for a particular group, goals that will be relevant to the needs of the population the group is intended to serve. The psychology interns in Situation 3 would be able to formulate group goals for their inpatients other than those requiring the members' long-term involvement in the group. Second, therapists will better recognize when a group referral is warranted. For example, the intake worker in Situation 2 would know whether a group could serve the needs of the man with authority problems, or another individual afraid of driving over bridges, or still another who cannot sustain a long-term intimate relationship. Third, practitioners will be helped in identifying the distinctive contribution group therapy can make in a given setting. For example, on the unit providing treatment for persons with depression, a number of interventions are designed to relieve symptoms. A program director's awareness of the multiplicity of possible group goals will allow her to know that the group need not duplicate the contributions of other modalities.

Target Areas of Change

While the number of goals that can be pursued in a therapy group is virtually limitless, any given goal will for the most part fall under one or more of four target areas of change: interpersonal change, intrapsychic change, skill acquisition, and symptom relief. With some approaches to group therapy, change in a given target area will be conceptualized as leading to change in another. According to some approaches, for example, intrapsychic change is expected to lead to interpersonal and symptomatic change. In this case, the intrapsychic change is primary in that it is the object of interventions. The interpersonal and symptomatic changes are secondary in that they follow change in another target area. The distinction between primary and secondary changes is important because clarity about primary targets of change will help the therapist to plan effective interventions. An awareness of secondary targets of change enables the therapist to recognize the number of ways in which the effectiveness of an intervention can be measured.

Interpersonal Change

Through group participation, members can increase their capacities to have fulfilling, successful relationships. Chapter 1 gave an example of a therapy group whose members exhibited various behaviors that would be likely to alienate them from others. Our protagonist, Renata, exhibited an excessively cautious style of relating that created a sense of distance in her relationships. Over the course of the group, Renata showed more spontaneity in her relationships with other members, a spontaneity that would be expected to transfer to her relationships outside the group. Another member, Maureen, who showed a high level of intrusiveness in her approach to other members, might exhibit increased sensitivity to members' levels of willingness to disclose private aspects of themselves. The reader may also remember Oscar, whose condescending demeanor created trouble for him. Over the course of his group participation, Oscar might show a manner of interacting that is less peremptory and more respectful.

Is there any evidence that group therapy can foster interpersonal change? The relatively small number of studies addressing this question have generally supported the notion that group therapy participation can lead to healthier, more effective relationships. For example, an early study by Beard and Scott (1975) compared inpatients with chronic mental illness who participated in group therapy with those who did not, emphasizing the examination of communications. Relative to the control subjects, participants in the therapy group showed greater flexibility in social behaviors, a more accurate understanding of social situations, and a greater capacity to obtain feedback to correct their distorted ideas. Byrnes, Hansen, Malloy, Carter, and Curry (1999) found that adolescents in a group therapy program showed a reduction in rates of criminal charges (reflecting a decrease in antisocial behaviors). Carbonell and Parteleno-Barehmi

(1999) observed that participation in a 20-week psychodrama group led to less self-reported withdrawal in middle school girls who had experienced chronic stress or traumatic life events. Shechtman and Ben-David (1999) found that children participating in a 10-week group showed less aggressive activity relative to controls. Kilman et al. (1999) found that participation in a 3-day weekend group helped women with attachment difficulties report improved interpersonal styles and more secure attachments relative to controls.

Intrapsychic Change

A second area of possible change is intrapsychic. Here the effort is to effect a positive change in cognitive/emotional process and structures or in their organization and interrelationships. An axiom of the approaches emphasizing intrapsychic change is that for external change (such as in interpersonal behaviors) to occur in a way that is reasonably lasting and generalizable to circumstances outside the group, such change must take place in tandem with internal change. The nature of the internal change sought is critically dependent upon the particular model a therapist uses. However, for many approaches, part of the change sought is making unconscious aspects of the self conscious so that they can be integrated into the self.

For many approaches that emphasize intrapsychic change, conflict resolution is an important type of integration frequently enabled by group participation. A conflict occurs when two psychological elements create such an unendurable tension for the person that one element is banished from consciousness. For example, anger toward and dependency upon authority figures can create an intolerable tension for many people because the anger is seen as interfering with the person's ability to maintain the dependent tie. Consequently, the person may suppress his or her anger or the dependent urges. Conflict resolution can occur as the person comes to discover that, for example, anger need not lead to the destruction of the caring dimension of the relationship. Within group therapy, an important element is the recognition that arises that other members share in the kinds of experiences members find so dreadful. As Alonso and Swiller (1993) note, "Shame and guilt flourish best in the darkness of isolation" (p. viii).

In the vignette in Chapter 1, group members helped Oscar achieve awareness of the sense of insecurity about himself that underlay his patronizing interpersonal style. Possibly Oscar would develop upon this awareness by learning more about the conscious and unconscious bases of the insecurity. So, too, might Renata develop an awareness of the elements underlying her excessively cautious interpersonal style. For both Renata and Oscar, the newfound consciousness of the motives behind the self-protective style would make self-protection less necessary. Both Renata and Oscar will have "made friends" with the emotional elements they sought to banish, a change that (at least in theory) would lead to a more open posture in their relations with others.

Of all the areas of targeted change, that of intrapsychic change has been least subject to outcome evaluation, possibly because of the difficulty of measuring internal as opposed to external change. In fact, appropriate methodologies do exist. For example, several instruments with a psychological battery such as the Rorschach Inkblot Method and the Thematic Apperception Test provide considerable information about personality functioning (Stricker & Healey, 1990). However, the administration, scoring, and interpretation of data are extremely time-consuming. Frequently, investigators have sought to measure the consequences or effects of intrapsychic change, consequences such as reduced symptomatology or altered interpersonal behavior. For example, one team of investigators (Ends & Page, 1957) contrasted the success of inpatient male alcoholics in maintaining sobriety after participating in a psychoanalytic group, a client-centered group, a learning theory group, or a discussion group. Psychoanalytic and client-centered group participation led to a greater decrease in drinking episodes. However, the client-centered group members had lower hospital readmission rates than the psychoanalytic group over an 18-month interval. Investigators have surmised that if the group has been organized to foster certain internal changes that would lead to various external effects and the external effects occurred, then the internal changes must have taken place.

An example of a well-designed outcome study in which internal change was targeted was undertaken by Piper, McCallum, and Azim (1992), who investigated the effects of a short-term group for individuals who were having pathological grief reactions to a loss on a variety of aspects of their functioning. Group members participated in 12 sessions in which they explored the unconscious conflicts underlying their loss reactions and to resolve them successfully. Relative to a control group, the investigators found positive changes in the group members both at the end of treatment and at the 6-month follow-up. Positive symptomatic changes included diminished depression and increased self-esteem relative to control groups. Group members also exhibited enhanced interpersonal functioning such as an improvement in relationships with their family of origin.

Skill Acquisition

To function effectively within the environment, people require a large repertoire of skills; such skills can be acquired in the context of a therapy group. The targeted skills may be of a highly general nature such as problem solving or affect management, or they may be more specific such as smoking cessation, weight control, or the management of psychotic symptoms in the community. Groups that are designed to train members in a skill are typically based upon a deficit view of psychopathology (Kibel, 1987). Such a model embraces the notion that the difficulties individuals encounter in life, that is, their psychological problems, are due to developmental deficiencies. The group experience is designed to provide learning experiences to help people incorporate into their repertoire of coping abilities the essential adaptive skills they were unable to acquire in the course of normal development.

The success of skill acquisition groups is often assessed through determining whether members can exhibit the skill at a higher level of proficiency than when they entered the group and relative to a control group. Of interest also is whether members can retain the skill at a considerably later interval. However, often the assumption is made that the benefits of acquiring a skill are various. For example, the acquisition of improved problem-solving skills has been assumed to reduce the number of failures an individual may experience in everyday situations. Because failures may precipitate symptoms, a long-term effect of problem-solving group participation is symptom reduction, although symptom reduction is not the primary target of change.

Within the outcome literature, abundant evidence shows that groups targeted toward skill acquisition can achieve both their primary and secondary goals. The effectiveness of problem-solving groups has received considerable support. For example, Coche and Flick (1975) investigated the relative effectiveness of problem-solving training with inpatients of mixed diagnoses in an acute-care facility. Inpatients were assigned to play reading or problem-solving groups[1] or to typical hospital care without a group experience. In the problem-solving training group, members learned to use a five-step process of clarifying problems and identifying and choosing solutions. When compared with inpatients in the alternate groups, patients in the problem-solving group were able to "widen their horizons and think of more possibilities of resolution" (p. 27). Coche and Douglas (1977) found that relative to no group treatment and poetry reading controls, the problem-solving group produced greater improvement in members' impulse control, self-esteem, and feelings of competence.

Other skills that have been shown to be strengthened through group participation are: greater assertiveness (Zappe & Epstein, 1987) empathic listening (Fromme & Smallwood, 1983), initiating interactions (Fiedler, Orenstein, Chiles, Fritz, & Breitt, 1979), attention focusing (Massel, Corrigan, Liberman, & Milan, 1991), expressing negative feelings, compromising and negotiating (Douglas & Mueser, 1990), and discriminating appropriate from inappropriate self-disclosures (Foxx, McMorrow, Bittle, & Fenton, 1985).

Symptom Relief

A third area of potential change is in symptom relief. In considering a particular behavior or emotional reaction as a symptom, we are placing it within a diagnostic framework such as the *DSM-IV*. Because mental health settings frequently place great focus on symptoms (both because they often activate the need for treatment and establish its reimbursability), symptom reduction is a goal that has legitimacy to others. Both for this reason and for the reason that symptoms are relatively easy to measure, many studies have been done investigating the effectiveness of group therapy in diminishing a wide range of symptoms.

The evidence that group therapy can provide symptomatic reduction is overwhelming. Just to provide a small sampling, group therapy has led to the lessening of *depression* and *anxiety* in inpatient

---

[1] Assignment was not random. Every other week patients were assigned to the problem-solving training group and during the intervening weeks, patients were assigned to the control groups. While this procedure is not random, it is not evident that the assignment method introduced a variable, other than treatment, that would distinguish the groups from one another.

populations (e.g., Talbot et al., 1999; Zerhusen, Boyle, & Wilson, 1991) and outpatient populations (Kush & Fleming, 2000), and in persons suffering these symptoms in connection with various physical disorders. Examples of the latter are *irritable bowel syndrome* (Toner et al., 1998), *herpes* (Drob, Bernard, Lifshutz, & Nierenbergt, 1986), *metastatic breast cancer* (Fawzy, Fawzy, Arndt, & Pasnau, 1995), and *HIV infection* (Kelly et al., 1993). Other symptoms that have been shown to be treated effectively by group therapy are *obsessive-compulsive symptoms* (Fals-Stewart, Marks, & Schafer, 1993), *sexual dysfunction* (Stravinski et al., 1997), *post-traumatic stress syndrome* (Lubin, Loris, Burt, & Johnson, 1998), *substance abuse* (Eriksen, Bjornstad, & Grotestam, 1986), *paranoid ideation* (Talbot et al., 1999), and *social phobia* (Heimberg et al., 1990).

Perhaps more surprising than the psychological relief provided by group therapy is its capacity to provide physical relief. For example, participation in a group was shown to lead to lessened gastrointestinal symptoms in irritable bowel syndrome patients (Toner et al., 1998) and decreased mortality rates in persons with metastatic breast cancer (Fawzy & Fawzy, 1994; Spiegel, Bloom, Kraemer, & Gottheil, 1989).

The literature, however, is not wholly supportive of the value of group therapy. In some studies, group therapy was not associated with targeted symptom relief (e.g., Beutler, Frank, Schieber, Calvert, & Gaines, 1984) or improvement in health (e.g., Cunningham et al.'s 1998 finding of no difference in survival for breast cancer patients in group therapy relative to a control group). While we know that group therapy is effective with a vast range of symptoms, there may be some moderater variables that limit its effectiveness with certain patient populations under certain conditions. For example, cardiac patients with fibrillators did not show a diminishment in depression and anxiety as a function of participation in a therapy group relative to a waiting-list control group (Slovak, 2000). Although the literature has documented distress in this patient population (e.g., Pauli, Wiedemann, Dengler, Blaumann-Benninghoff, & Kuehlkamp, 1999), the psychological symptomotology may not have been at a threshold level in the particular sample used in the study to enable the demonstration of an effect. What is currently needed is an investigation of the particular conditions under which group therapy is most likely to be effective, particularly relative to other interventions of demonstrated efficacy.

Beyond the Four Target Areas of Change

Any effort to list the types of change that can be instigated by group therapy is necessarily incomplete. While this fourfold scheme of areas of changes covers many group therapy circumstances, other types of change may be appropriate for certain patient populations and treatment contexts.

For example, Yalom (1983) describes a model of group therapy for inpatients in short-term treatment. For the brief time members are in the group (sometimes only a single session!), interpersonal change is not a realistic goal. Establishing symptomatic relief as the goal would deprive group therapy of a distinctive role, given that many other interventions in the hospital are directed toward alleviating symptoms. Yalom proposed as an appropriate goal for an inpatient therapy group the cultivation in group members of a positive attitude toward therapy. If members have, upon leaving the hospital, a favorable attitude toward therapy in general, and group therapy specifically, they will be disposed toward engaging in more substantive work on an outpatient basis, work that may avert the need for further hospitalization.

The therapeutic objective that Yalom established for his group model, the objective of cultivating in members a positive attitude toward therapy, is highly compatible with the needs of a particular group of patients in a given setting for a delimited time frame. Yet, this objective does not fit neatly into the fourfold classification of target areas of change offered earlier. Indeed, while the classification scheme will comprehend many group situations, potential therapeutic objectives meeting the demands of this clinical situation will lie outside this scheme.

Another type of change sought relates to behavioral indicators of a general condition of well-being. For example, frequency of hospitalization, use of prn (*pro re nata*) medication doses, or visits to a medical practitioner for somatic complaints would fall into this category.

While many approaches to group therapy will embrace one of the four areas of change as primary and the others as secondary, in some cases, two or more areas may be primary. For example, there is a particular model of group therapy, social skills training, that focuses upon skill acquisition in the interpersonal realm. Within this model, the interpersonal and the skill-acquisition objectives blend together, with neither component being more primary than the other.

Summary

Therapy groups may be directed toward various types of changes. The main types of change are intrapsychic, interpersonal, skill acquisition, and symptom reduction. These areas are by no means mutually exclusive. In some groups, a change in one realm will instigate change in another. In other groups, change in two or more realms may proceed simultaneously. There are still other types of change that lie outside the list.

The empirical literature provides support for the conclusion that therapy groups have the potential for effecting change in multiple target areas. How the therapist develops goals within any particular target area is the topic of our next section.

Selection of Appropriate Goals for a Therapy Group

Groups are most effective when the therapist has a clear idea what the group is expected to accomplish. With such clarity, the therapist can arrange many of the specifics of the group such as length of session, frequency of meeting, and so on to ensure that these features are compatible with the group's goals. The therapist can also develop a set of interventions that are consistent with the group goals. Because the choice of goals determines so many other decisions about the group, it is typically the first component of the group design to be established. *Group design* is the specification of all of the features that define a group, including goals, characteristics of members, therapeutic processes, the time frame, and the elements of the contractual agreement between patient and therapist.

Hence, one of the most important steps a therapist can take in ensuring that a group experience will be helpful to its members is to think out with great care the group's objectives. In identifying goals, the therapist must be much more explicit than in specifying the target area of change. That is, to say that the group aims to reduce symptoms or to promote intrapsychic change is to say too little. Each target area of change has innumerable goal possibilities. For example, if the target area is intrapsychic, the therapist might design the group to help members work toward the development of more mature defenses, increased capacity to distinguish between internal experience and the outside world, increased self-esteem, and so on.

A group therapist may set upon a single goal or a set of goals. If the therapist is pursuing multiple goals, the therapist should be aware of the interrelationships among the goals. For example, suppose that in a short-term group experience, the therapist establishes two goals: (1) diminishing anxiety and (2) helping members to become aware of those feelings that he or she deems unacceptable. These goals are potentially but not necessarily incompatible. Certain methodologies may increase the member's anxiety as he or she becomes aware of disturbing feelings. By being aware of the possible conflict between these goals, the therapist can choose a methodology that avoids the conflict. The therapist is also well served by distinguishing between primary goals corresponding to primary targets of change and goals that are realized as a consequence of the achievement of the primary goals. The importance of the primary goals is that they will have the major (if not exclusive) role in determining interventions.

A critical step in establishing a goal for a group is to consider the entire context in which the group takes place. All group therapists operate within some context. For a group therapist working within an institution, the context is likely to be more apparent than it is to the practitioner operating in independent private practice. For the former, there is a known patient population, a set of other modalities included in the treatment package, the orientation of the unit, the values of the institution at large, and so on. For a therapist who is interested in beginning a therapy group in private practice, contextual factors are also important. For example, the mental health needs of the community that is served by the therapist, the reimbursability of certain types of services, and the therapist's competence level in running groups of various types are all important dimensions of the context.

The group therapist must also consider context so that the goal is compatible with the context. If the goal and the context are compatible, then the environment in which the group takes place is likely to be supportive. For example, taking into account the mental health needs of the community in establishing a group focus is likely to increase the chances of a robust flow of referrals to the group. In contrast, a group designed with oblivion to context is unlikely to find a nurturing home. In fact, in some instances, the environment will actively undermine the group's work, as can be seen in the following case example:

Dr. Wellington, a psychodynamically oriented therapist, took a position as staff psychologist on a short-term crisis unit. The unit was designed to assist patients in a speedy return to their levels of functioning prior to hospitalization. Key interventions were medication and problem-solving training of various types.

Dr. Wellington, noting that many of the patients were organized at the borderline level, developed a group to assist them in acquiring more mature defenses. When members would see others in all-good or all-bad terms, she worked to enable them to recognize the defensive component of their polarized experiences.

Staff observed that members appeared to enter the group sessions with much trepidation and leave with intensified hostility. When certain staff approached Dr. Wellington with concerns, she assured them that these reactions are a natural part of the therapeutic process. Over time, however, referrals to Dr. Wellington's group dwindled until Dr. Wellington was forced to rethink her stance.

Dr. Wellington is a therapist who, in planning her group, focused on only one feature of the therapeutic context to the neglect of many others. She considered the tendency of individuals at this level of functioning to use the primitive defense of splitting. (Splitting is a defense mechanism identified by object relations theorists [see Kernberg (1976) for a more extensive discussion of this concept] involving the defensive perception of others and of self as all good or all bad. This defense serves to protect the individual from the pain that can be experienced when the good and bad aspects of self and of others is experienced simultaneously.) A most important feature that she ignored was the time frame of the group. The goal of facilitating members' acquisition of more mature defenses is one that requires time beyond what is available in a short-term hospitalization. In fact, patients generally require hospitalization because they have lost access to the defenses that enabled their premorbid or usual level of functioning. Borderline patients at the time of hospitalization tend to show a developmentally early presplitting defensive style (Kibel, 1981). In fact, these patients must reacquire splitting before they can move on to more mature defensive styles. On a short-term basis, a more reasonable goal would have been to assist members in reaccessing their premorbid defenses. Such a goal would also have been more compatible with the mission of the unit, to restore patients to their previous levels of functioning.

Another dimension not addressed by Dr. Wellington is the theoretical orientation of the unit. On a surface level, there would seem to be an incompatibility between Dr. Wellington's psychodynamic effort to foster intrapsychic change and the unit's effort at skill building. While it is not necessarily the case that Dr. Wellington must work within a problem-solving paradigm, in fact, doing so may lead her to duplicate others' contributions, she must at least develop an approach with accompanying goals that is congruent with the unit's approach. Moreover, Dr. Wellington must help others on the treatment team to appreciate that the therapy group makes a contribution that is at once compatible but distinctive. It is not sufficient to design a context-sensitive group; the therapist must enlist the support of others in the context for the group that has been designed.

The example of Dr. Wellington provides the reader with an awareness of some of the variables that ought to be considered in identifying a reasonable set of goals for members to pursue in the course of a group. In the sections that follow, particular attention will be given to variables that must be explored in any treatment context: member, time, and therapist variables.

Member Variables

A group design should encompass a survey of all the features of the target population from which members will be drawn. What are potential members' needs and resources? Will their group attendance be voluntary? Are there ethnic/racial/social-class features that will affect their group work? What are their symptom patterns? All of these aspects of the population from which members will be drawn are important, and many will be taken up later in this text. However, in this section, we will consider a variable that has particular importance because it is a moderator variable—that is, a variable whose level affects the operation of other member variables. For example, if a member has a given symptom, how the member experiences that symptom will in part be determined by that member's status on this variable.

This key variable, the developmental level of personality organization (McWilliams, 1994), refers to the degree of maturity of basic personality processes such as reality testing, impulse control, affect modulation, defensive functioning, capacity to have intimate, fulfilling relationships, and so on. While each individual may show some variability across these functions, the person's developmental level would be his or her modal level of functioning in the various areas. While developmental level of personality organization is a continuous variable, for ease of exposition and comprehension, this continuum has been segmented into three categories: psychotic, borderline, and neurotic. Given any of the four target areas of change, the goals that are likely to be appropriate will vary depending on the extent to which the target population resides in each of these three categories.

To get a flavor for how the individual's level of personality organization may affect what goals may be appropriately pursued by the person in group therapy, the description of three individuals will be presented, each at a different developmental level. Following each description will be a discussion of the kinds of goals with the target areas of change that would be appropriate for each person.

Psychotic Level: In the following case, the potential group member shows a low level of development across many personality processes:

> *Frank is a 31-year-old man who lives in supervised housing. He suffers from auditory hallucinations, which are under fairly good control with medication. He says that with the medication, he still hears voices occasionally, but they don't bother him. He has an organized delusion about a group of people who are intending to harm him. In part, because he is uncertain about who is in this group, his interactions with others are minimal in his group home. Frank has a proneness to alcohol abuse, although for the past 6 months he has achieved sobriety. Frank has a fairly positive relationship with his caseworker, who finds Frank to be an endearing, earnest person. He feels that if Frank could make some headway in trusting others, he could hold a job, an accomplishment that would affect his self-esteem immeasurably. The caseworker has begun to discuss with Frank the possibility of joining a group.*

The caseworker identified Frank's difficulty with trust, an exceedingly common characteristic of persons at this developmental level. This difficulty has ramifications for potential goals in the intrapsychic and interpersonal target areas of change. From an intrapsychic standpoint, individuals at this level have a proneness to use primitive defenses that lead to serious distortions of reality. For example, *projection* is a defense by which individuals impose upon the outside world their own negative feelings and impulses. Certainly, Frank's persecutory delusion could be understood as a consequence of his extravagant use of projection. An appropriate goal for Frank, and for persons organized at his level, would be to acquire defenses that would involve less of a distortion of reality. Such an achievement would require greater tolerance on Frank's part of his own negative feelings so that he would not experience such an urgency to rid himself of them. By relieving others of the responsibility to be the bearers of his own negative contents, Frank would be freed up to have more trusting, positive relations with others.

As suggested in the previous discussion, Frank's achievement of the intrapsychic goals of the treatment would be likely to lead to favorable interpersonal changes. However, there are primary interpersonal goals that could be established for Frank as well. Oftentimes, persons at this developmental level lack the most basic relational skills such as initiating contact, expressing feelings and ideals, perceiving others' reactions, terminating contact, and so on. Group therapy can provide individuals at this level with the practice and feedback opportunities to acquire a new repertoire of social behaviors. Whereas the entire group may work toward the mastery of this repertoire, individuals may focus on identified areas of weakness. For example, Frank might address his tendency to conclude automatically that others wish to harm him. An individualized goal for Frank would be to learn how to collect and evaluate evidence to assess others' trustworthiness.

To some extent, with individuals at this developmental level, the target areas of interpersonal change and skill acquisition overlap considerably. Any of the interpersonal changes specified previously, such as initiating contact, could qualify as the development of a new skill. Yet, persons at this level show other deficits in relation to various activities necessary for adaptation to the environment (Bellack, Gold, & Buchanan, 1999). Registering information, organizing and remembering it, making judgments, solving problems, controlling emotional reactions, and delaying gratification are all skills that persons in this category benefit from cultivating.

Frank's symptoms are representative of those of persons at his developmental level. Hallucinations and delusions are examples of positive symptoms, which are behaviors whose presence contributes to a psychotic diagnosis. However, another symptom that is prominent is anxiety (McWilliams, 1994). These individuals are vulnerable to intense experiences of anxiety not only in response to the delusions and hallucinations but also to the chronic apprehensions about their own existence and identity. The most everyday stressors can challenge these persons' senses of themselves. Negative symptoms, also characteristic of this developmental level, are behaviors that represent an insufficiency in some adaptive activity. Examples are difficulty in abstract thinking, emotional withdrawal, apathy, and poor rapport (Andreason & Olsen, 1982).

In recent years, the effort at symptom reduction has been aimed at negative rather than positive symptoms. The reason for this emphasis is that many in the mental health community see antipsychotics as the treatment of choice for positive symptoms. However, group therapy has been used extensively to treat negative symptoms, particularly those that have a social component, such as withdrawal and apathy.

Frank's substance abuse, which represents a major problem for persons at this developmental level (Kosten & Ziedonis, 1997), is also a possible object of group intervention. However, the likelihood of substance abuse in this patient population also creates the need for the group therapist to establish and enforce a clear policy about the use of alcohol and other substances prior to group meetings.

Borderline Level: Individuals organized at this developmental level exhibit a lower level of impairment than psychotic individuals in certain key areas such as relation to reality. However, as highlighted in the following case illustration, they have great instability in their reactions to themselves and to others. This instability compromises their relationships and their capacities to enjoy a reliable sense of well-being:

> *Ernestine, a 22-year-old African American woman, had been referred for treatment by her Baptist minister, who had recently completed his religious training. He was frightened over the intensity of Ernestine's reactions to his behavior. Ernestine, a member of his congregation, approached him several months prior to the referral for spiritual counseling. Initially, the relationship seemed to be a warm and supportive one. However, the minister noted with some uneasiness a steady increase in the number of telephone calls he received from her requesting comfort for various losses and rebuffs.*
>
> *On one occasion, his failure to respond with alacrity to one of her messages on his answering machine led her to deliver fierce accusations about his level of commitment to his ministry. The anxiety evoked by this episode*

intensified upon his return from a weeklong vacation. Ernestine came in saying that she was worried she may be pregnant. She indicated that she was so distraught by his departure, she thought of killing herself. Instead, she comforted herself by spending time with a young man whom she had previously ignored when the minister was available. The minister felt he was in over his head and referred her for a psychiatric evaluation.

Ernestine's lability of feeling and instability of perception that were so disturbing to the young minister are hallmarks of persons at this developmental level.[2] The individuals are somewhat more aware of reality as others experience it than persons organized at a psychotic level. However, they exhibit erratic internal experience and behavior that is the result of their use of primitive defenses such as splitting to maintain whatever precarious sense of well-being they are able to achieve. Splitting entails the separation of positive from negative perceptions and feelings of others and self. For Ernestine, the good minister that comforted her was someone other than the depriving and abandoning minister who evoked her rage. Ernestine's acting out, in which she translates her internal impulses and feelings into behavior to avoid an intense and sustained experience of them, is also highly characteristic of this group.

Through her group participation, Ernestine would benefit from pursuing the intrapsychic goal of the acquisition of a defensive system that would preserve rather than undermine her positive relationships with others. For example, rather than separate the good minister from the bad minister, Ernestine would develop a more integrated perception of him as a person with negative and positive characteristics. Another intrapsychic goal is for Ernestine, through a greater tolerance of her own negative feelings, to exhibit a lessened tendency to engage in the acting out that so jeopardized not only her well-being but also her relationships.

Interpersonally, these individuals show a more substantial repertoire of skills than persons at the psychotic level. These include initiating contact, terminating contact, expressing feelings, and so on. However, relative to higher-functioning persons, they exhibit marked difficulty coordinating these behaviors in ways that will further their

---

[2] For individuals such as Ernestine who have a histrionic presentation, the lability will be very conspicuous. There are other personality styles (e.g., obsessive) that are less expressive. Hence, the lability will occur on a more internal level.

adaptation to any particular social situation. Ernestine exhibited such difficulty in her interaction with the minister. While she was able to enter a helping relationship with him, her demanding behaviors ultimately overwhelmed and frightened him. An interpersonal goal for Ernestine would be to gain an appreciation of the impact of her behavior on others and to acquire new ways of relating that would advance relationships rather than lead to their destruction.

A variety of goals in the area of skill development are highly relevant to this group of individuals, including improved impulse control, affect modulation, problem solving, and decision making. This population shows a wide range of symptoms, any of which could be a specific focus for their group participation. While affective symptoms and their management are very common objects of treatment in group therapy, difficulties in thinking and relation to reality, which are less of a concern in this population than those organized at a psychotic level, are more infrequently the basis for symptom-oriented goals.

Neurotic Level: Persons at the next developmental level are distinguished from earlier levels by their more mature defensive system, a system that allows for a more accurate perception of others and a greater capacity to accept responsibility for difficulties:

Roy is a well-educated and successful businessman in his mid-30s. Part of his success was attributable to his excellent interpersonal skills. Coworkers saw him as considerate, engaging, and reliable. He perceived himself as far less successful in more intimate relationships, and his recent past was a good illustration. For some time, his long-standing girlfriend had been suggesting entering into a more committed relationship, but he felt greater uneasiness about taking this step. He felt trapped because he was certain that if he did not take the requested step, she would leave him. During this period, he noticed his burgeoning interest in another woman. He began to see both women, each in a clandestine way. However, one evening when he was with one woman in his apartment, the other came to visit. Each woman, feeling angry and betrayed, ended her involvement with him.

Roy sought out therapy and ultimately group therapy, because he recognized that his inability to make a decision led him to embark on a course of action destructive to all participants. He recognized that he did not understand his indecision. He also feared that his unawareness would lead him to repeat such episodes.

Roy can be distinguished from Frank and Ernestine in the level of insight that he brought to therapy. He showed a capacity to recognize that the difficulties in his life were not the result of the actions or characteristics of external figures (such as the women he was seeing) but of his own concerns, apparent or hidden. Such a capacity does not preclude his engagement in less mature modes of responding. For example, his flight into the new relationship bore some resemblance to Ernestine's embarkment on a new relationship after the departure of the minister.

Through his group participation, Roy would benefit from pursuing the intrapsychic goal of understanding and resolving conflicts related to establishing an intimate tie with others. Through group participation, he might come to recognize some unconscious fears about the risks of establishing an intimate tie with another and challenging these fears in terms of their likely basis in reality. For individuals at his developmental level, the conflicts that need to be addressed in treatment often have a more specific character than for persons at the earlier levels. In an interview, it is not at all unusual to hear, "I can't understand why I can have so many close friends and not be able to find a relationship with the opposite sex" or "I do fine with my co-workers but I can't get along with my boss."

Persons organized at the neurotic level typically have a wide range of skills and a capacity to use them in a coordinated way with sensitivity to the demands of the social situation in which they find themselves. Nonetheless, potential group members are likely to show less effective interpersonal behaviors in certain situations. For example, some persons who are capable of asserting their needs may be less able to do so when the other person is angry. The goal would be to help the individual to learn more about the challenging interpersonal circumstance and to function more successfully in it than they had prior to group participation.

In a similar way, any skills-training groups are likely to have a more specific character than groups for psychotic or borderline groups. Whereas impulse control might be the skill cultivated in a group of borderline-level members, group members organized at the neurotic level might address the management of specific impulses such as the impulse to eat, to smoke, to gamble, and so on.

Persons organized at the neurotic level have the array of symptoms that can be seen in a borderline-level population. For example, both Ernestine and Roy experienced some measure of depression, the amelioration of which could be a goal of their group participation. Probably the central difference between borderline-level and neurotic-level patients is the perspective each has on their symptoms. Neurotics are more likely than borderline-level persons to see the locus of responsibility for symptoms within themselves. For example, Roy realized that his mishandling of his relationships led to his loss of relationships. They also recognize that the amelioration of a symptom can be effected only by their own efforts. The borderline-level person is more likely to see the symptoms as being controlled by external factors.

The implication of this distinction is that it is simpler to establish a goal of symptom amelioration for neurotics than for borderline-level individuals. For the latter, the goal must be not only the treatment of the symptom but also the cultivation of the motivation to address the symptom through psychological work. Because neurotic-level individuals have a much greater capacity to enter into a therapeutic alliance and greater motivation to engage in psychological work, the goal of symptom reduction can be pursued more directly.

The developmental level of personality organization has been discussed in some detail because it is a prime concern for the group therapist designing a group format for a given population. This awareness will aid immeasurably in helping the therapist to develop an appropriate group design for an individual population. However, once a group design has been developed, many other variables must be considered to determine if a given individual is suited to a group. For example, does the group member have personal goals that are compatible with the goals of the group (Schoenholtz-Read, 1994)? If a group is organized to foster intrapsychic change and a potential group member wishes only to have relief from anxiety, then there may not be a match between the group and the individual. Whereas the present chapter focuses on the development of goals in terms of the group design, in Chapter 8 we consider how a given candidate might be evaluated for a particular group.

Temporal Factors

In this era of managed care, prospective group members often can feasibly pursue therapy only for a limited time. In deciding upon a set of goals for a group, the therapist must consider how much time is likely to be available for the group to do its work. Some goals inherently require a long-term participation in group therapy, while others can be achieved over a relatively brief period. The therapist has to make a realistic appraisal of what is possible in a given time frame. In doing so, it may be of benefit to use MacKenzie's (1995) tripartite scheme for categorizing groups on a temporal basis into crisis intervention (two months or less), short-term group therapy (8 to 25 sessions), and long-term group therapy (beyond 6 months). MacKenzie notes that crisis intervention groups can work toward goals associated with the person's return to his or her usual level of functioning. Such groups are helpful to basically healthy individuals who have faced challenging life events. MacKenzie also notes that in time-limited therapy, it is possible to accommodate individuals in greater distress and with problems of a more long-standing nature than in crisis intervention groups. Finally, longer term treatment is helpful to two types of individuals. The first type is an individual who requires time-unlimited support and containment to avert regression and hospitalization. The other type is a person who has severe difficulties (e.g., persons organized at the borderline level) but who can eventually leave treatment and function adequately.

Sometimes the research literature can be useful in assisting the therapist in recognizing what goals can be reached within different time frames. For example, does intrapsychic change require long-term group participation? Earlier in this chapter, an outcome study by Piper et al. (1992) was described in which the effects of a 12-week group on the resolution of loss-related conflicts were studied. As noted earlier, the investigators found that members received a variety of benefits that lasted over a six-month period. This finding establishes that certain intrapsychic goals can be fulfilled in a short-term time frame. In the areas of skill training and symptom reduction, the greater amount of research provides more direction about the needed time frame for certain goals to be realized. For example, studies on cognitive-behavioral groups have generally shown that between 12 and 20 sessions are needed for significant symptom reduction to occur (Brabender & Fallon, 1993).

What if a research base does not exist to guide the therapist in designing a group faced with a temporal limit? To some extent, a trial-and-error process may be necessary in which a goal is divided into subgoals and an experimental process undertaken to see how many subgoals can be achieved within a given time. For example, social skills training groups take a complex interpersonal behavior

such as initiating a conversation and divide it into component behaviors. Any one of these behaviors may constitute a goal for a
member's participation. In some populations, it is not uncommon
for an individual to have brief but frequent intervals of therapy.
Each interval offers an opportunity to work on a new component
behavior of a larger social skill.

The tenure of members' participation also has relevance to another aspect of goal setting: the extent to which goals are highly
variable from member to member or are shared goals. All other factors being equal, the less time the group has, the less individualized
the goals of the group can be. When goals are shared, a given intervention will have relevance for multiple members of the group. In
the 12-session loss groups run by Piper et al. (1992), the therapist
was able to make interpretations about loss-related reactions that
were applicable to each member of the group. The success of the
group in such a short-term time frame was likely the result in part of
its delimited focus.

The Therapist

Different theoretical orientations are associated with different target areas of change. For example, psychodynamic/psychoanalytic
orientations emphasize the importance of intrapsychic change. Behavioral approaches are more likely to emphasize symptomatic
change and, in some instances, skill acquisition. When therapists
come to the enterprise of designing a group, their theoretical orientations are going to be very important in determining what target
area of change seems more worthwhile to pursue. Theoretical orientations should inform the decision of goal setting because otherwise
the therapist may work without conviction. This does not mean that
the therapist should be heedless of the empirical literature showing
whether a particular approach guided by a given theoretical orientation leads to the fulfillment of a therapeutic goal. However, there is
no compelling support for theoretical monotheism within the empirical literature: Many approaches have been shown to be effective.
Therefore, the goal that one should pursue should be based both on
a consideration of what theoretical orientations are most compelling
and on the empirical research.

The personality of the therapist is also important in goal setting.
Different goals involve different types and levels of activity on the

part of the group therapist. In this context, activity refers to interventions that can be witnessed by others, not the mental activity of the therapist. For example, skill acquisition tends to involve a high level of activity on the part of the therapist, some of which is teaching. Some therapists' temperaments and personalities are going to be more suited to this kind of therapeutic activity than others. Unfortunately, in North America and abroad, the study of the person of the group therapist has been a relatively neglected area (Dies, 1993).

Broader Therapeutic Context

Earlier in this chapter an example was given of a therapist who neglected to consider the theoretical orientation and goals of the unit of the psychiatric hospital in which she was designing a group. The theoretical orientation, goals, and values of the setting are of paramount importance in deciding upon the goals for a particular therapy group. For therapists who have been operating within a given treatment context for a protracted period, this process of considering context may be automatic and barely conscious. For the therapist who is coming into a context from another environment—for example, a therapist who has been hired to run therapy groups in a residential treatment center and performs only that function— the process must be much more explicit. Failure to consider the context will lead any group, however well designed otherwise, to founder.

Summary

In this chapter, we discussed the importance of the group therapist's having a clear understanding of the goals of a group he or she plans to lead and conveying this understanding to potential members. Many goals toward which group work can be directed fall under one or more target areas of change: interpersonal change, intrapsychic change, skill acquisition, and symptom reduction. Often, change in one area will precipitate change in another. There is empirical evidence that therapy groups can effect change in all four target areas. However, probably because of the greater ease of measuring some types of change relative to others, the most substantial evidence exists in the area of symptoms relief and skill acquisition.

The therapist's establishment of the goals of the group should rest upon a variety of factors such as the features of the target population (particularly the developmental level of personality organization), the time frame, the personality and intellectual characteristics of the therapist, and the context of treatment. The establishment of goals in the design of the group can be done at a sufficient level of generality to allow latitude for their tailoring to the needs of individual members.

CHANGE PROCESSES

Development of the Group

Now that the reader has a sense of the kinds of goals that can be pursued in a group, the question of "how" arises. How does a group therapist move the group toward its goals? Chapters 3 and 4 describe the resources available within the group that the therapist can mobilize. Chapter 3 takes a longitudinal perspective, outlining how a group changes over time and the implications of these changes for a group accomplishing its objectives. In Chapter 4, from a more cross-sectional view, we examine the potential resources available at any point in time. Chapter 5 explores the role of the therapist in unlocking and capitalizing upon the resources.

Basic Developmental Concepts

Whether it is a therapy group, a group of children in a third-grade class, or a team of scientists collaborating on a nuclear fission project, a remarkable aspect of any group is its capacity for growth or development. Consider, for example, the exchanges in a therapy group that had been meeting for two months:

> *The therapist announced that she would not be able to meet with the group for the next two weeks on their usual meeting night. She posed a question: Would members be able to meet on another night? The ensuing discussion was brief. After some preliminary efforts to find an alternate day, one member strongly put forth the sentiment that the group, having met for two months, could use a break. Other members seemed to go along with this notion, but neither embraced it nor put forth a competing proposal.*

This group response can be contrasted with that of the same group that had now been meeting for eight months:

> *Upon being informed by the therapist that she could not meet with the group on that day the following week, members discussed whether the group should be rescheduled to another night. One member said it would be good to get a break from the tension associated with some of the difficult issues the group had been addressing. Another member said she thought that a break would be too disruptive to the group's work. Another said she was afraid that if there were a break, she would "play it safe" the week before it; otherwise, if she took a significant risk, she would be left with the fallout for several weeks. Members then began a very focused discussion of alternate dates and arrived at a viable plan for maintaining the continuity of the group.*

The reader can see that the group responded very differently to the same problem at two different points in time. In the first instance, the group assumed a rather dependent stance, allowing one especially assertive member to take control of the discussion. In the second instance, different points of view were expressed. The resultant solution seemed much more the product of members' collaboration than in the first instance. Most observers of these two sessions would see the second group as exhibiting greater maturity than the first.

Social scientists, including clinicians, having observed all types of groups, have found that the potential for development is a universal attribute of groups in much the same way that development is a potential of each human person. Development has both quantitative and qualitative aspects. From a quantitative perspective, observers of group development have noted that over time groups become more complex (Agazarian & Peters, 1981). For example, the group we considered achieved greater complexity in that members were better able to allow different and opposite elements to enter the group's discussion. Over time, groups also tend to become more independent. Whereas in the earlier session of our example, group members were willing to defer to one member's wishes, in the later session decision making was far more collaborative. Also over time members become more engaged with one another and less prone to avoid important issues (MacKenzie, 1983).

While the mature group may differ from a newly formed group on a variety of variables, these differences do not do justice to all aspects of developmental phenomena. For example, there is a period in the life of a group after the group has been meeting for more than a brief duration in which members appear to be more dependent upon the leader than when they entered the group. Whereas members' earliest manifestations of dependency may be subtle, as the group progresses they become direct and aggressive. Hence, development or growth cannot accurately or comprehensively be understood only as a continuous linear progression along one or more dimensions. Rather, an intensive study of groups over time has led many (e.g., MacKenzie, 1987)[1] to believe that the group's growth is much like the psychological growth of the person in that it is organized in stages. A stage is a period of a group's life that is defined by a given distinctive set of internal and external boundaries. The notion of a boundary is one that is extremely important to the understanding of therapy groups and, hence, will be discussed in some detail.

Boundaries of the Group

The concept of *boundary* is one that has been incorporated into group developmental theory from general systems theory (von Bertalanffy, 1950). General systems theory is a "scientific model that describes the organization, workings, and interrelationships of living systems" (Brabender & Fallon, 1993, p. 185). General systems theory applies to group therapy because all groups are living systems (Agazarian & Peters, 1981; Durkin, 1981). A group is defined by its boundary with the external environment. For example, suppose a therapy group for adolescents whose parents have recently divorced was organized in a school setting. The *external boundary* will determine who is and who is not included in the group. For example, the external boundary would establish that children whose parents were not divorced could not be included in the group.

From stage to stage, the external boundary changes in its permeability. *Permeability* refers to the extent to which information can pass from the group to the broader environment and from the broader environment to the group. For example, suppose members of a school-based group became angry at the therapist and acted rebelliously in class following a group session. In this instance, the

---

[1] MacKenzie (1987) examined four time-limited outpatient therapy groups and found that the variables of self-revelation and psychological work changed in nonlinear ways over more than 20 sessions.

external boundary between the group and the broader environment would be conceptualized as having a high level of permeability. In some periods in the life of a group permeability is extremely high, whereas in others very little information leaves or enters the group.

Concept of Subgrouping

Also significant, however, are the shifts that occur in the internal boundaries from stage to stage. According to general systems theory, as groups mature, they increase in complexity, a phenomenon alluded to earlier. Increasing complexity occurs through a process of differentiation and integration. Differentiation is a process by which the group system divides into subsystems or subgroups, thereby establishing the *internal boundaries* of the group. For example, members could subgroup on the basis of their political beliefs, religion, or race. From a developmental perspective, however, the subgrouping that is most germane to the group's growth is its subgrouping in relation to key conflicts that sequentially emerge in the group. These conflicts are basic issues people have in relation to other people. Should I trust the people in this group? Should I depend upon them? Should I allow myself to become intimate with them? As each of these issues emerge, members inevitably take different positions on them. Individuals who perceive themselves as having similar positions on these issues will come together as a subgroup (Bennis & Shepard, 1956). Through their connection with one another in a subgroup, members achieve the solace of being validated by others. This validation fortifies members in exploring and expressing more fully the nuances of their positions.

The polar positions that emerge in the group on each issue exist not only within the group but within each group member. For example, at one point in the life of the group, members will question whether they should accomplish the goals of the group by looking to the leader for protection and gratification or whether they should operate more independently. Typically, a subgroup will emerge of those members who take a strongly dependent stance and another of those who eschew dependency upon the leader, a position known as *counterdependent* (Bennis & Shepard, 1956). Whether a given member allies with one position or the other, both positions have some representation within the psychological life of each group member. Both the longing to depend upon another and the wish to be self-sufficient are universal elements of human psychology. Hence, the conflict that exists at the level of the group is mirrored within each person. Within general systems theory, this phenomenon is known as an *isomorphy,* in which a structural or functional feature is repeated within every system in a hierarchy of systems. The individual group member is a subsystem of the subgroup. The subgroup is a subsystem of the group as a whole. The group is a subsystem of some larger system (to use the earlier example, the school system). This is an example of a *hierarchy of systems* and embedded subsystems.

If members have represented within themselves both positions, why do members not identify with both positions? In other words, why do subgroups form? Subgroups form because they serve a defensive purpose. While some members may be able to accept the presence of both sides of a conflict within themselves, others cannot. One side of the conflict may be a psychological element that is unacceptable to the individual. For example, some people cannot feel good about themselves if they experience themselves as having anger. Other people find their wish to feel close to another person as discrepant with their view of what they ought to be. By seeing these unacceptable elements as residing not within themselves but within a subgroup of the group, these members are able to deny their presence within themselves.

As subgroups form in relation to basic issues, the process of differentiation continues within each subgroup (Agazarian, 1997). For example, members who have taken a counterdependent stance in relation to the leader will in natural course begin to recognize differences in their positions. Some may begin to perceive that they are less adamant about the perils of depending upon authority than others in the subgroup. Members of a subgroup might recognize that among themselves they have different ways of being self-sufficient. As members within a subgroup distinguish themselves from others, they become better able to identify with the position of the other subgroups. For example, members of a counterdependent subgroup achieve greater ability to identify with the positions of members in the dependent subgroup.

Movement toward Integration

The differentiation within each subgroup culminates in the dissolution of the subgrouping structure. That is, members gradually come to accept that within themselves there are facets and elements that resonate to the position of the alternate subgroups. They thereby no longer need the subgrouping structure to defend against heretofore threatening psychological elements. This dissolution represents a developmental achievement for the members of the group because it signifies that members have acquired tolerance of a greater range of their own psychological contents than when they had entered the stage. This shift is effected not only through the process of differentiation but also through the process of integration. *Integration* is the reconciliation of diverse and contradictory psychological contents.

This developmental achievement has consequences that are at once intrapsychic and social. The intrapsychic consequence is that individuals are able to use more of their internal resources for adaptation than for defending against parts of the self that are unacceptable to the self. Suppose a group member is in a problem-solving group in which the learning of new skills is at the core of the treatment. Such a group member would be able to take greater advantage of the instruction within the sessions if he or she were to be relatively unfettered by the internal demand to deny psychological elements that are part of his or her psychology.

The social consequence is that the group member need not use other people as defensive opportunities for the placement of aspects of the self that are perceived by the self as negative and unacceptable. This defensive use of others is referred to as projective identification (Goldstein, 1991; Ogden, 1979). *Projective identification* involves projecting onto another a part of the self that is unwanted and then treating the other in a manner consistent with the projection. Such treatment may induce in the other feelings and behaviors consistent with the projection. For example, if Carlos finds his own sadistic impulses to be intolerable, he may see Janine as being sadistic, treat her as a sadist, and succeed in maneuvering her into feeling so. While Carlos has divested himself of something unwanted, his relationship with Janine has inevitably taken a toll. To the extent that Carlos is relieved from the burden of using others in the service of his self-protection, he is freed to have more positively toned relations with Janine and others around him.

Importance of Considering Group Development

Later in this book, the reader encounters a number of models of group therapy. Regardless of what model a group therapist uses, he or she does well to keep the developmental status of the group in mind for several reasons. First, a developmental perspective enables the therapist to have realistic expectations concerning the resources members are able to summon in working toward group goals. To elaborate on an earlier example, suppose as part of the application of a model, a problem for the group to solve during the course of a session needed to be identified. The therapist may be required to decide whether to set the problem for the group or to allow the group to establish the problem. If a consensual decision about the problem were important to the group's work in the session, then it would be important for the therapist to realize that the group is unlikely to make a considered selection early in its development. Therefore, in a young group it might be preferable for the therapist to formulate the problem. As the group gains in maturity, it may be possible to turn this activity over to the group.

A second value of a developmental awareness is that it helps the group therapist to anticipate possible obstacles to the group reaching its goals so that these impediments can be addressed effectively. Consider the following circumstance:

> *A cognitive behavioral group therapist seemed to hit a snag in a group she was conducting in an adolescent group in a residential treatment center. Members had been dutifully completing their homework assignments and were enjoying the group. Gradually, however, they seemed to become less cooperative. They came late, missed sessions, and did homework rarely. As one session drew to an end, one member said sarcastically, "My automatic thought is not to come back. I don't feel I'm getting anything out of this."*

The cognitive-behavioral model, which is discussed in Chapter 11, does not make formal use of developmental stages. Yet, the cognitive-behavioral practitioner who keeps group developmental principles in mind will know that there is a stage in the life of the group when members violate the norms that the therapist is seeking to establish. This cognizance is an antidote the possible discouragement the therapist might feel about either the motivation of the group members or the effectiveness of cognitive-behavioral techniques. Moreover, the therapist may achieve greater empathy for the experience of group members. From this empathy may come some well-timed comments that convey to members the therapist's sensitivity to the issues with which they are struggling. The therapist might even incorporate her understanding of the key group-level issues into her cognitive-behavioral interventions (Rose, 1990; Satterfield, 1994).

Third, a knowledge of the stage in which the group is residing helps in understanding the meaning of events in the group (Rutan & Stone, 2001). To the extent that the group therapist ascertains accurately the meaning of an event, the therapist is likely to respond with greater effectiveness. Consider the following example:

> *The group is meeting in its last session prior to the holiday break. One of the group members brings a mug with a bow affixed to it for every member. The therapist's mug says "#1 Doc." The therapist wondered about the meaning of this gesture.*

If, based on other data, the therapist had developed a formulation about the stage in which the group was residing, it may help the therapist to decode the meaning of the gifts. For example, early in the life of the group, this act may reflect the member's eagerness to observe social convention. If the group had matured somewhat more, and the therapist had recognized this fact, the gesture might be correctly regarded as an act of opposition vis-à-vis the therapist, who, the patients might recognize, would see the presents as lying outside the parameters of the group. Still later, the presents might signify a yearning to shed the boundaries of the relationship in pursuit of total intimacy. At the group's end, the presents may represent a defensive effort at hiding feelings of disappointment in the group experience.

Fourth, within some theoretical approaches, the extent to which that the group moves from stage to stage or remains fixed within any given stage may enable the therapist to determine the effectiveness of the group as a working environment. Using the group's passage through different stages as a measure of the group's effectiveness is most appropriate when the goal of the group is to help members resolve interpersonal problems. Moving to the next developmental stage signifies the group's success in addressing the problems of the prior developmental stage. Each member has some, albeit varying, participation in this success. Moreover, the greater the number of stages through which the group passes, the greater the array of interpersonal problems that are addressed.

If a group fails to move beyond a given stage, a phenomenon known as *fixation,* or if the group retreats to an earlier developmental stage, a phenomenon known as *regression,* some attribute of the group's working environment may be hindering the group from progressing. At least three questions must be answered to elucidate the meaning of a group's failure to make stage-to-stage movement:

1. *Have the most critical external boundaries of the group been relatively stable over the course of the group?* For example, have there been changes in membership? I spent many years conducting inpatient groups that lasted for eight sessions. By design, all members would begin the group in the same session and end the group in the same session. Generally, the group was able to proceed through several developmental stages (Reed, 1986). Yet if one or more members were precipitously discharged early in the group, this membership instability would significantly retard the group's progress. Having a similar effect are other sources of instability such as canceled sessions, failure of the group to start and end on time, relocation of the group, or the absence of one member of the cotherapy team.

2. *Does the therapist have a reaction in a given stage that impedes the group's development?* Chapter 5 takes up the topic of therapist reactions in some detail. However, for the present it might be noted that therapists may have a variety of subtle or obvious reactions to the group that will affect the group's work. For example, suppose in a given stage the therapist reacts with fear or anger to members' escalating expressions of dissatisfaction with the therapist. Even as members express their displeasure with the therapist, they remain dependent upon him or her. Therefore, members monitor the therapist to ensure that the therapist can withstand the group's attack. If the therapist provides sufficient evidence of not finding members' reactions endurable, members may avoid any further direct expressions of hostility. Therefore, they deprive themselves of the opportunity to developmentally advance.

3. *What is the modal developmental level of the members in the group?* Groups composed of members functioning at a very low level of interpersonal relatedness will proceed through the early stage slowly (Rutan & Stone, 2001). For individuals with impoverished interpersonal capacities, the first two developmental stages involve those conflicts having the greatest significance for their

everyday interpersonal difficulties. Demonstrating this point was a study of a group of outpatient schizophrenics (Kanas, Stewart, Deri, Ketter, & Haney, 1989). The investigators discovered that over a period of 12 sessions, the group remained in the first stage of development. Yet they also observed that the group had made progress in addressing issues of trust that are paramount in Stage I. In fact, it is precisely in this stage that members' progress would hold greatest value for their everyday lives. A group of higher-functioning patients would be expected to proceed through the earlier stages of development more quickly than lower-functioning patients and spend more time in the later stages of group development. Hence, the developmental expectation of the members must be predicated on the therapist's knowledge of their interpersonal capabilities. When the members fail to meet the therapist's expectation, barring the possibility of an initial incorrect assessment of their interpersonal abilities, the therapist must consider whether the group environment is one that adequately nurtures the group's growth.

Stages of Group Development

Within the group therapy literature, the reader will find many characterizations of group development. Variability among existing schemes is the result of a variety of factors, including the context in which developmental observations were collected, the theoretical orientation of the observer, the time frame, the goals of the group, and so on. Yet, the commonalities among most of the existing theories are considerable. A most important commonality is the assumption that there are group-level phenomena that transcend the internal experiences or behaviors of the individuals in the group (Agazarian, 1997). Another critical commonality is the notion of invariance of sequence. While groups vary from one another in their rates of passage through individual stages, the order of the stages is constant.

The developmental stages that will be described combine various developmental approaches. Five stages will be presented. The first four stages apply to ongoing groups whose members enter and leave the group at different times. All five stages apply to time-limited, close-ended groups that have a fixed beginning and ending date common to all group members.

Stage I

In the earliest stage of group life, members are not truly a group. While they presumably have a common purpose—the improvement in their psychological and social lives and the amelioration of psychological difficulties—they are nonetheless merely a collection of individuals. Becoming a group is the task of Stage I.

However, becoming a group demands that the group as a whole begins to address a conflict between the wish for members to establish relationships with one another and the wish to remain disconnected. In the following vignette, both psychological trends are present:

An outpatient group was in its third session. One member, Jill, opened the session saying to another member, Desiree, "You know, most of us have opened up in here. You haven't said much of anything. I really have no idea why you're here. I thought maybe you were here just as an observer, but tonight you look down so maybe now is a good time to start talking." The group member initially appeared disarmed but then shrugged and said, "I went to the movies Saturday night. Ever since then I have felt like crying. It was a movie about a woman who reminded me of myself. She was always going to bars and was desperate. She finally met this guy and it seemed that something might work out finally, but then she noticed that he was doing some odd things . . . something just didn't seem right. So she started following him to see what he was up to. In the last scene, you see her looking through a window, the window of his home. . . . He's there with his family . . . a very cozy scene . . . and she's outside alone . . . total desolation."

Desiree then began to cry. Jill responded, "I think you should feel hopeful given that you are in this group now. You should feel good, too, because you're not like all of the people out there who aren't doing anything about their problems . . . they're the ones out in the cold!"

Jill proceeded to inquire about the details of Desiree's life, particularly her efforts to meet men and her failure to establish a lasting relationship. Other members provided various sorts of advice to Desiree. Suggestions of alternate ways of meeting men were provided. Tom shared some notions he garnered from his AA participation. Several members consoled Desiree by revealing that they had much the same difficulty.

As the session progressed, Desiree appeared to be more rather than less distraught. Toward the end of the session, Jill turned to the therapist and said, "Isn't there something you can do to help?"

Many features of this vignette are characteristic of Stage I and reflect the trends outlined earlier. The desire on the part of members to come together and forge a group is seen in a variety of ways. That all members came to the group, that Jill monitored who had spoken and who had not, that Desiree spoke about herself despite her reticence, that members identified their commonalities with Desiree, that Jill distinguished between motivated people in the group and the unmotivated people outside—all were indications of members' desire to invest themselves in the group and one another. Yet there are abundant indicators of members' wishing to maintain their insularity. For example, group members continued their ministrations despite Desiree's escalating distress. The group's exclusive focus on Desiree and their placement of her in the subordinate position of being the patient of the group were both means of avoiding placing themselves in the more vulnerable peer positions. Tom's introduction of AA rhetoric, a form of intellectualization, may have been an effort to set himself apart from others. It may also have been an effort to soothe himself with a familiar frame of reference as he was confronting unfamiliar and anxiety-arousing events.

During this stage, the therapist's ability to convey empathy in relation to the competing yearnings to both connect and stay apart can be enhanced by a clear understanding of the multiple bases of these urges. Certainly, the desire to connect is rooted in the social nature of the human person (Scheidlinger, 1964). Bonding to others enhances the likelihood of survival. More specific to the therapy group, however, is each member's expectation that the group will ameliorate difficulties. Jill bears testament to this as she says to Desiree that she should be hopeful that she has begun the group. As members begin their participation in the group, they obtain support for the expectation in that they soon learn, as did Desiree, that other members have similar experiences, a source of validation that can relieve members of considerable anxiety. This discovery of commonalities is such a regular, expectable part of group life that Yalom (1995) termed it *universality*. He saw its operation as having major therapeutic value for many types of groups. The phenomenon of universality is discussed more fully in Chapter 4.

The wish for separateness is born out of a desire to protect the self from many of the perils of human contact such as loss of identity, rejection, loss of control, being misunderstood or criticized, and having one's ideas and feelings disconfirmed by others. Desiree may have had a direct experience of some of these perils. For example, she may have felt patronized by members as they bestowed upon her advice that she had likely heard many times before. As she revealed, being the recipient of all of the input only made her feel worse.

Beyond these factors, however, members have another strong motive to avoid connecting with others as equal partners pursuing a common task. However, appreciation of this factor requires some grounding in psychodynamic group theory. Sigmund Freud, a major contributor to our understanding of groups through his classic work. *Group Psychology and the Analysis of the Ego* (1921/1955), held the notion that the unconscious lives of members in the group have a powerful role in influencing members' behavior and conscious experience. He believed that the relationship members establish with one another occurs through their shared positive (or libidinal) attachment to the leader, who is unconsciously perceived as a parental figure.

Wilfred Bion (1959) elaborated on Freud's ideas by positing that the group has an unconscious life that is apart from that of any individual group member. This group unconscious life can interfere with the explicit task of the group. When the group is successful in focusing on the explicit task of the group, it is in its *work group* mode. The work group is distinguished by orderly and logical processes in pursuit of its goals. However, when the group is being controlled by an unconscious fantasy, the group is in a basic assumption state. Bion used the term *basic assumption* because the group acts on an unconscious assumption that the group gratifies a shared need state of members.

Bion delineated three basic assumption states: *dependency, fight/flight,* and *pairing.* Bion did not see these states as occurring in any particular order. However, other observers of group life, Bennis and Shepard, felt that the basic assumption that emerges depends upon the maturity of the group. The earliest basic assumption to emerge is the dependent state. (The other two basic assumption states will be discussed in the context of later developmental stages.) Bion described the dependent basic assumption state as one in which the group expects to have all of its needs met by an all-powerful, all-knowing parent. The assumption is activated in the group setting because the group in its ability to surround and encompass the group member is unconsciously seen to be like the mother who encompasses and surrounds the infant. The group members under the sway of this basic assumption state expect to work to get their needs met no more than does the infant. Members see their mere presence in the group as sufficient to have their longings satisfied.

The activation of this basic assumption state has implications for how members treat one another and the therapist at this time in the group's life. Unconsciously, members do not expect to accomplish their goals through the assumption of responsibility for their problems and through their own efforts in addressing them. They imagine that whatever help will be forthcoming will proceed from that figure who most approximates a parent, that is, the therapist. Stated briefly, they expect that the therapist will cure them. This notion explains many of the behaviors that have commonly been observed in the group's earliest stage. For example, members frequently give only passing attention to one another's comments and riveted attention to those of the therapist. Tendencies to place blame on external figures, to rationalize difficulties, and to offer bromides rather than genuinely grappling with others' concerns are all typical flights from work that occur in the earliest stage. They occur in the service of the notion that if any help is to come, it is to come from the therapist.

In the vignette, group members made Desiree into the patient of the group and tried to cure her. When the group is a basic assumption group, it is extremely common for group members to converge upon the most vulnerable members in this fashion. Members identify with this member's high level of need. As the whole group participates in the "cure," all members are vicariously cured. Furthermore, by underscoring the fragility of the member, the group unconsciously endeavors to tempt the therapist into being more forthcoming with his or her curative resources. It is as if the members are saying to the therapist, "See how much we need?"

Having considered the nature of basic assumption groups, the reader is in a position to appreciate the implication of the dependent basic assumption group that emerges early in a group's life for members' wishes to stay disconnected from one another. As noted previously, group members did not treat Desiree as a peer. They related to her in terms of the function she could perform for the group. Apart from this function, group members remained separate from Desiree and Desiree from group members. Indeed, such separateness is demanded by the basic assumption state. Members hold little interest in one another because they collectively believe that whatever help is to come will come from on all-powerful caretaker.

The resolution of the dependency issue comes in the next rather than the present stage. Because both stages form a couplet in which members are occupied with authority-related issues, some theorists (e.g., Agazarian, 1997; Bennis & Shepard, 1956) regard them as substages of one large stage. Yet most theorists see them as separate stages both because of the distinctive behavioral features of members in each period and the significant accomplishments of members in each. In Stage I, members achieve some modicum of trust and comfort in relating to one another. Members see they can identify with one another's experiences. They begin to understand some of the group's processes and develop more accurate expectations of one another and the therapists. All of these accomplishments lay the groundwork for the critical work the group will do in Stage II.

Implications for Intervention: In Chapters 5 and 6 the activities of the therapist are discussed in some detail. For now, however, a few implications will be drawn for what the therapist might be doing at each stage so that the reader can appreciate the importance of developmental sensitivity on the part of the therapist.

As the group addresses the conflict between connection and isolation, work and flight, the therapist's attempt is to help the group resolve the conflict in the direction of involvement. Across all theoretical approaches, the therapist's strategy is to provide members with a positive experience of relating to others. One especially critical means is for members to have a common sense of purpose in the group, which is accomplished through careful preparation of members with respect to the group's goals and processes. (See Chapter 8 for further discussion of this point.) In most types of groups another prime means is the therapist's support of members' identifying with one another:

HAROLD: I just feel like a loser, like being here means I can't fend for myself.

THERAPIST: Jeb, didn't you say something like that earlier in the session?

When presented with Harold's utterance, the therapist has many options, including challenging Harold's assumption that being in therapy means that one has failed. However, the forging of positive connections has a priority in the group's early life; otherwise, members will lack sufficient attachment to the group to commit themselves to psychological work with one another. Not uncommonly, the commonalities that members identify will be exaggerated. The therapist's allowing members to enjoy the relief that inevitably attends the carving out of common ground, no matter how great or little its foundation in reality, is important to the group's developing cohesion.

In structured groups members forge a positive connection to one another by participating in activities and exercises in which they have the opportunity to experience themselves as productive in their interactions with one another. For example, members who are placed in an interpersonal problem-solving group learn to do brainstorming. Members practice the uninhibited generation of solutions to a given problem identified by the group. This experience is often exhilarating for members: They see, usually to their astonishment, the multitude of solutions they can develop by working together. Such experiences bolsters members' enthusiasm for continued group participation and also challenges their fears about involvement. For example, members who had expected to be criticized by other group members may discover that they receive little or no input from other members that lowers their self-esteem.

In exploratory groups, the members' more active recognition of the negative pole of their feelings about being in the group occurs. The therapist can help members describe their fears by staying alert to subtle expressions of them:

MAXINE: I find that when I talk about the need I feel to check things over and over, my family thinks I'm crazy. Even the nurses on the floor look at me funny when I feel I have to go back to my door and make sure that I closed it.

THERAPIST: So maybe you were wondering if we could understand this part of you?

MAXINE: [giggles] I had images of everyone just being Dumbfounded . . . you know, sitting in absolute silence.

THERAPIST: And maybe others had some real doubts about whether members could understand.

Members' active identification of the fears that underpin their hesitation to immerse themselves fully in their relationships with one another is extremely useful. It suggests that these fears are not so great as to be beyond articulation. Moreover, once the fears are labeled, members are far more able to compare the anticipations with their actual group experiences. In these ways, verbalizing the presence of fears almost always leads to their diminishment.

Stage II

The waning of Stage I and the emergence of Stage II are often seen in an increasing irritability and contentiousness among group members. This shift is often a noticeable one because during Stage I members typically make a great effort to be agreeable and to minimize their differences with one another. The following vignette from the same group illustrates this development:

> *In the group's eighth session, Jill was still concerning herself with Desiree's reticence. Jill said admonishingly, "I just feel you're not trying to help yourself. You come here every week and just sit. Unless you're just a voyeur, you're not going to accomplish anything." Tom said, "Why don't you leave her alone. If she just wants to sit, if she just wants to listen, that's okay. You're not her personal manager." Jill responded, "I'm not trying to be! But I've been in therapy a long time and I do have a sense about how it's suppose to go." Blake retorted, "Maybe you don't even need to be here then. . . . If you're such an expert, you should be running your own group." Dorothy injected, "If it weren't for Jill, this group would be a sinking ship." Desiree said, "Yea, even if I don't talk, having her here makes me feel better. . . ." [Then to Jill] "I'll try to talk more." Tom fired back to Desiree, "Okay, you're on your own then."*

Jill's behaviors in the group had placed her in a leader position. In their response to her, members were able to articulate their stances in relation to authority and recognize others whose positions were similar to their own. Dorothy and Desiree, in their defense of Jill's behavior in the group, were taking on a compliant position toward Jill's authority. Dorothy's comment, while in defense of Jill, was an attack upon the effectiveness of the therapist. In the Janus-faced aspect of her behavior, the compliance and the defiance, she illustrates how the group-as-a-whole conflict about authority (as well as other issues) exists within each member. Dorothy and Desiree also articulated their sense of dependency upon Jill for their well-being and security in the group. Jill, acting on her beliefs about how therapy should go (presumably, what would please the therapist), joined Dorothy and Desiree in assuming a compliant stance toward authority. However, Jill was more active in her compliance in that she strove to influence others to be compliant. Tom and Blake, in their challenge of Jill, the perceived surrogate leader, took on a defiant stance toward leadership; they openly challenged her authority. In doing so, however, they obviously aroused the anxiety of the compliant subgroup, whose members derived a sense of security from the activity of authority in the group.

In some groups the initial attacks upon authority may not be directed toward another member of the group. Particularly in the circumstance where group therapy takes in broader treatment environments that are shared by members—for example, an inpatient unit—alternate candidates are often identified by members as targets for their negative feelings (Brabender, 1985, 1988). In running groups in an inpatient setting, I observed that those members who were disposed to take an oppositional stance toward authority were more likely to do so toward other staff members. For example, they would complain about the psychiatrist on the unit who did not spend enough time during the individual session or the psychiatric technician who curtailed the group member's phone calls. This is often a propitious development: Members' anger toward authority can be both intense and primitive and is usually difficult for an individual group member to bear (Jackson, 1999). Individuals who are objects of such attacks may be tempted to flee the group. While different theoretical approaches provide different strategies to spare members from being the recipients of others' strong expressions of anger, all are in agreement that the therapist can neither take a laissez-faire stance in this circumstance nor join the group in the attack (A. P. Beck, 1974).

Another means that many groups use to express dissatisfaction is acting out. Acting out is the behavioral expression of impulses or feelings as a means to avoid their emergence in consciousness. Members engage in behaviors that they see as being at odds with the expectations and requirements of authority figures. Arriving late, missing sessions, failing to make timely payments, violating confidentiality, and socializing with members outside the group (in a group where this activity has been outlawed) are examples of common acting-out behaviors. All of these behaviors enable members to express hostility without having to experience it, at least in its full intensity.

As the group continues to progress through this stage, criticism of the therapist becomes more and more direct. Members' increasing frustration in relation to the longings of the dependent basic assumption state lead them to find their attacks on substitute figures less fulfilling. Furthermore, in the process of airing their dissatisfaction, members become more confident in their expression of negative feelings. At such times the group approximates what Bion (1959) referred to as a fight/flight basic assumption group in which members act on the unconscious belief that its survival depends upon the elimination of a common enemy, who in Stage II is the person of the therapist. The form this elimination will take varies from group to group. Flight will be an emphasis when group members feel too vulnerable to take on the leader. When members feel sufficiently powerful, fight will be the emphasis. Bennis and Shepard (1956) described a moment in the group's life called the *barometric event* in which, in a fight mode, all members participate in a symbolic act challenging the therapist's power. In the inpatient setting I had an opportunity to see a variety of barometric events. For example, in one session when I and my cotherapist arrived, all members were seated on the floor. These members were literally trying to bring the leaders down. Yet, not all groups will muster such dramatic and unified expressions. In other cases one outspoken member challenges the therapist's authority by making a strong, sustained attack on some aspect of the therapist's style while other members give silent assent. The key element is that members achieve some solidarity in the expression of dissatisfaction with the therapist.

Work in Stage II holds many potential benefits for members. Members learn to handle differences among themselves in a far more effective way than they had in Stage I. This ability is essential for the work members do in the later stages. Members at the completion of this stage have to a large extent abandoned the expectation that a magical cure is forthcoming from an omnipotent caregiver. In what Foulkes (1964) referred to as the decrescendo of reliance upon the leader and the crescendo of self-reliance, members take responsibility for their group, their difficulties, and their progress in therapy. They move from a position of dependence to one of interdependence upon each other (A. P. Beck, 1974; Cohen & Ettin, 1999). Individual members who have particularly maladaptive stances toward authority have an opportunity to modify them. An example of such modification is provided by those group members who take a passive-dependent stance toward authority. These members fear that any expression of negative feelings toward authority will lead to some untoward consequence such as retaliation by the authority figure. They have the opportunity to compare their catastrophic fantasies to reality by witnessing the effects of their own manifestations of displeasure toward the therapist or those of the other group members.

Implications for Intervention: In Stage II, the therapist's task is to provide a safe environment for members to address conflictual feelings toward authority figures. In some types of groups the thorough exploration of the feelings enables members to better resolve authority-related conflicts. In other types of groups such feelings are given sufficient attention to enable the group to move on to other types of work. A particularly big challenge for the therapist during this stage is responding to the acting-out behaviors such as lateness and absences that are especially prevalent in the early period before the feelings have fully flowered and been acknowledged by members. Across many theoretical orientations therapists will assist members in recognizing the message hidden in the acting-out behaviors. For example, a therapist noticing that two members are absent, two members arrived late, and other members are frequently looking at the clock might say something like the following:

> *In the last session, people commented that that group seemed to be a bit slow . . . and there was a sense of uncertainty about whether it will provide any solutions to problems. We haven't really gotten back to that topic today. However, I wonder if the lateness, the absences, and the clock-watching might not be different ways of showing disappointment in the group.*

One important aspect of this comment is that it is made on the *group-level.* The psychological element that is the focus of the comment is attributed not to any one individual but to the group as a whole. The power of such an intervention format is that it enables members to acknowledge what ordinarily would be highly threatening if not unacceptable psychological contents. Once the therapist makes such an intervention that allows for the direct emergence of feelings, the way the therapist helps the group to frame cognitively this affective experience will depend crucially upon the therapist's theoretical approach. As explained in Chapter 5, however, what is essential is that the therapist does have a theoretical framework to offer members to organize what can oftentimes be new and frightening feelings and impulses. The therapist must also have a readiness to protect members whom the group may seek to attack. For example, the therapist in our vignette should have been monitoring the hostility directed against Jill closely. Were this hostility beyond what Jill could bear, the therapist should intervene to alter the group's dynamics. A common strategy is to interpret the displacement, that is, to point out that the group's hostility toward the therapist has been placed upon Jill (Kirman, 1995).

As members become more aware of shared feelings in relation to authority, their capacity to join with one another in their expression is crucially dependent upon how the therapist responds. To the extent that the therapist exhibits withdrawal, retaliation, or extreme solicitude, the members will recoil from the challenge to authority that is essential for a move to a peer-centered group. By exhibiting an accepting attitude toward the group's challenge, the therapist will facilitate the group in taking an important developmental step.

Stage III

The feelings following the group's survival after a unified attack upon the leader are ones of joy and euphoria. Members feel an enhanced sense of their own power and regard for the other members of the group. In this stage members become much more of a genuine focus of one another now that they are free of their nearly exclusive focus on the authority figure of the therapist. This capacity to attend to other members is seen in their more accurate grasp of one another's comments. Consequently, members have an enhanced sense of being heard by one another and thereby find the total group experience more satisfying. Nonverbal behavior, most particularly eye contact, reveals the shift from authority to peers. As Agazarian wrote, "In the phase of authority [Stages I and II in this model], eye contact is nearly always triangular: Members talk to each other and at the same time keep an eye on the therapist. As soon as the group enters into this phase of intimacy, these sidelong glances all but disappear and groups members' focus is on the relationships themselves" (1997, p. 262).

While members' attunement to one another is heightened, this attunement is almost entirely toward that in the other member that is positive and that with which they can easily identify. The benefit of this focus is that members see their own positive qualities through the eyes of the other group members. Not surprisingly, then, this is a period in the life of the group when self-esteem runs high. Members also receive validation for a wider range of experiences than they had previously.

Out of the closeness that members feel for one another comes an effort to extend the group beyond its usual time and space boundaries:

> *Tom said to Dorothy, "I have seen you driving on the expressway both coming here and leaving. . . . You must live in my area." Dorothy said, "Oh, yes."*
>
> *"Then you've seen my jalopy that has done just about its last highway merge. . . . Say, I don't suppose you could give me a lift sometimes?" Tom continued, "I'd really like that. We could get a head start on the conversation." Other members laughed and seemed to take delight in the notion of Tom and Dorothy's drive together. Soon, however, the plan was changed to Desiree picking up each member in her van. Blake said, "Since this is my favorite group of people, I am thrilled at the prospect of spending a bit more time together." Blake went on to describe some very painful interactions with significant figures in his life outside the group. Members supported him in seeing these figures as uncaring and untrustworthy.*

This group attempted to extend the group through ride sharing. Another common boundary crossing involves members' meeting before and after the session in the parking lot. Members also show increased punctuality and higher attendance rates. Self-disclosures such as Blake's increase as members become more trusting of other members' possession of some of the more intimate details of their lives (Garland, 1981; Jackson, 1999). All of these behaviors suggest that the group has achieved greater cohesion, which Yalom describes as "the attraction that members have for their group and for other members" (1995, p. 67).[2]

---

[2] Bion posited a third basic assumption state, the Pairing Basic Assumption group. This group acts on the unconscious belief that a savior from the group will emerge through the union of two or more members (Bion, 1959). Under the sway of such a state, members become acutely interested in the pairings of members and any implication of sexual interest of one member for another. It is in Stage IV that the phenomena of the pairing basic assumption state can be seen. To some extent, the interactions between Tom and Dorothy might be regarded in this light. Yet, as most writers have described the kind of intimacy of Stage IV, it seems to be something more akin to the experiences of *amae* described by the Japanese psychoanalyst, Takeo Doi (1963). Good *amae* is the experienced wish for emotional closeness to others that is rooted in the infant's desire to be held and nurtured by the mother.

What is often missing from members' interactions is information that would enable members to make positive changes in their interpersonal lives. For example, whatever contribution Blake makes to his problems with significant people in his life is likely to remain unarticulated. Moreover, members' understanding of Blake's situation is likely to be incomplete because members do not attend to the aspects of his experience that may differentiate him from at least some other members of the group.

As has been pointed out in the literature (e.g., Agazarian & Peters, 1981; Bennis & Shepard, 1956), this stage tends to be short-lived because it is predicated upon the denial of differences and negative feelings, an exorbitant level of denial that is difficult for members to maintain. Nonetheless, group members do achieve an intensified sense of closeness that fortifies the group in its difficult work ahead.

Implications for Intervention: The biggest challenge for the therapist is how to respond to the boundary violations typical of this period. For some therapists, the sense of being a killjoy of the group's exhilaration may deter the therapist from responding appropriately to the group's challenges to the frame of the group. The therapist may also hesitate to discourage what in some cases may appear to be initiative taking by group members (for example, when members organize a catered group session). However, to ignore rule breaking and other boundary violations will prevent the therapist from preserving the group as a safe place for work. How the therapist responds will be determined by a variety of factors, such as the group contract, which is described in Chapter 7, and the theoretical orientation. Yet across approaches it is through the therapist's behavior that he or she models observation of the group rules. The therapist is likely to be aided in reinforcing the group boundaries by those members who feel some discomfort with the group's movement toward complete intimacy.

During this period, the therapist begins the cultivation of the resources that have become available with the group's shift from a leader-centered to a peer-centered group. Members now have greater attunement to one another, even though the focus is on one another's positive qualities. This very feature makes it a particularly propitious time for the therapist to point out opportunities for members to give feedback to one another and to shape how it is delivered so it is maximally constructive. Because the feedback is likely to be immediately bolstering rather than threatening, members can achieve comfort with the feedback process before they are confronted with the more balanced feedback of Stage IV.

Stage IV

In this stage, the group's greater maturity enables members to achieve a higher level of balance between positive and negative feelings toward one another and a more individualized perception of each group member. This transition occurs for a variety of reasons. Members' efforts to deny the reality of differences simply become too strained as time passes and evidence of other group phenomena accumulates. Moreover, a subgroup of members experience considerable anxiety in Stage III in relation to the group's newfound closeness (Jackson, 1999). These members will work actively to move the group to a position in which members are more clearly recognized as separate entities and their individual identities are more fully acknowledged. They will be skilled in articulating to members the dangers of too much closeness:

> *Marta's verbiage was like liquid putty filling up the cracks in the group. Early in the life of the group, the group appreciated Marta's chatter, which was generously offered whenever an awkward silence fell on the group. Later in the group when hostilities emerged, Marta's offerings seemed to diffuse some tension. The therapist privately observed that Marta's verbal productions were such that equal weight was given to essential and nonessential details. Consequently, members were unable to distinguish what was important, and her comments were generally met with benevolent but sometimes wearied silence.*
>
> *Yet in one session Marta was strikingly different. She came into the group tearful because she had lost her job. Her employer informed her that she was too scattered. Members began a line of questioning that was directed toward uncovering some unfairness in the employer. Clearly, many group members wanted to see him as a bad person. Marta was able to accommodate them, and as she sculpted a negative impression, her spirits appeared to ascend. The group's line of inquiry was interrupted by Tom, who said in an unusually self-conscious tone, "I don't think you're doing her any favor." With perplexity Dorothy said, "I don't know what you mean." Tom challenged, "I think you do. If her employer said she was unkind, we wouldn't believe it. If*

he said she was . . . I don't know . . . irresponsible . . . we'd have a hard time believing that too . . . but the boss said she's scattered . . . and well . . . she is." [To Marta] I mean, you are." Desiree cautioned, "But maybe this isn't the time . . ." Marta responded, "No, if it's true, I want to know now. I don't want to fail again."

In this stage, you have the fullest emergence of a process that is critical to most major models of contemporary group therapy: feedback based upon members' immediate experiences with one another. Because over the course of the group's development members have become increasingly attuned to one another and able to attend to both the positive and negative aspects of their own reactions, they are able to offer one another detailed, useful feedback on one another's styles of relating.

In the vignette, the group was now in a position to offer Marta observations of both her behavior and their reactions to her behavior. Such information could lead her to make changes that would positively affect the likelihood that she would experience fulfillment and success (e.g., sustaining employment) in relationships outside the group. While members can offer feedback earlier in the life of the group, once the group arrives at Stage IV, the comments tend to be much more specific and, hence, useful.

Groups also distinguish themselves during this stage in their capacities to monitor their own boundaries. For example, it is in this stage that members' violations of the time boundaries (e.g., tardiness, absences), are noted and challenged by other group members. Groups also begin in this stage to exhibit a mature decision-making process. The reader will recall that early in a group's life decisions tend to be made hastily with consideration of few points of view. With its greater ability to recognize differences the group has a greater ability to look at the different sides of an issue. Moreover, the changed relationship with the therapist enables the group to engage in a more mature decision-making process. Early in the group's life, the group does not want to make decisions because of a hidden expectation that the therapist should make the decisions. At this time, the group's relationship with the therapist is more collaborative. The group sees the therapist as someone with special skills. However, because members no longer regard the therapist as a parent who will direct action, they look more and more to themselves for direction.

Implications for Intervention: The task of the therapist during this stage is to help the group realize its potential as a mature working group. This stage is the first one in which the group can clearly recognize and explore differences among members. The therapist's interventions are geared to ensuring that these explorations proceed in a way that furthers the goals of the group. For example, during this stage members such as Marta receive information about the aspects of their interpersonal styles that may alienate others. The therapist must help the group to work with differences in a way that is constructive. For example, the therapist can sculpt members' feedback to one another so that it is noncondemnatory, specific, and inclusive of multiple member perspectives.

Another aspect of the group's maturity is its capacity to make a considered decision. The group therapist can nurture this capacity by providing members with opportunities to make decisions. For example, Agazarian and Peters (1981) allow members to decide not whether a new member enters the group but when the event occurs. Groups may deliberate on the application of group rules when certain behaviors fall into a gray area. For example, in a group in which the therapist had established a rule that there would be no socializing outside of groups, members might be allowed to decide whether conversation among members would be permitted. These issues, because they typically pertain to the definition of group boundaries, have a high level of importance. By giving members responsibility to deliberate and resolve such issues, the therapist increases their sense of stewardship over the group.

During this phase of the group's life, a challenge for some therapists is in accepting the group's newfound autonomy. Some therapists may experience this transition as a loss (Brabender, 1987). To promote the group's more dependent posture, the therapist may inject him or herself unnecessarily into the group's process or emotionally withdraw from the group altogether. These therapist behaviors hinder the group's development. However, such tendencies can be identified and usefully explored in supervision.

Stage V

The developmental stages that have been discussed refer to a sequence of conflicts and issues that the group as an entire system faces over time. While a member's termination from the group may activate a number of the issues outlined in this section, an impending termination launches a group developmental stage only when all group members terminate together. This simultaneous termination of members occurs in a time-limited group in which all members begin and end the group in the same session. An argument could be made that the group's terminal period does not represent a developmental stage per se because the phenomena that are observed during this period do not necessarily represent a natural unfolding from the prior stages. Rather, these phenomena have been precipitated by a temporal boundary that has been imposed upon the group. Nonetheless, a group that has proceeded through the first four stages of group development will approach its ending in a way that makes use of the accomplishments of the prior stages. For this reason, this fifth stage is appropriately considered in this sequence of stages.

As the group approaches its ending, it faces the loss of the supportive structure of the group and the loss of specific relationships with one another. Members may have other specific losses, too. For example, some members may draw a conclusion, accurate or otherwise, that certain goals they had established for themselves in the group will not be realized. Some experience the absence of expected progress as a loss.

Loss is a human experience associated with various painful affects, so it is natural that the specter of loss invites the emergence of defenses (Roller, 1997). In this last stage, members frequently subgroup around their use of particular defenses. Idealization and devaluation of group experience are common defensive strategies. With idealization, frustration, disappointment, and anger about the group experience are lessened as members see the group, its members, and the therapist as all-perfect. The use of idealization can be heard in such statements as, "This is the finest group of people I've ever known" in the absence of other balancing statements. While idealization assists members in defending against anger-related affects, devaluation, another common strategy, helps members to minimize their sadness about the loss of the group. Members who devalue the group may focus on any of its perceived insufficiencies—for example, the group didn't accomplish anything, the members were superficial and not insightful, the therapist was incompetent, and so on.

While devaluation and idealization are common ways to quell the disturbing affects of loss, another means is to deny the loss altogether. Members say to one another, in essence, "We don't need to feel anything in relation to a loss because there is no loss occurring." The interplay of denial, idealization, and devaluation can be seen in the following vignette:

> With only two sessions remaining in the 24-session group, members had fallen silent. The therapist wondered aloud whether the group's newfound reticence showed how difficult it is to face the pain of saying good-bye. Tom said, "I've been thinking about that . . . the saying good-bye business . . . and it just doesn't seem necessary to me. I know you may not be available [to the therapist] but that doesn't mean the rest of us can't get together every week. Desiree exclaimed, "That's a fabulous idea." Jill said, "It just wouldn't be appropriate. This was not designed to be a social club. The deal was that we would learn about ourselves in here so we could have good relationships out there." Dorothy said, "I'm not sure I would be comfortable meeting without the therapist. But I would like to get holiday cards from all of you so you can let me know how you're doing." Marta said, "Maybe we could schedule annual reunions." Blake said, "That sounds nice but I just can't promise how I'll feel a year from now. Maybe we're just clinging to something that has run its course."

In this vignette, when the therapist made the ending of the group a focal event for members, a defensive effort got under way to prevent the group's ending. When that effort failed, members tried to frame the ending so it would be less absolute.[3] The use of denial was bolstered by idealization and devaluation. Tom established that the group must continue because what had been achieved among members could not be established elsewhere. To release the group from the constraint of needing the therapist's agreement, he devalued the therapist, making her contribution expendable.

This vignette also points to another conflict that often emerges prominently in the group's last stage: conflict over change (Piper et al., 1992). Leaving the group activates members' desire to change themselves, the fear of doing so, and the worry that perhaps they cannot. These negatively toned feelings lead a subgroup of members to conspire to make therapy relationships permanent

---

[3] Rutan and Stone (2001) point out that sometimes therapists are lured into extending the group. They generally find that some members who said they wanted to continue did so under coercion. These authors counsel the therapist to hold on to the originally agreed-upon date. If necessary, a new group can be formed, even with the original members and, possibly, with an open-ended departure date.

social relationships. Yet typically a subgroup will emerge that opposes this effort. Members such as Jill will remind the others that such a transformation in members' relations would fly in the face of the group's original mission. Members such as Dorothy may see the risk inherent in such a movement. Members such as Blake may point out the unreality of the group's scheme for continuing its life. This subgroup will be the voice of the wish to change, the same wish that led members to join the group.

Members' progress in earlier stages will be of particular benefit at this time. Their developed capacities to experience ambivalence in regard to a range of conflicts and tolerate the tension of the ambivalence will support their relinquishment of their defenses in favor of having a rich emotional experience during the group's ending.

Implications for Intervention: In this stage, both interpretive and supportive elements are likely to be helpful to the members of many types of groups (MacKenzie, 1996). Interpretive efforts should be directed toward enabling members to have a greater awareness of all elements of their response to the loss of the group to enhance members' ability to deal with losses in their future. The therapist can assist members in recognizing the defenses that they resurrect against the experience of loss. Idealizing or devaluing the group, attempting to extend the group, and distracting themselves from the ending of the group are all means that members use to fend off some feeling in relation to the loss of the group, means that can be identified by the therapist. Yet the awareness of their defenses may not be sufficient for members to have a fuller psychological experience of the ending of the group. Members may also need to recognize the unconscious beliefs or fantasies that sustain the use of defenses against loss reactions (Brabender & Fallon, 1996). By carefully listening to the fabric and flow of members' exchanges, the therapist may hear such fantasies embedded in the material:

> *Minnie was someone to whom the group could look for very candid but sensitively delivered feedback. However, in the last session her comments about other members were uncharacteristically positive and somewhat superficial. None of the members seemed to take notice of this shift. At one point she noted, "I never met such a perceptive group of people," even though several sessions ago, she had upbraided other members for their lack of sensitivity. Then, she suggested that members exchange e-mail addresses or consider*

organizing a chat room after the group.[4] *The other group members greeted this session with relieved delight and began to work out the logistical details.*

The belief that may have underpinned Minnie's idealization of members as suggested by the sequence of group events was, "If I don't express any negative thoughts about members, the group won't end." A corollary to this belief is, "If I express not only my positive but also my negative reactions toward members, I may effect the ending of this group." The therapist could continue to test out this hypothesis as new material emerged in the group. However, once the therapist feels some confidence that the hypothesis is capturing an aspect of members' experiences, that hypothesis can be shared with the group. As in individual therapy, the descriptive power of the hypothesis can be determined not by members' agreement or disagreement with the hypothesis but by the extent to which it spurs productive work. For example, this work may take the form of members' reflections on the pressure they feel to inhibit the expression of dissatisfactions in intimate relationships lest the other party become disaffected with the relationship. An on-target hypothesis may also create a dynamic change in the group—in this case, the diminished use of idealization.

Members' greater awareness of the beliefs that undergird their defensive efforts during the group's termination enables the testing of these beliefs. This process may be more or less explicit. For example, in a cognitive-behavioral group in which members routinely have homework, members may be given the assignment of expressing a complaint in a relationship and observing the consequences of this expression. Alternately, within the group session itself, members may simply consider how likely it is that the therapist would continue the group based on whether members derided the group in the group's final sessions.

By labeling defenses, identifying the beliefs underlying the defenses, and encouraging the reality testing associated with beliefs, the therapist helps members have a greater appreciation of their full set of affects in relation to the group's ending. While earlier in their lives members may have been unable to tolerate certain emotions

---

[4] The ethical issues associated with group therapy on the Internet are considered in Chapter 9.

associated with loss, these reactions now become more tolerable because they can be shared with the other members of the group.

The supportive aspect of the therapist's activity entails helping members crystallize learning and planning for the future. Members can consolidate learning through review of their progress over the group's life. For the very last session, MacKenzie (1996) suggests the use of a go-around in which each member shares his or her observations of, and reactions to, the other members of the group. MacKenzie writes:

> *Often specific critical incidents in the group's life are reviewed. Most of these center around an experience of confrontation or anger that was worked through. Sometimes they refer to powerful bonding experiences that took place early in the group. Members often talk of their hope for others as they address issues that were not fully explored in the group.* (1996, pp. 56–57)

MacKenzie's quote also refers to the other supportive aspect of the therapist's activities. By encouraging members to focus on what they have achieved, the therapist helps members realize what work lies ahead. Members can use their final sessions to plan how this work might be accomplished. In an inpatient group members might place such work on their agenda for an outpatient experience. In an outpatient group members might contemplate how they could continue to address problems outside of therapy by using skills acquired in therapy. Members might also anticipate obstacles to realizing therapeutic gains and how these obstacles might be overcome.

The preceding suggestions for intervention apply most fully to the circumstance in which all members of the group are terminating at the same time. However, many of these therapeutic strategies also apply in the circumstance in which a single member departs from an ongoing group. Particularly when a member has been in a group for a long period, his or her departure is likely to activate many of the issues of this developmental stage. By assisting that member in reviewing his or her own progress in the group, members prepare for their own eventual termination. However, the departure of a member from an ongoing group may stimulate other reactions than those occurring when all members leave together. If the member is perceived to be ready to depart, members may feel some envy toward him or her or apprehension about their own progress in the group. If group members perceive the member to be leaving prematurely,

Table 3.1   **The Stages of Group Development**

Stages	Conflictual Issues	Characteristic Behaviors
I	To become a group or remain separate	■ Focus on external situation (members' lives outside the group) ■ Avoidance of genuine affect ■ Placement of particular members in patent position ■ Intellectualization ■ Effort to identify commonalities
II	To become an authority-centered or peer-centered group	■ Argumentativeness among members ■ Expression of dissatisfaction with authority figures outside the group ■ Increasing questioning of the group's efficacy ■ Absences, tardiness, various forms of rule violations
III	The wish to achieve complete, total union in the presence of differences among members	■ Greater eye contact among members ■ Increasingly personal self disclosures ■ Denial of differences among members ■ Denial of negative feelings toward members of the group
IV	The wish to maintain individuality and connection with others	■ Greater balance in the expression of positive and negative feelings (relative to Stage III) ■ Greater capacity to give more specific, individual feedback ■ Mature decision making ■ Use of the therapist as a specialist rather than as an omnipotent figure
V	To hold onto the positive internal tie to the group while reckoning with the separation and the full range of feelings associated with loss	■ Use of idealization and devaluation in relation to group experience ■ Effort to avoid the loss by redefining relationships

there may be worry over whether the group will be adequate to help him or her or guilt over a sense of having failed the departing member. While some of these reactions may be explored while the member is in the process of departure, others may be more easily addressed after the patient has left. Whether the termination is for the entire group or individual members, whether a member is terminating prematurely or following a successful and complete group experience, this event provides valuable and distinctive opportunities for learning.

Like every other stage of development, the therapist may have reactions that can potentially interfere with the group's fully pursuing the work of this stage. For example, the therapist may have difficulty accepting any disappointments the members may express in relation to their group experience (Rutan & Stone, 2001). The therapist may thereby fail to recognize the group's defensive idealization of the group while imagining that the totality of members' response is contentment and unwittingly quash other types of expressions (Brabender, 1987). Hence, as in the other stages, the therapist must monitor his or her own reactions to ensure that they are used to advance rather than obstruct the group's development.

Table 3.1 summarizes the five stages of group development, their issues, and their characteristic behaviors.

Final Considerations on Developmental Stages

In this chapter we considered a particular model of developmental stages. As stated earlier, many developmental models are proposed in the literature, and the scheme presented here emphasizes the common features of a number of them. Most of the models have emerged in clinical contexts and have not been subjected to rigorous empirical testing. Empirical support for the existence of developmental stages can be found in the literature (see MacKenzie's review, 1995), and such research continues to accumulate (e.g., Ellsworth & Hoag, 2000). Nonetheless, the available research is not specific enough to provide strong support for one model over another. Furthermore, it is possible that different models have varying descriptive powers based on context. For example, A. P. Beck (1974) delineates nine phases of group development. This model, which has some empirical support, may have less suitability for a short-term inpatient situation than for a long-term outpatient situation.

The reader should regard any developmental model as a conceptual tool. As such, it assists the therapist in attuning him or herself to the various phenomena occurring in the group that might not be evident without it. Earlier in this chapter, the more specific advantages of having a developmental frame of reference were delineated. Nonetheless, group developmental models are inherently limited because they are general. They guide therapists to recognize what groups have in common; they provide little assistance in helping the therapist recognize what distinguishes each group from other groups (Brabender, 2000; Elfant, 1997). Groups develop distinctive ways of solving the problems that each stage presents. For example, one group may use humor; another may be highly disposed to intense emotional expressiveness. Without these individual variations, our groups would be far less intriguing. A comprehensive consideration of the life of the group requires that the group therapist attends both to what groups have in common, such as the stages, and to what distinguishes groups, one from another.

Summary

Like individuals, groups mature over time. Group development, much like individual development, is organized into stages. During each stage, in the language of general systems theory, a group has an external and internal boundary configuration that is characteristic of that stage. The external boundary, which pertains to who is and is not in the group, has varying levels of permeability depending on the stage of development. Internal boundaries pertain to the connections members establish with one another within the group. Within any stage a conflict that is at once intrapsychic and interpersonal arises in which members have different positions. Members join together into subgroups based upon their similar positions and their wish to disavow other possible positions. Because the conflicts vary from stage to stage, the subgrouping structure does as well. The work of each stage is the exploration of that stage's conflicts. Through this activity, the group as a whole and the members within it can move toward the resolution of the conflicts in a way that is likely to enhance their intrapsychic and interpersonal functioning.

A group's progress through the development stages is not guaranteed. Groups can become fixated at any stage or regress to an earlier stage. In considering why a group may fail to progress, the therapist might attend to a variety of factors, including the stability of group membership, his or her own reactions to the group process, and the modal developmental level of members. Groups have also been observed to act in ways to ensure their own destruction, a phenomenon referred to as the antigroup (Nitsun, 1996).

Five stages of group development were presented. In Stage I, the conflict between the wish to come together and form a group and the wish to remain isolated is activated. The wish to become a group is rooted in the social nature of human beings as well as the longing to achieve the goals of the group, such as the amelioration of suffering. The effort to remain isolated is undergirded by the apprehensions of the perils of human contact as well as by the yearning to have all needs met by an all-powerful caretaker. In Stage II, members struggle with emerging negative feelings toward the authority figure and their fears about the consequences of expressing such feelings. Stages I and II constitute a couplet and culminate in the group's expression of negative feelings toward the therapist, an expression that effects a shift from a leader-centered to a member-centered group. In Stages III and IV, the group is occupied by members' conflictual feelings over how differences and similarities are handled in the group. Should members ignore differences and boundaries to achieve a level of intimacy that is total, or should each member's individuality be acknowledged and protected? In Stage IV, groups exhibit features of maturity such as the capacity of members to give one another balanced, in-depth feedback and the engagement in systematic decision-making processes. In Stage V, members grapple with conflictual feelings associated with the experience of loss.

To highlight certain aspects of the developmental stages, the thinking of Wilfred Bion was introduced. Bion described the ever-present tension between the work group, in which the group systematically pursued its explicit goals, and the basic assumption group, in which members' behavior is under the sway of an unconscious fantasy. Three basic assumption groups were delineated: dependency, fight/flight, and pairing. Following Bion, many theoreticians have noted that the particular basic assumption group that gains ascendancy depends on the stage in which the group is residing.

The utility of a developmental perspective on group life was noted. A developmental conceptualization can help the therapist to have realistic expectations about what a group can do at any point in its life, to anticipate obstacles to members' reaching their goals, to elucidate the meaning of events in the group, and to evaluate the group's effectiveness. At the same time, the therapist must recognize that the unfolding of every group is in many respects unique. To do justice to the phenomena in the group, the therapist must not impose a theoretical framework upon group events in a way that obscures each group's particular mode of functioning and changing over time.

Mechanisms of Change

Over the hundred-year history of this modality, a great deal of thought has been given to the question of what occurs in group sessions that is helpful to its members. While ideas on this question emerged as early as the first decades of the century (e.g., Lazell, 1921; Marsh, 1935), it was not until 1955 that an effort was undertaken to account, systematically and comprehensively, for these factors. Corsini and Rosenberg combed 300 articles to construct a list of 10 factors. These factors, many of which will be discussed in later sections and in some cases by different names, were *acceptance, altruism, universalization, intellectualization, reality testing, transference, interaction, spectator therapy, ventilation,* and *miscellaneous*. In 1963, Berzon, Pious, and Farson developed a nine-factor scheme based on their analysis of members' responses to the question of what the most important event in a session was. Their system overlapped considerably with Corsini and Rosenberg's system.

Irvin Yalom extended this work with his publication of *The Theory and Practice of Group Psychotherapy* in 1970, now in its fourth edition. Yalom, along with his colleagues Tinklenberg and Gilula (1968, an unpublished study cited by Yalom, 1995), studied 20 successful group members who had been in group therapy a minimum of eight months and had completed therapy or were about to do so. These group members were asked to perform a Q-sort. They were given various statements about possible aspects of their group experience, with each statement printed on a separate index card. Examples of such statements are: "Belonging to and being accepted by a group"; "Group members telling me what to do"; and "Admiring and behaving like my therapist." Members were asked to sort the cards into piles based on degree of helpfulness.

4

Chapter

From the results of this card sort, he identified the following factors: altruism, cohesiveness, existential factors, family reenactment, catharsis, instillation of hope, guidance, identification, self-understanding, universality, and interpersonal learning. Yalom made an extremely important contribution in identifying a therapeutic factor unique to group therapy and underscoring its importance. This factor is interpersonal learning. Research has borne out his assertion of the criticality of this factor. As the reader may remember from the meta-analytic studies on the effectiveness of group therapy, the give and take of members' reactions to one another is key to a number of approaches; it is that which enables the potential of group therapy to be realized.

Following this classification scheme, several others were developed that had great similarity to the prior systems but also had their own distinctive qualities. For example, whereas Yalom's system was developed in relation to his own interpersonal approach to doing group therapy, Bloch and Crouch (1985) developed a system that was, by design, atheoretical. It could be applied to groups run according to a variety of theoretical approaches. However, there was another important development: Practitioners began to appreciate that certain factors are more germane to some clinical situations than others. For example, Jerrold Maxmen identified a subset of the commonly recognized factors that have, based on inpatients' self-report, considerable importance for them. Included in these factors are instillation of hope, group cohesiveness, altruism, and universality. However, other studies cited by Yalom (1995) have shown that for outpatients, catharsis, self-understanding, and interpersonal input, followed by cohesiveness and universality, are most important. In this chapter we integrate the contributions of the prior writers and those of many other contributors to the theoretical and empirical literature on mechanisms of change. Moreover, a categorizing scheme of the potentially useful processes and elements in group therapy will be presented, which may help the reader to think about the relationship between these processes and elements and the goals of the group. Bloch and Crouch (1985) proposed a set of two categories: *intrapersonal,* or factors that might operate in individual therapy and therefore do not necessarily involve a group for deployment, and *interpersonal,* or group-specific factors. In this chapter, a tripartite distinction is made among (a) individual factors; (b) interpersonal factors, and (c) group-level factors. Whereas the second set of factors may pertain to dyadic relationships (i.e., relationships between two people), the new third category includes the processes that can and often do encompass most or all members of the group. Their discussion of these factors is based upon the work of Yalom (1995), Bloch and Crouch (1985), and many other contributions. Indeed, the literature on therapeutic mechanisms is among the most extensive in the group literature.

Before we turn to the elements themselves, an important clarification is in order. While the literature labels many of the mechanisms or processes "therapeutic," none of them are inherently therapeutic. They are therapeutic only insofar as they move members toward fulfillment of the goals of the group. In fact, for each of these mechanisms there is some group therapy circumstance in which the factor's activation may serve as an impediment to members' progress in a given area. Some examples of the antitherapeutic sides of these mechanisms are given in a later section. The important point is that in considering the likely impact of any factor and to know whether to support the factor's activation, the therapist should examine the factor in relation to the group goals.

Types of Mechanisms

In this discussion, the interpersonal and group-level mechanisms will be discussed first since they pertain uniquely to group therapy.

Interpersonal Mechanisms

Among the interpersonal mechanisms that can be deployed by group members are interpersonal learning, altruism, identification, and self-disclosure.

Interpersonal Learning: The operation of this all-important factor is seen in the following vignette:

Segment 1

Bruce was an immediately likeable group member who, upon his entrance into the group, electrified it. He had a capacity to generate jokes with the alacrity of a late-night talk show host. After several sessions of his presence in the group, members declared that the group was far more entertaining than prior to his membership. They described their excitement prior to each session. Particularly valued was his talent for affectionately poking fun at those idiosyncracies of members that others had found vexing but seemingly impossible to address.

One evening Beatrice opened the session by dolefully telling the story of her discovery that her teenage daughter had stolen money from her and had eloped with her [the daughter's] boyfriend. Uncharacteristically, Bruce did not make a joke, but he did interject a comment suggesting that her passivity led others to treat her in disrespectful if not abusive ways. Beatrice paused for a moment, appearing nonplussed, and then a flash of recognition crossed her face.

"You are confusing me with Eleanor. That's what the group told Eleanor only two weeks ago. You've been here . . . I don't know how long but it's more than a little while. And you don't really have us straight. It's all part of your glib manner that everyone seems to love," she said angrily.

For the first time since his entrance into the group, Bruce appeared astounded at this reaction and seemed uncertain which tack to take.

"Well, I'm sorry, I was just trying to help . . . I know you're not Eleanor. . . . I mean I thought we said that to you, too, but perhaps in my vagueness to make you feel . . . I don't know . . . but I am sorry."

Jerry turned to Beatrice and noted, "We've been in group a long time and I haven't seen you this angry at another member very often."

"Well, of course, I'm angry at my daughter, but yes, I am upset that he confused me with Eleanor because I think he's done it before. . . . [Turning to Bruce] I'm not really sure that you know who each of us are . . . or remember that much from week to week. We're nonentities to you."

With exasperation, Dina [to Beatrice] responded, "Of course, he knows who we are. It's just your standards . . . no one can do it well enough . . . no one can be sensitive enough to suit you. I mean, he's a great guy . . . Bruce is . . . and if you keep it up much longer, I don't think he'll be here much longer!" The therapist observed to herself that all of the members were sitting on the edges of their seats waiting for Bruce to respond to the suggestion that he might leave the group.

Comment: At this point, members' involvement in the session is characterized by three features. First, their feelings have been stimulated. Beatrice feels angry about Bruce's mistake. Bruce feels embarrassed and guilty about Beatrice's confrontation of him. Dina feels angry about Beatrice's confrontation of Bruce and apprehensive about his possible departure from the group. Second, members are highly engaged in the session. While they are finding aspects of the session distressing or anxiety arousing, clearly they do not find the session to be dull, boring, or tedious. Third, the focus of members is on their relationships with one another as they unfold within the immediate session. This focus is to be contrasted with one in which members' focus is external to the group. For example, the group might have followed a different trajectory in which it delved into the parenting difficulties of Beatrice and other members.

All of these three features are related to one another. That strong feelings aroused in the group command interest is a very predictable, regular feature of group life. However, this interest becomes that much more acute when the feelings concern the situation at hand. One could imagine an alternate scenario in which the members who are parents express strong feelings about the behavior of their progeny. While some members may have been highly absorbed in the discussion, others who were not struggling with parenting issues may have been quite indifferent. In the present example members' interest is naturally elicited because each member has a stake in the discussion and its outcomes. The captivation of members' attention because of the group's focus on internal issues is accompanied by the evocation of members' feelings. In this instance they are likely to care, one way or another, about whether Bruce remains in the group. Many group therapists have witnessed a session that was lackluster because of members' preoccupation with an outside topic (the "there-and-then" in group therapy terminology) transform itself into a hotbed of affects as members turn their attention to the "here-and-now,"[1] the internal and immediate issues of the group.

The power of the here-and-now in group work has been demonstrated repeatedly. Kurt Lewin, a major contributor to the understanding of small group dynamics, spent years studying how groups develop the capacity to work effectively. Lewin and his colleagues at Massachusetts Institute of Technology were asked to conduct workshops with the goal of developing leadership skills in participants to enable them to address and lessen racial tensions. The workshop sessions, held in Bethel, Maine, were conducted during the day, and in the evenings the leaders and researchers met to process

---

[1] The term "here-and-now" was coined by Jacob Moreno, the founder of psychodrama, a major approach to group work.

their observations. During the day the participants talked about situations outside the group—clearly within the realm of the there-and-then. Then, on one occasion a daytime participant happened to stay on into the evening and was permitted to attend the evening research meeting. The participant gave feedback to the researchers about his evaluation of the accuracy of their observations. Gradually, more and more participants attended the evening meeting. The evening meeting became a more vibrant workplace than either the daytime meeting or the earlier format of the evening meeting. The vibrancy was directly due to members' active here-and-now processing of their interactions with one another. It was no longer a discussion group; it was an experiential group.

Lewin recognized the importance of feedback in effecting change. As Jacobs (1974) notes, the term *feedback* was coined by the physicist Weiner (1948), who defined it as the alteration of a system's input through its output in the form of an informational (or feedback) loop. Lewin, drawing upon his observations of groups, applied the concept of feedback to systems studied by the social sciences.

If we compare the meetings in Bethel, Maine, to the therapy group meeting in the vignette, we see an important difference. The participants in the research project were trying to *understand* their interaction with one another. While the therapy group members no doubt had understanding as a long-term goal, members were primarily interested in expressing their emotional reactions. What has been learned about groups involving the expression of emotional reactions in the absence of understanding is that they fail to be beneficial and can even be detrimental to participants (see Beutler et al., 1984, and Pattison, Brissenden, & Wohl, 1967, with inpatient groups and Lieberman, Yalom, & Miles, 1973, with short-term growth groups).

While there might be many ways in which a group can achieve an understanding of its affective experience, the following segment demonstrates one unfolding that is inconsistent with this group's mode of operation:

Segment 2

The therapist noted that some strong feelings had been expressed and sensed that there was an uneasiness and apprehension that the expression of feelings might lead to some negative outcome such as a member, perhaps Bruce, leaving the group.

"You're not going to leave the group are you, Bruce?" Eleanor asked mildly.

Bruce quickly replied, "And miss the opportunity to be scolded by Beatrice? Wouldn't dream of it! Besides, I always feel better after getting my 'comeuppance'!"

Eleanor smiled, and several members moved back in their seats.

The therapist said, "So perhaps one worry can be put aside. But we still have some strong feelings here that we've yet to explore."

Bruce nodded, saying, "I still want to follow up on what you said when you nailed me. . . . I think it's on the money . . . at least in a way. It's not that I don't care about you. . . . I think about you all after we leave and during the week. But when I'm here, it's sort of a rush for me. I get exhilarated and that can make it hard for me to hear everything you say or noticing who says it. At times, I avoid using your names so I don't get them wrong."

"Maybe," Jerry said, "it's because you are so on . . . if I were as entertaining as you, I think I would find it irresistible not to be garnering laughs every moment."

"There's a cost though," noted Eleanor. "When the show is over, you go home alone. And at that point, the audience is . . . just a blur."

"Right," said Bruce, "That's why I'm here. That's it exactly."

"So when you're boring us, we'll know you're making progress?" Jerry asked.

"Yeah, and when I'm quiet," Bruce added.

"I feel guilty that I lashed out at you," Beatrice said. "Probably whoever would have been the first one to speak to me would have gotten decapitated."

Jerry said, "That may have been true. Most of us have come in here that way one time or another. But when Dina said that thing about your high standards . . ."

Interrupting, Dina said, "Maybe I was lashing out then. . . . I thought Bruce might leave and I . . ."

"But wait . . . I still think there's something to that. . . . In fact, when you [Dina] spoke, I had the thought that maybe you were actually responding to what happened last week when Beatrice got irritated that you said that you felt sympathy for Eleanor. She said 'sympathy' is condescending."

"Yes, I felt stupid."

"That's sort of similar to what happened here tonight." Jerry continued, "Bruce wanted to be helpful but [to Beatrice], he didn't get it exactly right so it felt all wrong to you. And if someone uses a word that's not quite on target, same thing. Sometimes I avoid interacting with you just because I

won't meet your standard. But when I do, I feel cheated because I so value your perceptiveness."

"I'm the one who is cheated," Beatrice said, almost to herself.

The therapist noted, "I think what we are seeing here tonight is extremely important. Yet, it is certainly not new to the group. Beatrice and Bruce came to the group wanting to connect with other members and yet, discover that there are obstacles to doing so in a way that is truly satisfying."

Comment: Taken together, the two segments suggest a two-step process. In the first step the group members expressed a great deal of strong affect toward one another. Although the members made observations of one another, these observations lacked the specificity to be helpful to members. In the second step the level of intensity of feeling declined, and members were able to invest themselves more fully in the enterprise of understanding their experiences with one another. Group members achieved understanding in a way that was consonant with the goals of the group and the theoretical orientation guiding the group. In Chapters 10 through 13, the reader learns that such understanding can be achieved in a variety of ways. The means by which understanding is achieved are not nearly as important as the achievement itself.

The alternation between the two steps is part of the natural rhythm of a group session. Without the initial affective aspect, the session is listless. It lacks the capacity to engage members' attention sufficiently to enable learning to occur. However, affect in the absence of a cognitive frame is mere overstimulation.

New members of therapy groups will commonly express perplexity with more seasoned members' focus on their relationships with one another. "My problem is not with members in this group; my problem is with the people in my life out there," the member will lament. The senior members will, with varying levels of weariness, explain a concept central to the usefulness of interpersonal learning. This is the concept of the group as a *microcosm*, or little world (Yalom, 1995). Like the world in which all of us live, it is populated with individuals with a diversity of relational styles. That is, the interpersonal patterns that any member exhibits within the group are generally representative of that member's patterns in his or her life outside of therapy. As such, whatever learning the member achieves about these patterns in the group is likely to raise awareness about his or her interpersonal style in general. One of the most significant tasks of the developing group therapist is to learn how to nurture a process of interpersonal learning. In Chapter 10 we discuss the interpersonal approach in some detail and describe the various interventions at the therapist's disposal to foster interpersonal learning. As is noted, the members in many types of groups are likely to focus on topics external to the group. The therapist must support their focus on one another, on themselves in relation to others and their own group process. Once members explicitly turn their attention to matters inside the group, the therapist must both monitor and participate in this group process to ensure that it is a constructive one for all participants.

Continuing Questions on Interpersonal Learning: The possibility of interpersonal learning is at the crux of what is unique about group therapy. Despite its centrality, the research that has been done to evaluate the technology of this mechanism is relatively limited. A variety of questions remain to be answered by future research.

What elements of interpersonal learning are most important? For example, is it more helpful for a person to learn about his or her behavioral patterns, the motivational underpinnings of those behavioral patterns, or others' reactions to the behavioral patterns? One study (Flowers & Booraem, 1990) demonstrated that therapists' interpretations in 10- to 30-session psychodynamic groups were associated with positive outcomes if they provided members with, in decreasing order of importance, information on their behavioral patterns, the reactions of others to these behavioral patterns, or the possible historical bases of these patterns. Interpretations of the motives underlying behavior appeared to increase symptomatology over the course of treatment. The investigators explained this finding as the result of the power of interpretation of motives to increase members' anxiety levels. They considered the possibility that in long-term groups, motivational interpretations may produce more favorable responses.

Another important dimension is the valence of feedback (Jacobs, 1974). The valence of feedback is the extent to which the feedback is experienced as positive or negative. Jacobs and colleagues found that members of a therapy group perceive positive feedback as more credible than negative feedback (e.g., Jacobs, Jacobs, Gatz, & Schaible, 1973; Pine & Jacobs, 1991). Because it is unlikely that people will alter their behavior on the basis of feedback that they find of questionable validity, this finding would seem to suggest the greater usefulness of positive feedback. However, negative feedback was found to be more credible when it followed positive feedback; positive feedback was perceived to be less accurate when it followed negative feedback. Perhaps members feel that when the positive feedback is offered first, there is a caring dimension to the relationship. In this context the negative feedback is seen as constructive rather than attacking. Altogether, these findings suggest that group therapists would do well to ensure that positive feedback is plentiful in a group. Moreover, positive feedback may be especially vital early in a member's involvement in the group and even perhaps early in each session.

One important variable that has not been explored sufficiently is the cultural background of the member and the extent to which providing positive versus negative feedback is common within a culture. In a culture emphasizing politeness and civility, exchanges of negative information may be more threatening than in a culture that accords individuals greater latitude of expression.

When is feedback most useful? Some research suggests that the timing of feedback may be important. Tschuschke and Dies (1994) found that individuals who benefited from group tended to receive considerable feedback relatively early in the life of the group. Persons with poor outcomes tended to obtain an increasing amount of feedback over the course of the group. These investigators hypothesized that feedback, to be effective, must be assimilated. Assimilation requires time. Individuals who obtain feedback late in the group may not have sufficient opportunity to integrate the feedback with their preexisting understanding of themselves. But why do some members receive feedback unremittingly? An alternative explanation is that members who do not improve are ones who do not implement the feedback they have received and consequently continue to receive it. To evaluate this finding more fully, research should focus on the characteristics of the feedback as they remain the same or vary over the course of the group.

Are there any steps that should be taken to guarantee that the interpersonal learning achieved in the group will be transferred to experiences outside the group? In the study mentioned earlier, Flowers and Booraem (1990) found that group members exhibited more favorable outcomes when the links between their patterns of behavior in the group and those outside the group were identified. How might such links be identified? A member may enter a group session complaining about some difficulty he or she encountered outside the group. For example, the member may say, "People where I work are so touchy. I was told by my supervisor that my coworkers were complaining that my teasing is offensive. I'm just trying to make the mood a little lighter." At this juncture the therapist should question whether this member engages in similar teasing behaviors in the group. Both their complexion and impact upon members could be discussed. The member might be given alternative behaviors that could be piloted in the group and used in the outside environment. The specification of alternative behaviors brings in another change mechanism, guidance, which can be paired with the interpersonal learning mechanism.

Can the positive effects of feedback be augmented by technology? The primary use of technology has been in the videotaping of groups. Videotaping segments of sessions may enhance members' recognition and understanding of their interpersonal patterns. Videotaping offers a measure of distance. It allows individuals to get outside of themselves and see themselves as others do. Videotaping also allows for playbacks. Members can thereby observe details that may have been ignored upon first viewing.

Research on the usefulness of videotaping has produced mixed results. Robinson and Jacobs (1970) had group leaders replay segments of a session enabling hospitalized group members to see behavioral patterns that the group leaders saw as significant for those members. The cotherapists gave a commentary on the behaviors, highlighting both positive and negative features. Relative to a control group, the videotaped groups showed a diminishment in maladaptive behaviors and increase in positive social behaviors. However, other studies (e.g., Martin, 1971) have failed to show positive effects and have even shown negative effects. Jacobs (1974) attributes these negative findings to the failure of the group leaders to provide a cognitive framing for the videotaped material. This interpretation is consistent with Yalom's (1995) emphasis that interpersonal learning must entail both affective stimulation and the cognitive organization of affective material to lead to positive change.

Given the ever-increasing reliance of our society upon technology, efforts to employ video techniques in the change process are likely only to increase. Somewhat fancifully, perhaps, Ettin (2000) forecasted, "As the twenty-first century comes to a close, small screen, sequential response, computerized group treatments will become passé, having been replaced by new home entertainment systems equipped with sophisticated holographic imaging technology. It will be possible to chose from a voice-activated list of group therapists from around the world and cross historical eras" (p. 4). In the meantime, there is a great deal of work to be done in exploring the ethical and legal dimensions of such technological applications. Some of these dimensions are explored in Chapter 9.

Altruism: This process is deployed when any member attempts to respond helpfully to another member. Members' ways of being altruistic are various. In the prior vignette a number of Jerry's comments appeared to be altruistically based. For example, when Beatrice says in a self-critical way that she "lashed out" at Bruce, Jerry notes that every member at some time has come in poised to be judgmental of, and hostile toward, other members. Given the content of his comment, his intent seemed to be to reduce the harshness of Beatrice's self-evaluation. While perhaps less effective, Bruce's initial effort to assist Beatrice in seeing what enduring interpersonal behaviors contributed to her predicament with her daughter also constituted altruistic behavior.

Altruism is of potential benefit to both the altruist and the recipient of the altruism. Recipients of altruism have an experience of being cared for by others and being valued by others. The altruists themselves are able to experience the caring dimensions of their own person. An individual's awareness of his or her goodness can be particularly important when the individual's self-regard has been compromised by guilt or hostile feelings toward others. This form of altruism does not necessarily require that the recipient of the altruism feels helped (Kibel, 1981). For example, although Bruce would be unlikely to feel that he had been successful in assisting Beatrice, he might at least derive satisfaction from feeling he attempted to be helpful.

However, another benefit of altruism to the altruist is the sense of self-efficacy that attends the act of being helpful to another. This aspect of altruism can be extremely important to people whose circumstances have led them to see themselves as unable to act competently (Maxmen, 1973). For example, individuals requiring inpatient hospitalization frequently imagine that they are bereft of any resources to take care of their own needs, let alone some else's. They are then surprised and heartened to discover that they can be capable of offering others valued advice, soothing, or some other commodity that appears to enhance the well-being of others. This benefit of altruism places a greater demand that the recipient of the altruistic act either appreciate or use in an obvious way the ministrations of the altruist.

Altruism is a factor whose importance may vary considerably depending on the context of treatment. Outpatients do not see altruism as of great importance to their progress in the group (Yalom, 1985). On the other hand, inpatients see altruism as a critical feature of their group participation (Macaskill, 1982; R. Marcowitz & Smith, 1983; Maxmen, 1973). Furthermore, models of inpatient group therapy place great emphasis upon the therapeutic use of altruism. For example, Jerrold Maxmen's Educative Model (Brabender & Fallon, 1993) taps the self-efficacy aspect of altruism. Members who are new to the inpatient group and in many cases not ready to self-disclose are given opportunities to be helpful to others. By seeing evidence of their own competence, these members are encouraged to deepen their levels of group participation.

Identification: There is no more basic a human propensity than identification. It is a process that begins in infancy (an argument could be made that identification occurs on a prenatal basis as the fetus engages in such activities as sucking the thumb) and that leads to the development of the psychological structures necessary for adaptation to the environment (Fenichel, 1945). Identification is taking in the outside and making it part of one's internal self. Initially, the internal self is one's physical self, but increasingly, external input leads to the development of psychological mechanisms for adaptation.

Because identification occurs quite naturally in human interactions, it is ubiquitous in therapy groups. Identification leads to changes in the identifying person that admit of degrees. It can be a short-lived phenomenon. For example, one member may imitate for a brief period the laughter of another group member whom she admires. Conversely, identification can lead to relatively permanent changes in behavior. This level of alteration is seen in the following case example:

> *For weeks, Audrey had been intrigued with Andrea because she sensed in her a kindred spirit. She noticed that Andrea was reticent; yet she saw in her an inner strength. Audrey was aware that Andrea was peeved lately. On several*

occasions she had answered members' questions in a rather testy tone of voice. Then one evening Pete said to Andrea, "What's been bugging you?"

Andrea hesitated and then said in a crisp tone, "I have been feeling frustrated because lately it's always a few members who are dominating our meetings."

Pete said, "Maybe we should give each person five minutes. Then we would be sure that each of us gets our share . . . you included."

Another member said, "But maybe some of us need to talk some nights more than other nights."

Pete shrugged and said, "Okay, I withdraw my suggestion."

"It's not so important to me that, say, I get the same amount of time as everyone else. Of course it's going to be true that some of us may need more time on any given night than other members do. But what bothers me is that on some nights, we come in and two people will go back and forth as if there's no one else here. Even if someone wanted to say something, it's like you'd be interrupting a private conversation."

Pete, looking abashed, chortled, "Guilty as charged."

"No," Andrea rejoined, "I'm not saying that you did anything wrong. I feel it's [nodding at the therapist] her responsibility." The group became very still. Audrey was flabbergasted but agreed with Andrea. She resented the therapist's permitting other members to go on and on. Yet she never would have expressed this criticism. She sat in suspense to see what would happen next.

"So you see me as not doing my job," the therapist probed.

"Not doing it completely enough," Andrea responded.

"Perhaps others feel that way," the therapist noted.

Other members indicated that indeed they did feel dissatisfied with the therapist for the reason Andrea gave and for other reasons. Audrey was surprised that the therapist looked so calm as members were describing their unhappiness with her. It appeared that Andrea was going to suffer no ill consequence for having directly criticized the therapist. Audrey imagined herself telling the therapist about some of her less endearing behaviors.

Audrey engaged in an act of learning in the session; she learned that the expression of negative reactions toward a figure of authority need not lead to an act of retaliation by that authority figure. Yalom refers to this process as vicarious learning because it is learning based not on action but on observation. This process of identification is different from mere *imitation* in that the latter notion refers to a copying of another person's behavior. Identification requires an internal, psychological alteration. It can also be distinguished, as Rutan and Stone (2001) do, from internalization, which involves an alteration in an internal mechanism enabling a new way of responding to the environment. If over time Audrey's fears about the consequences of expressing various reactions to authority figures, if her representation of authority figures shifted in the direction of seeing them as less threatening, then a process of internalization was at work.

In our example of Audrey and Andrea, Audrey's activity of identification was presented as a conscious one. This was done primarily for ease of exposition. While identification may have conscious elements, it is often largely unconscious. Audrey's registration of Andrea's interactions with the therapist may have been entirely outside of her awareness.

As Crouch, Bloch, and Wanless (1994) note, while many approaches may allow for identification, some models, such as psychodrama, do so in a way that is more formal and explicit. The technique of *doubling* entails a double playing the inner life of the protagonist, who is the principal of the psychodrama. The protagonist can see and make part of his or her own self the capabilities of the double to express his or her experience. Likewise, within psychodrama there is an audience that observes the enactment of the psychodrama. The purpose of the observation is to enable the learning that occurs via identification.

There is some evidence in the literature on the usefulness of identification. Jeske (1973) had group therapy members press buttons each time they experienced themselves as identifying with another group member. Group members who were categorized as having improved, as measured by their degrees of positive change on the scales of the Minnesota Multiphasic Personality Inventory, made twice as many identifications as those who did not improve. This result suggests that the therapist should attend to evidence of the extent to which members are identifying with one another. Sometimes this information is obtained from verbal behavior ("You remind me of myself") or nonverbal activity. Dugo and Beck (1984) note that members' identifications with one another have particular importance early in group life: Members who can identify with no other member are at risk for prematurely leaving the group.

Self-disclosure: This mechanism of change refers to a group member's communication of information that he or she regards as personal.

Self-disclosures can both indicate and produce therapeutic progress. Such disclosures indicate progress when they reveal that the member has established a deeper level of trust in the other members of the group than he or she had previously. Most seasoned group therapists have witnessed the almost magical event when an excessively cautious group member offers, for the first time, some personal detail. While the substance of the communication may be relatively unimportant, the event is important because it signifies that the communicator's fear that interactions with others will be dangerous has lessened.

Self-disclosure can effect change in both the disclosing person and the group as a whole. Often there can be an immense sense of relief at having articulated that which was felt to be too shameful to reveal to others. Self-disclosure can lead to others talking about similar experiences (a phenomenon referred to as universality, which is discussed more fully in a later section), often resulting in a diminished sense of aloneness. Self-disclosures provide the opportunity to receive feedback from others:

> *Finally, Doris got the courage to tell members that she thought others were repelled by her facial tic. The members indicated that while the tic was rather noticeable to them at the point at which they were getting to know her, they found it much less conspicuous after a time. One member said she was only mindful of it when there was overt conflict in the group. The member noticed that at such times, Doris's tick appeared much more frequently.*

Doris may never have received this potentially helpful feedback had she not invited members to give it through her self-disclosure. Finally, research has shown that mutual self-disclosures create a sense of intimacy in relationships, particularly when the self-disclosure concerns emotions rather than factual information (Laurenceau, Barrett, & Pietromonaco, 1998). Moreover, self-disclosures about the here-and-now are more likely to increase group cohesion than self-disclosures about the there-and-then (Slavin, 1993).

Do members who self-disclose more than other members derive more from the group? Tschuschke and Dies (1994) found that inpatient participants in a psychoanalytic group who had more favorable outcomes (reflected in an outcome score combining a variety of measures) engaged in more disclosure over most of the course of the group relative to individuals who had less favorable outcomes.

However, the latter individuals tended to disclose more toward the end of their group participation both relative to the more successful participants and to their own original levels of self-disclosure. Once again, we may be seeing the contribution of the cognitive component of interpersonal learning. Members who disclose a great deal at the end of the group may not have an opportunity to achieve full understanding of the disclosure itself, members' feedback on the disclosure, or both. This finding highlights the importance of the therapists' attunement to the developmental status of the group.

Group-Level Mechanisms

The next class of factors are those that refer to mechanisms that members see as operating beyond the dyad and often extending to the entire group. These mechanisms are universality, reenactment of family of origin, and cohesion.

Universality: Universality is a recognition that one's experiences are part of the human condition and, therefore, that one is neither alone with them nor distinguished by them. Universality can take a variety of forms in a group. Which type may be emphasized in a given group depends upon a variety of factors. Members may establish universality with respect to painful feelings associated with a traumatic circumstance in their lives. For example, suppose members of a short-term loss group share a sense of abject despair in response to the death of a child. They will come to recognize that as intolerable as the despair may be, it does not separate them from all other human beings.

Another level of universality occurs when a member shares some aspect an experience that threatens his or her self-esteem. Consider in this regard the following exchange between two group members:

HELEN: Ever since Tammy has entered the group, I have been feeling—and it makes me sick to say this—envious. I'm glad she's not here tonight so I can get this thing off my chest. She is so pretty and seems so innocent. I just want to tear her down. And I don't respect myself very much for that level of pettiness either.

JOYCE: I can't believe you're saying that.

HELEN: I know . . . I'm a worm.

JOYCE: No . . . I didn't meant that at all. I was shocked just because I have been having the same reaction. She's all perfection. And I can't stand it . . . it makes me feel mean toward her. Sometimes when she is speaking, I sit here privately mocking her . . . then I despise myself.

HELEN: Exactly! But you're a nice person so if you feel that way, it must not be . . . *that* awful.

Envy is an affect that can be extremely disturbing to the person experiencing it and highly undermining of that person's good opinion of himself or herself. Discovering that another person is also beset by the same troubling feeling diminishes self-criticism. That these forms of universality are beneficial was demonstrated in one study that focused upon the reactions of Harvard undergraduate students who shared concealable stigmas such as being gay, having bulimia, or being members of a family that earned less than $20,000 a year (Frable, Platt, & Hoey, 1998). In the presence of others whom they saw as similar with respect to stigmatizing characteristics, the students showed higher self-esteem and a more positive mood than those who were not in the company of similar others.

A third level of universality is that in which a member gains access to, and accepts, some hitherto disavowed aspect of the self by increasingly realizing that the aspect in question is simply part of human psychology. For example, if another member, upon listening to Helen, Joyce, and others share their reactions, becomes aware of envious feelings, then this achievement may have more than a palliative effect. It might enable the individual to reorganize her sense of self by integrating aspects that she had previously seen as too threatening into her self-awareness.

Many factors bear upon which level of universality is possible in a given group. Theoretical models and types of groups vary in the extent to which they cultivate members' establishment of universality on each of the three levels. In contrast to therapy groups, many support groups operate strictly on the first level, that in which members share painful reactions in relation to some stressor. Many models and types of groups make use of the second level of universality in which members share esteem-challenging reactions. In fact, both the first and second levels of universality will occur in most groups where there is the opportunity to share reactions rather spontaneously with one another.

The third type of universality is likely to be seen in those psychodynamic groups that place an emphasis upon members becoming conscious of unconscious elements of their personalities. These approaches have intervention strategies for existing members in moving toward achieving universality on this deeper level. For example, the object-relations approach, which is described in Chapter 11, employs the group-as-a-whole interpretation. A relatively new approach to group therapy, systems-centered group therapy makes use of the natural proclivity of members to form subgroups (Agazarian, 1997). Members are supported in forming subgroups in relation to whatever conflictual issue is besetting the group. The subgroups in which members place themselves are based upon their common access to a particular psychological content and their lack of access to another. While in the safety of their subgroup, members gradually gain access to the formerly repudiated content. By always enjoying some level of universality, by never being placed in a position of isolation in the group, members can move to deeper levels of self-discovery and universality.

Another factor affecting the level of universality a group achieves is the tenure of members' group participation. When group participation is relatively brief, the first two levels of universality may be all that are possible. When I led eight-session inpatient groups, much discussion occurred early on about the distress members experienced in relation to stressors, which members saw themselves as sharing. For example, members frequently complained about relatives and friends who were very nonempathic about their struggles. Somewhat later in the group's life, members would move to an exploration of disturbing reactions that they perceived to be less externally driven, such as their senses of being too dependent upon persons in authority for direction or too unable to modulate their impulses. While occasionally the group could move to the third level of universality, it was by no means the emphasis of the group. A group that affords members the opportunity to get to know each other over a considerable duration is more likely to move to deeper levels of universality. Over time, trust increases and the strength of defenses against the recognition of a variety of human experiences diminishes.

Corrective Recapitulation of the Primary Family Group: Since the early days of group therapy, there has been a realization that a special aspect of the group situation is its resemblance to a family situation. Therapists occupy the position of parents and the group members of siblings. Within individual therapy the activation of sibling dynamics is difficult to achieve because the person to whom the patient is relating, the therapist, is in a position of authority. Hence, the therapist is likely to be seen as a parental figure. The potential of group therapy to bring to life not only parental but siblings dynamics (as well as siblings in relation to parents) adds to the richness of the group situation.

The resemblance between the group and the family can and has been used in the therapy group in two ways. The first is an explicit analysis of each member's early family relations with parents and siblings as suggested by the relationship with the therapist and other group members. For example, the therapist might draw a connection between a member's response to a member who has recently joined an ongoing group to that member's possible response to the birth of a sibling (Shapiro & Ginsberg, 2001). A second use of the resemblance between the family and the group is more general. It assumes that the various tenors of early relationships with a family member will affect the individual's internal schemas of contemporary relationships, including relationships with group members. Group therapy activates these schemas in their variety and creates opportunities for their updating.

While many if not most therapy groups draw upon the implicit use of family reenactment, far fewer use the reenactment concept explicitly. Group therapists are disinclined to do so because such explorations must be made on a highly individual basis. Delving into a member's history leaves other members uninvolved. Furthermore, the empirical literature provides very limited evidence that historical interpreting is associated with more positive outcomes. Finally, while groups and families have similarities, the dynamics of each differ somewhat from one another. Trained observers of families and juries rated the importance of various features in their impact upon the efficiency and effectiveness of the groups' functioning. Certain factors, extremely important to family process, were relatively unimportant to the process of a group, and vice-versa. This research suggests that one cannot assume a one-to-one relationship between familial relationships and group relationships.

On the other hand, dealing with conflicts related to family on a symbolic or implicit level within the here-and-now process of the group brings all members into the discussion. Research suggests that such a present focus can address issues related to familial relationship (Tschuschke & Dies, 1994). For example, members who entered the group with representations of themselves and their parents as enmeshed achieved more separateness between parent and self-representations. Interestingly, some members exhibited these shifts after relatively brief intervals of group participation.

Cohesion: The reader can get a sense of the meaning of group cohesion and how groups differ on this variable by considering the following two vignettes:

Vignette 1

A therapy group had been meeting for two years, and most of the members were the original members. The therapist noticed that all of the members had gathered in the waiting room before the group was scheduled to begin. When the session began, Paul expressed anger toward Erika for implying at the end of the last session that he used women in his life, including women in the group. He indicated that her comment bothered him all week. Erika noted that she, too, had thought about the group and worried that she had gone too far in her comments to Paul.

For much of the session, group members focused on both Paul and Erika, noting that Paul's tendency to become distractible and unresponsive when the women in the group expressed vulnerability made it appear to others that he was simply using them. He responded to them only when they were in a position to give rather than to receive. A number of men in the group identified with Paul and recognized that it was not so much that they did not want to give but that when the women in the group exhibited vulnerability, it stimulated similar feelings in them. They felt that if they were to show this vulnerability, they would be repulsive to the other group members, especially the female members.

The group, however, pointed out to Erika that often the demands she makes upon other people were excessive, particularly her demands on men. If others' attention flagged for even a second, members noted, she seemed to feel utterly abandoned by them. Erika then acknowledged to the group that she expected men not to pay attention to her. She merely waited for it to happen. Several men and women in the group recognized that they, too, were inclined not to give others an opportunity to give to them because of their often-unwarranted expectation that disappointment would follow. In the midst of this energetic discussion, the therapist looked at her watch and noticed that the group had run five minutes over its scheduled ending time.

Vignette 2

A group composed of adolescent boys had been meeting for about two months. All of the boys had been referred to the group because of academic problems that were thought to be due to emotional concerns. Although the group began at 7:00 P.M., members straggled in until 7:45. The therapist announced at the beginning of the group that two members were not going to be present for that session. A third member never showed up and never called to cancel. At the beginning of the session, members talked about not knowing what to talk about in the group. Finally, one member spoke about some conflict he was having with his parents over their establishment of curfews on weekday nights, which he saw as totally unjustified. After he was done talking, no one responded. Another boy spoke about his anger over having to come to the session and his resentment that his mother had bribed him with the use of the family car over the weekend. When he was finished talking, no one responded. Another boy asked the therapist for tips on how to prepare for the college boards. The therapist said that maybe someone in the group had some ideas. When no one had any ideas, the youth said it didn't matter because he intended to cheat anyway. The session was to end in five minutes and the boys sat in sullen silence waiting to be freed of that week's obligation to be in the group session.

DEFINITION OF COHESION: In a variety of ways, the group in the first vignette showed a far higher level of cohesion than the group in the second vignette. The members in the first group seemed to want to be in the group. Unlike the members of the second group, they arrived early and showed no readiness to depart. Furthermore, the members of the first group had made a long-term commitment to the group. Cohesiveness was seen in the group members' willingness to grapple with the painful feelings emerging in their relationships with one another. Paul came to the group wanting to examine further the distress he felt in relation to Erika's feedback. Erika also showed a willingness to confront her ready disappointment in others, especially men. In the second group, members did not seem to have established relationships with one another; they appeared to be motivated by a longing to be relieved of group participation. Although this reaction was shared among group members, they could not yet work together to achieve this end by, for instance, staging a protest. A third manifestation of cohesiveness in the first vignette was the group's presence in the minds of its members outside of sessions. Between sessions both Erika and Paul reported thinking about the content of the session and their interactions with one another.

Now that the reader has an intuitive sense of group cohesion, a more formal definition is in order. *Group cohesion* is a felt bond among members. It is a sense of camaraderie or togetherness that members feel in relation to one another and the group as a whole, and a commitment to the goals of the group. Group cohesiveness is the counterpart in group therapy of the therapeutic alliance in individual therapy (Kaul & Bednar, 1986).

A primary way in which group cohesiveness has been studied is through its measurement as the perceived attractiveness of a group to its members. The use of this definition of cohesiveness makes it relatively accessible to investigation. Each group member can rate the group-as-a-whole and the other members on the dimension of degree of attractiveness. Higher ratings of attractiveness would correspond to higher levels of cohesiveness. Despite its convenience, this way of thinking about group cohesiveness eliminates a core aspect of this property (Evans & Jarvis, 1980; Rutan & Stone, 2001). Webster's *New Collegiate* dictionary defines *cohesion* as "Molecular attraction by which the particles of a body are united throughout the mass" (1981, p. 216). What this definition captures is that cohesion is a kind of magnetic field into which members are irresistibly pulled. It exists at the level of the group, not at the level of the individual. In fact, members may feel attracted to the other members or the idea of being in this particular group, yet the group may never cohere.

THE EFFECTS OF COHESION: Are cohesive groups more effective in meeting the goals? This question has been investigated in two situations. The first is in task groups that do not have a therapeutic aim. For example, a recent study (Langfred, 1998) focused on the supervisors' ratings of the effectiveness of army units in the Danish military in accomplishing highly operationalized tasks. Findings on work groups generally support a positive relationship between group cohesion and the effectiveness of the group. Summarizing such studies, Johnson and Johnson (2000) write:

As cohesiveness increases, absenteeism and turnover of membership de-crease, and the following increases: member commitment to group goals, feelings of personality responsibility to the group, willingness to take on dif-ficult tasks, motivation and persistence in working towards goal achieve-ment, satisfaction and morale, willingness to endure frustration and pain on behalf of the group, willingness to defend the group against external criti-cism or attack, willingness to listen to and be influenced by colleagues, com-mitment to each other's professional growth and success and productivity. (p. 110)

However, cohesion is a complex variable in that its effects are moder-ated by other variables. As Langfred (1998) demonstrated in his pre-viously cited study, the influence of cohesion occurs in relation to the work norms of the group. In Chapter 7, we consider the topic of norms in some depth. For the present, suffice it to say that group norms are those work-related behaviors that are seen as acceptable by the group. One group, for example, may see high levels of productiv-ity on the part of each member as necessary for each member to be seen as a good citizen of the group. Slackers may earn the group's dis-approval. In another group work-oriented behaviors may be deni-grated. For example, one could imagine a class of high school students in which earnest efforts to master the material in a given class bring scorn rather than praise. The point about cohesive groups is not that they are more effective in pursuing any externally imposed task but rather that they are more effective in pursuing a task they embrace. The aforementioned high school class may have as its goal socializa-tion (despite the faculty member's having another goal). If highly co-hesive, the group will be much more effective in pursuing the goal of socialization than if the group were deficient in cohesion.

The research on cohesiveness in therapy groups is more limited in part because of the inherent difficulty of investigating therapy groups relative to groups that occur in a work setting. However, a well-designed study by Budman's research team (Budman, Soldz, et al., 1989) provided some support for the generally positive relation-ship found between level of cohesion and productivity (or in this case, member improvement). These investigators studied 12 groups, each lasting 15 sessions. Outcome was measured by a set of global scales and target problem measures. The investigators found that co-hesion established early in the group is associated with higher levels of improvement than either low levels of cohesion or cohesion established later in the life of the group.

However, like the results with work groups, therapy groups do not invariably show a rise in productivity with an increase in cohesion. Roether and Peters (1972) found an inverse relationship between level of cohesion and offender rearrest rates in a group of sexual offenders who were required to attend group therapy. Given the circumstances of treatment, question may be raised as to whether these group members embraced the treatment goals of the therapists, a necessary condition for cohesion to enhance productivity.

How Cohesion Works: How can we account for the power of group cohesion to facilitate a group's progress toward its goal? Irvin Yalom, writing from an interpersonal theory perspective, identifies three aspects of group cohesion. First, group cohesion leads the individual to take seriously any discrepancy between the member's self-esteem and his or her public esteem (or others' regard for that member). Further, cohesion compels the member to use the awareness of that discrepancy for positive change. For example, suppose the individual's public esteem is higher than her self-esteem and that the latter is exceedingly low. If the member does not feel a sense of belonging to, or solidarity with, the group, she is likely to devalue the group's valuation of her and cling to her negative self-perception. If the member does value the group, then she is likely to adjust her self-regard in the direction of the group's view of her. She would thereby experience an increase in self-esteem. However, the person's public esteem may be substantially lower than his or her self-esteem. Presumably, the individual is engaging in behaviors that produce negative reactions in others. In a group lacking cohesiveness the member can simply dismiss the group's perceptions. In a cohesive group in which the member feels a strong sense of connection to others, a sensitivity to other members' negative reactions will foster that member's engagement in interpersonal change.

A second factor is members' willingness to share negative reactions toward others and to tolerate others' negative reactions toward themselves. When we share with another our negative reaction to him or her ("I am feeling irritated with you."), it generally increases the tension level in that relationship. It also stimulates catastrophic fantasies about how the recipient of negative reactions is likely to respond. For example, a worry may be evoked that the other person will respond with more hostility than the person expressing the negative reaction. Because of the discomfort produced by such fears, a reluctance to express negative reactions in relationships is not unusual. The cost of the failure to express negative reactions is that problems fail to be resolved and relationships remain superficial as members relate to one another guardedly. In groups lacking cohesion members are not motivated enough to bear the anxiety associated with expressing negative reactions in order to obtain the long-term benefits of doing so. In a cohesive group, however, members' commitment to their relationships with one another leads them to risk their short-term comfort for the sake of the long-term advancement of the relationship.

An intuitive grasp of this point may be achieved through an example from a dyadic relationship. Suppose two individuals spent an evening on a blind date. Neither party felt a marked attraction to the other. One party irritated the other by cracking gum during the movie. However, the irritated party refrained from complaining about the irksome behavior because of the lack of commitment felt toward the other person ("I'll just ignore it. . . . I'll probably never see him again anyway"). On the other hand, in a relationship that was expected to have some longevity, the motivation would be higher to address the offensive behavior. As in the dyad, members of groups are willing to subject themselves to dangers and discomforts for the long-term benefit of relationships when cohesiveness is present.

A third benefit of cohesion identified by Yalom is good member attendance. Members of cohesive groups are not inclined to leave their group precipitously, that is, before they have had an opportunity to profit from their group involvement. The connection between group cohesion and attendance has been shown in a number of research studies. For example, Piper and colleagues (1983) studied 45 participants in experimental groups. They found that members' levels of commitment to the group, an aspect of group cohesion, were positively related to members' group attendance. Members who expressed a low level of commitment tended to drop out early in the life of the group. They also found that the significance or value a member placed on other members of a group was positively related to the member's promptness in arriving for sessions.

Beyond the factors identified by Yalom, an additional factor is the depth of cognitive processing of information received by a member in the group. In cohesive groups the communications among members are subjected to greater processing than in noncohesive groups because members place a higher value on those communications. In vignette 1, Paul thought all week about Erika's comments. Perhaps he reviewed other experiences with women to determine if her observations could be generalized to his life outside the group. Perhaps he pondered his motives underlying his group behavior. From investigations in the area of cognition, we know that the number of associations that are made to an idea determine how memorable that idea will be (Wilhite & Payne, 1992). Furthermore, as a member contemplates a bit of feedback, he or she is more likely to use it as a lens through which to perceive extragroup interactions. The feedback is thereby more likely to alter those interactions. Hence, by working more actively to assimilate the input, the group member is more likely to be altered by his or her group experience.

What might be concluded from the discussion of the mechanisms of cohesiveness is that this property of groups works in a variety of ways to enhance members' capacities to derive benefit from the group. Given its importance, the next chapter offers suggestions for interventions a therapist can make to enhance group cohesiveness.

Intrapersonal Factors

The following factors are ones that could occur in an individual therapy situation in that they do not necessarily draw upon the relationships among group members. However, the way the operation of these factors is experienced in group versus individual therapy may differ. An example of such a difference is seen in the first intrapersonal factor discussed, instillation of hope.

Instillation of Hope: Imagine a group member listening to a departing group member talk about the enormous benefits reaped from her participation in the group. Such a testimonial might be expected to intensify the member's commitment to being in the group because the member is now hopeful that the therapy will work. Hope is a process that encompasses goals and the awareness of viable routes to those goals and the belief that one has the capability to pursue the route to the goal (Snyder, Cheavens, & Sympson, 1997; Snyder, Ilardi, Michael, & Cheavens, 2000). A hope-bolstering event of receiving an endorsement of the treatment within the treatment itself is unique to group therapy. As in the other modalities, however, hope is strengthened by the member's own awareness of his or her progress as the treatment proceeds. Oftentimes, simply entering treatment brings about a relief from suffering. The group situation also creates a sense of mastery in having contained the fears about group participation sufficiently to be installed in the group. This achievement nurtures a hope of future achievements. That is, the member increasingly comes to see therapy as a viable route to enhancing his or her well-being.

The capacity of any therapeutic experience to increase an individual's hopefulness that his or her life will improve is critical to the success of the treatment (Piper, 1994). In the absence of hope, the individual is not likely to have the motivation to bear the negative aspects of treatment such as the cost and the need to focus upon behaviors and reactions that may be problematic. Indeed, research has consistently shown that hopeful people are more likely to achieve their goals than those lacking in hope (Snyder, 1994), even when the effects of factors such as intelligence and ability to perform the task are removed (Curry, Synder, Cook, Ruby, & Rehm, 1997). One possible explanation for their greater success is that high-hope individuals do not perceive difficulties in accomplishing a task as reflecting a lack of ability. Rather, they perceive setbacks and failures as information that they must modify their strategy (E. Rieger, as cited in Snyder, 1994). High-hope individuals have also been found to be more tolerant of discomfort (Snyder & Hackman, 1998). In the group therapy setting, then, hope could function to enhance a member's productive reflectiveness on the input he or she is receiving.

Unsurprisingly, perhaps, the capacity of a group to instill hopefulness is most crucial when members enter the group in a relatively hopeless state. For example, Maxmen (1973) found that inpatients rated instillation of hope among the more important mechanisms of change. For individuals whose entrance into a treatment situation intensifies their sense of inefficacy in coping with external stressors ("If I need hospitalization, I must really be inept in handling life"), the therapist should give special attention to how the group might increase their levels of hope. For persons who are entering treatment with a relatively high level of optimism about the future, hope can be less of a therapeutic focus.

How does the therapist recognize manifestations of hopefulness? As the findings of Snyder and colleagues suggests, hope shows itself in ways other than the articulation of positive expectations. Hope reveals itself in the presence of those processes that constitute hope. For example, early on in group therapy, as in all forms of therapy, it is typical to see rather considerable symptomatic improvement. Snyder et al. (2000) hypothesize that this positive change is the result of an increase in agentic thinking, the felt capacity to sustain energy toward a goal. Both the decision to enter therapy and the confidence of the therapist in his or her particular approach strengthens a sense of agency in the person. Writing in an object-relations vein, Shields (2000), drawing from Winnicott, points out that sometimes the very behaviors inside of the group that are viewed as troublesome by therapists are manifestations of hope. Behaviors that are disruptive and even patently antisocial may be rooted in a wish to provoke others into being emotionally forthcoming in a way that allows the troublesome person to continue his or her process of maturation. By being alert to such hidden manifestations of hopefulness, the therapist can extract constructive elements from behaviors that might others seem wholly vexing.

Guidance: This factor refers to didactic instruction group members receive from the therapist as well as advice members give to one another. Therapists sometimes find more salient the aspects of advice and guidance that do not appear to be in the service of the goals of treatment. For example, many therapists have witnessed the following phenomenon. A person expresses a craving for advice and direction, receives it in abundance from group members, ignores it altogether, and demoralizes the group. Therapists also witness members giving one another bad advice or delivering advice with such condescension that the person receiving it feels demeaned rather than assisted. However, more important than any of these considerations is the fact that for most groups the objective is not to assist members in negotiating a specific situation. Rather, the aim is for members to learn how to respond more adaptively to whatever interpersonal circumstances might challenge members. In receiving specific instructions from other members, the group member may fail to develop the resources to handle situations on his or her own. In short, advice and guidance are seen as undermining members' autonomy.

Yet most groups do have guidance as an essential, if not delimited, component of the treatment. During the member's preparation for group therapy, the member receives an education about this modality that broadly falls under the domain of "guidance." In the preparation, the prospective member may develop a certain understanding of his or her difficulties that may facilitate the therapeutic work in a lasting way. For example, in groups centering on interpersonal relations as a major target area of change, the prospective member may develop an appreciation of the notion that interpersonal difficulties often underlie symptoms whose interpersonal aspect may not be evident. This idea might be useful both in the member's group behavior and in cultivating an attitude of reflection in his or her life outside the group.

In group sessions, two types of guidance occur. The first is particularly likely to occur in a relatively unstructured group, that is, a group format in which members have a large role in determining what is expressed. This type is advice that members offer in relation to external problems. It occurs early in the group because, as discussed in Chapter 3, members often take refuge from their anxieties about being in group by looking outside the group. As members begin to experience the power and benefits of interpersonal learning, a process requiring a here-and-now focus, the members rather naturally diminish their advice giving.

The second type of guidance is characteristic of those groups that are designed to promote skill building in a specified area such as impulse control or problem solving. In such groups it is common for therapists to provide some instruction especially early in members' participation in how to master the skill. For example, members in a group focusing on problem solving will be presented with the steps of problem solving. They will learn techniques such as brainstorming en route to acquiring the problem-solving skill. In some instances skills are taught not only by the therapist but by the group members themselves. For example, it is not uncommon for first-time prisoners to obtain survival tips from more long-standing residents. Such therapeutic activity is rated very highly by imprisoned group members (Morgan, Ferrell, & Winterowd, 1999).

Skill-building groups also may involve the assignment of homework to members and the monitoring of members' success in executing it. Such assignments are particularly important in this era of managed care in which many practitioners compensate for the brevity of treatment by intensifying it and extending it between sessions (Kazantzis & Deane, 1999). The use of homework is discussed further in Chapter 5.

That these different types of guidance may be at varying levels of usefulness to members was suggested by a study (Flowers, 1979) in which groups of sex offenders who were given simple, direct advice, a description of alternatives, detailed instructions, or no group treatment. All groups showed greater change than the control groups. Furthermore, the groups that received specific alternatives and detailed instructions showed more change than the group that received advice.

Support for the usefulness of homework is provided by several studies. In one study (Neimeyer & Feixas, 1990) homework led to a greater lessening in the symptoms of unipolar depressed persons relative to a group not receiving homework. This effect was observed at the end of treatment. However, the difference between the groups did not hold at the six-month follow-up. Another set of studies demonstrated the benefit of daily homework assignments for the acquisition of social skills (Falloon, 1981; Fallon, Lindley, McDonald, & Marks, 1977). In general, however, the use of homework in groups has been an insufficiently researched technique.

Catharsis: At some time the reader may have had a particularly vexing day filled with an accumulation of insults, indignities, and aggravations. Perhaps upon arriving home in the evening the reader had what is commonly known as a "good cry" and felt a great relief afterwards. The intense expression of feeling with subsequent relief is the mechanism of catharsis. Earlier in this chapter we discussed the factor of interpersonal learning, which also involved the activation of learning. The difference here is that interpersonal learning involves the arousal and expression of affect that is then cognitively organized. In catharsis it is the pairing of affect, intensely expressed, and relief that is critical. Interpersonal learning may not involve relief; catharsis may not involve cognition.

The value of catharsis is unclear. Some studies suggest that the expression of hostility and affection leads to positive outcomes. For example, Koch (1983) performed an investigation in which investigators taped sessions in a day hospital group and analyzed them for type and intensity of affective content. The expression of hostility and loving feelings was associated with increased self-esteem and lessened anxiety. However, this study and others did not directly tap catharsis in that one critical component of catharsis, relief, was not considered. In considering the usefulness of catharsis, the group therapist should give some consideration to members' cultural contexts. In different cultures, emotional expressiveness has different effects. For example, in the United States, positive expressiveness of feelings on the part of parents enhances their children's social functioning (Halberstadt, Crisp, & Eaton, 1999). In Indonesia parents' expression of strong positive feelings is unrelated to their children's social functioning (Eisenberg, Liew, & Pidada, 2001).

Although most contemporary approaches to group therapy do not emphasize catharsis as it is defined in this chapter, there will be times in the life of a group when it will make an important contribution. I have seen members enter an ongoing group and maintain a tenuous, cautious style for a number of sessions. Then, in a given session the member expresses her or himself in an unbridled way and subsequently appears to have achieved a newfound tranquility in the group. This event is important in a variety of ways. The emotional expression is a signal to the group members that the new member has achieved a deeper level of trust in the group. It also demonstrates to the member that experiencing emotions in the group need not have negative consequences. Often such an experience can both signify and facilitate further the new members' integration into the group.

A new member can be integrated into a group in a variety of ways besides a cathartic event. The example is offered to show that catharsis may at different moments be precisely the needed experience to carry the group forward. This discussion highlights an important point about outcome research. Outcome studies can be enormously helpful in telling us which mechanisms of change, when emphasized in a group, are likely to lead to more favorable outcomes. Yet outcome research in its present level of sophistication cannot do full justice to the complexity of groups. There are events in the life of a group that may, under a particular configuration of conditions, serve as catapults to the group's development. As Yalom (1995) stresses, the mechanisms of change represent a rich array of resources. Any one of them is likely to be of value in some group context.

Self-Understanding: Self-understanding is another term for insight. It refers to the increased awareness of psychological elements within the person, the behavior the person exhibits, and their interrelationships. This mechanism frequently overlaps with a number of the other mechanisms covered, particularly interpersonal learning.

For example, other members may share their strong impression that Joe, another member, is angry in a session. As other members give Joe the evidence for their collective conclusion, he begins to recognize the feeling state. He also sees which of his behaviors convey anger. Joe's unique style of being angry in the group was to act confused about the conversation among members, as if the members were speaking nonsense. Joe's achievement of an awareness of a fended-off feeling and the social behavior that revealed the feeling constituted both interpersonal learning and self-understanding.

But as Joe becomes aware of his difficulty in accessing his anger, he also becomes curious about how he shields himself from it and why. As the process of the group unfolds, he uses his defense of confusion over both his own experience and other members' communications. Subsequently he comes to understand that an unconscious belief that his hostility will damage others leads him to mask from himself his anger. Later still, he realizes that his parents' appearing to be damaged by his even mild expressions of anger in his early life is connected to his inhibition in expressing negative feelings. All of these are forms of self-understanding.

A clearer grasp of the meaning of self-understanding can be obtained by contrasting it with a related mechanism, interpersonal learning. Because these categories overlap, the distinction cannot be made sharply. Interpersonal learning involves the achievement of self-awareness that is closer to the behavioral surface, that is, what members can directly see and hear. Although interpersonal learning may require some level of inference making, the inferences are at a fairly low level; they are closely linked to the data used in making the inferences. For example, members' articulation of their impression that Joe was angry was based upon certain behavioral manifestations. In contrast, self-understanding oftentimes involves the summoning of a higher level of inference than is required for interpersonal learning. Moreover, the inferences may be based on an examination of the behavioral data through the lens of a particular conceptual model of group process.

For example, my colleagues and I conducted a study involving interviewing therapists who had conducted therapy groups during their pregnancies (Fallon, Brabender, Anderson, & Maier, unpublished paper cited in Fallon & Brabender, 2002). Therapists reported that rarely did members talk about or even seem to realize their reactions to the therapist's pregnancy and upcoming leave (permanent or temporary). However, members would more frequently than usual talk about losses outside of the group. They would also speak about people-in-charge who had acted irresponsibly or failed to discharge their obligations completely. Therapists reported interpreting these expressions as symbolic of their reactions to the pregnancy: Members experienced the therapist as an abandoning parent toward whom they felt sadness and anger. Therapists observed that when they made these interpretations, group members were able to use them productively to consider the difficulties of bearing an immediate loss. In this instance therapists considered members' verbal productions through a psychodynamic lens. They used as a guiding notion that to spare themselves the pain of focusing on an immediate loss, members focused on losses that were more remote and hence more bearable.

Does self-understanding lead to positive change? Two sets of studies speak to this question. In the first set the mechanism of insight is used as part of a group treatment either in isolation or in combination with other factors. Roback (1972), examining changes in a group of hospitalized chronic patients meeting over 30 sessions, found that insight used in combination with interaction (i.e., interpersonal learning) produces more favorable outcomes than no group treatment or insight or interaction alone. Abramowitz and Jackson (1974) found that a group combining here-and-now statements with there-and-then statements produced slightly more favorable results in a group of students meeting for 10 sessions than either condition occurring alone or a placebo control condition. Meichenbaum, Gilmore, and Fedoravi-cius (1971) found that a behavioral desensitization group was more helpful to treat a focal speech anxiety but an insight-oriented group was more useful to persons whose speech anxiety was part of a more generalized anxiety disorder. These results suggest that insight can be useful especially when combined with other factors and when addressing specific types of presenting problems.

A second type of investigation concerns the variable of the psychological mindedness of group members. Psychological mindedness is the degree of insight or self-understanding that a group member has. Several studies have examined the link between psychological mindedness and outcome. Abramowitz and Abramowitz (1974) had student volunteers rated on psychological mindedness. The students were then randomly assigned to two insight-oriented or non-insight-oriented groups. In the insight-oriented groups, higher levels of psychological mindedness were associated with greater improvement; in the non-insight-oriented groups, no relationship existed between the two variables. Presumably, the psychologically minded members in the insight-oriented groups were generating insights that contributed to their improvement. Again, the importance of insight depends upon the type of group.

Piper et al. (1992) examined psychological mindedness in a therapy setting. Individuals having a pathological loss reaction participated in a 12-week psychodynamically oriented group. These investigators did not find a relationship between psychological mindedness and outcome. However, they did find that members low in psychological mindedness dropped out of the group early. Given that these members did not have the opportunity to benefit from treatment, psychological mindedness did have an indirect relationship to outcome.

Piper, Rosie, Joyce, and Azim (1996) investigated the relationship between psychological mindedness and outcome (based upon a host of measures, including self-report, observation by others, and so on) using inpatients participating in a day hospital treatment program in which group therapy was the primary modality. The groups appeared to involve a combination of elements including insight and interpersonal learning. The investigators found a strong relationship between psychological mindedness and outcome.

Apparently, members were using the insights they were capable of producing to their betterment.

While insight may not be useful in all types of groups and while some types of insight may be more useful than others in particular types of group, evidence of the usefulness of self-understanding as a mechanism of change is reasonably substantial.

Use of the Mechanisms of Change

The mechanisms of change represent resources available to the therapist. How does the therapist determine which mechanisms to deploy for any given group? While at some moment in the life of a given group the therapist may use all of the aforementioned mechanisms, typically, some will have far greater prominence than others. What are the factors that might determine the relative importance of these factors in any given group?

Group Goals and the Group Model

A major factor that determines which mechanisms are appropriately activated is what goals the therapist is attempting to accomplish through members' group participation. For example, if the goal is the acquisition of a skill, then the mechanism of guidance will figure prominently because skill acquisition almost invariably involves some degree of didactic instruction. Likewise, if the goal is the change in some interpersonal behaviors, then interpersonal learning will be the centerpiece of the group treatment.

There are often many paths to get to one destination. If the group therapist adopts an explicit model for conducting group treatment, that model will specify the various processes that move the group toward its ends. For example, the problem-solving model seeks change in the target area of skill acquisition. This model instructs the therapist to use an organized sequence of interventions that systematically deploy specified mechanisms of change. Initially *guidance* is used as members are taught the steps in problem solving. As the therapist helps a member to see the real problem underlying at apparent problem (e.g., bravado covering up a difficulty in self-esteem), *self-understanding* may come into play. *Identification* is summoned as the therapist models for members the brainstorming technique. The members' energetic participation in brainstorming may foster *cohesion* and *hope* (that potential solutions extend beyond what may have initially been evident to the member). Finally, helping members to analyze the long- and short-term consequences of various solutions falls broadly under the domain of *guidance*.

A therapist using an approach other than one of the available group models must determine which therapeutic factors are of greatest import and how they will be activated. These specifications constitute essential aspects of the group design. How the therapist stimulates the therapeutic factors is discussed in Chapter 5.

Tenure and Developmental Status of the Group

One suggestion from the research on the outcomes of various mechanisms of change is that the variable of time moderates the usefulness of mechanisms of change (Tschuschke & Dies, 1994). Whether a mechanism is beneficial, neutral, or detrimental depends on when it occurs over the span of sessions in the life of the group. It seems that for some mechanisms such as self-disclosure and feedback (a component in interpersonal learning) to be effective, they must occur early enough in the life of the group such that phenomena generated by their operation can be adequately processed. The developmental status of a group is also likely to be important. Group therapists have noted that early in the life of the group, factors such as guidance and a relatively superficial form of universality naturally occur. This developmental trend may be based on a group need: To become a group, members may require the nurturing that is part of guidance and a sense of likeness to other members. Later in the group, as trust deepens, interpersonal learning becomes a process that is less threatening to members.

Characteristics of Members

For several of the mechanisms reference was made to the type of patient population that perceives the mechanism as important. For example, inpatients are likely to perceive the instillation of hope as far more important than do outpatients. Such findings highlight a theme of this text: The design of the group should always be predicated upon the group therapist's consideration of the context of treatment. The level of functioning is also key. Certain mechanisms of change may involve more arousal of anxiety that would be tolerable to prospective members at a given level. Yalom (1983) points out how actively psychotic members require a great deal of support and that a vigorous interpersonal learning process might evoke panic and promote regression. Mechanisms such as self-disclosure and catharsis have a similar effect. With such populations emphasis is well placed on mechanisms that are likely to alleviate anxiety, such as altruism, low-level universality, hope, and guidance.

The ethnic and racial characteristics of potential group members should also have a bearing on the mechanisms of change that the therapist emphasizes in the design of the group. Some cultures, for instance, place a priority on containing affect rather than arousing and expressing it. Members organizing their group experience through the lens of this cultural value are likely to feel greater trepidation when feelings come to the fore than persons from a culture that takes a different stance on the handling of affect. Therefore, a member from a containing versus an expressive culture will see mechanisms such as catharsis differently. For the former, cathartic moments, while by definition providing relief, may also lead to shame as the person feels he or she deviated from a cultural prescription for decorum. For the latter, such events are likely to be far less remarkable, if at times even impactful.

The point is not that persons from cultures oriented toward restraint may not ultimately benefit from mechanisms whose operation heightens the group's level of affective stimulation. In fact, for such individuals such events may be highly useful. However, insofar as they lead the person to go against his or her cultural grain, they must be approached with far greater delicacy than for the group member engaging in intense affective expression on a regular basis. The therapist must ensure that the member breaking new ground has a level of trust in the group to sustain a feeling of acceptance during and following the experience. The therapist must also take into account that a substantial period of time will be required to explore fully the member's reactions and questions following an affective event. For example, for one member it may mean the opportunity to ask each of the other members how his or her perceptions of the newly expressive member have been altered as a function of the member's new behaviors. In the absence of sufficient time (as in the case of brief group therapy), the goal of increased affective expressiveness may be inappropriate. Hence, the mechanisms that produce such change should be given less emphasis than mechanisms supporting more viable goals.

Summary

This chapter focused on the vast resources available within a therapy group to enable members to change in positive ways. Three sets of mechanisms were described. First were those mechanisms that rely upon the interaction among members: interpersonal learning, altruism, identification, and self-disclosure. Given its importance to the major contemporary approaches, interpersonal learning was described in greatest depth. This process involved increased awareness of members of how they are experienced by others through the exchange of feedback. Interpersonal learning entails the activation of affect through explorations of here-and-now phenomena and the subsequent cognitive organization of the affective experiences. While some valuable research has been done on various elements of interpersonal learning, much more work needs to be done to realize the potential of this mechanism. Identification, the forerunner of internalization, involves taking into the self the experiences of another. Altruism, the attempt to help other members, is of variable usefulness depending upon the patient population. Self-disclosure, which is the communication of a personal part of the self to others, can have a positive impact upon outcome depending upon the conditions of the disclosure.

The second category included those mechanisms that involve the group as a whole: universality, corrective recapitulation of the primary family group, and cohesion. Universality, the realization that one's experiences are shared by others, can occur on various levels. It can be established with respect to painful feelings in response to trauma, conscious aspects of the self that challenge self-esteem, and elements of the self that have been heretofore banished from consciousness. Some level of universality is likely to be established in most therapy groups. Corrective recapitulation of the primary family group uses members' reactions to the therapists and each other to address, explicitly or implicitly, relationships with parents and siblings respectively. Cohesion, a sense of camaraderie among members, and a commitment to the group as a whole, is generally associated with positive outcomes and good attendance. The various mechanisms by which cohesiveness produces its positive effects (such as members' greater tolerance for offering and receiving negative feedback were described).

The interpersonal factors, while often occurring in individual therapy, can have a unique character when arising in the group. They are instillation of hope, guidance, self-understanding, and catharsis. Hope is instilled when members' anticipation that their lives will improve increases their forbearance of any discomfort from group participation. Guidance, which includes receiving instruction from the therapist and advice from the members, is more of a prominent component in skills training and early in group life. Pretraining, which is a part of group treatment, entails the mechanism of guidance. Catharsis, the intense expression of feeling followed by relief, while one of the less emphasized mechanisms in many contemporary approaches, can play an important role in certain moments in the life of the group. Self-understanding or insight has been shown to positively affect outcome either directly or indirectly by affecting attendance, especially when used in combination with other factors.

Which of these mechanisms is emphasized in a group depends on a variety of factors, such as the group goals and model, the tenure of the group and its developmental status, and the characteristics of the group members. The specification of the key mechanisms of change is a key part of the group design. To the extent that the therapist considers all relevant variables within the context, the design is effective.

ELEMENTS OF
GROUP THERAPY

The Role of the Therapist

5

Chapter

Thus far, we have considered the goals to which the therapy group may be directed and the resources available in the group to move its members toward the goals. How does the therapist identify and develop the resources relevant to a particular set of goals? How does the therapist create those ambient conditions conducive to the emergence of such resources or respond to obstacles to their full deployment? These and other questions relevant to the role of the therapist will be considered in this chapter.

Group therapists are by no means uniform in the manner in which they practice. Variability in ways of intervening is created by differences in the target area of change established by the therapist for his or her patient population and, more specifically, by the goals within a given target area. Furthermore, to the extent that a therapist adopts an established model of group therapy, that model will prescribe the activities of the therapist. Some therapists use treatment manuals that provide highly detailed instructions for the therapists' behaviors at each point in the session. Beyond the choices that the therapist makes in theoretical frameworks is the person of the therapist, who determines how to interpret his or her role in the group. Group therapists' behavior cannot but be informed by the emotional and cognitive characteristics that they bring to the therapeutic enterprise. Individuals differ stylistically on the extent to which they are action oriented versus reflective (Exner, 1993). Because of the traitlike quality of these personality characteristics, they generally exert their influence across situations. Hence, whether a group therapist exhibits a tendency to direct group members, interpret their behaviors, exhibit his or her own emotional reactions, and so on in part has to do with his or her own personality style. In fact, group therapists can be drawn ineluctably to particular models because a given model is compatible with their own habitual ways of being with others. The fact that a diversity of models is available is fortunate, given that not one but many models have been shown to help members to move toward the goals those models establish.

Despite the existence of differences among group therapists in how they fulfill their roles in the group, therapists of successful groups are likely to engage in certain activities. A heuristic scheme for classifying these activities was suggested by a large-scale investigation of personal growth encounter groups conducted by Lieberman, Yalom, and Miles (1973) and published in a text titled *Encounter Groups: First Facts*. The reader may recall that this study was discussed in Chapter 4. Although this study was done on a variety of types of encounter groups, it has relevance for therapy groups in that both types of groups share an emphasis on feedback, emotional expression, and the goals of fostering greater self- and social awareness (Dies, 1994). Because of these similarities, the field of group therapy has derived a great deal of knowledge from the study of experiential or encounter groups.

The investigation took place at Stanford University and used students, many of whom were enrolled in an experimental course titled "Race and Prejudice." Two hundred and ten students were distributed among 18 encounter groups representing an array of 10 theoretical approaches. Because a major focus of the study was the effects of the leader's behavior on members' reactions in the group and the extent to which members profited from group participation, experienced clinicians observed all of the group sessions and categorized the interventions of the leader. Did the leader self-disclose, pose questions, confront members, make interpretations, express empathy, or use other types of intervention? From a factor analysis of observer ratings, four leadership functions emerged: executive function, emotional stimulation, caring, and meaning attribution.

This scheme, while having attracted great interest in the group therapy literature, has not received consistent support in research studies as a conceptual framework (Tinsley, Roth, & Lease, 1989). Nonetheless, the scheme has attracted interest because it is a helpful pedagogical tool for thinking about the diverse activities of the therapist. Another competing scheme that distinguishes between task and relationship activities lacks the richness to be useful to students. Therefore, the Lieberman, Yalom, and Miles framework is described in some depth. However, this framework is modified somewhat for two reasons. First, while therapy and experiential groups are similar, they are by no means identical. Certain types of interventions are more characteristic of a therapy group. Second, changes in the theory and practice of group therapy since the 1970s should be reflected in any classification of therapist activities.

Executive Function

When performing the executive function, the therapist provides the group with a structure that enables it to come into being, to maintain itself, and to proceed toward its goals. In this capacity the group therapist has been likened to the conductor of an orchestra who auditions and selects performers, establishes rules for their continued participation, selects pieces, creates a rehearsal schedule, and directs musical activities during practice. The processes associated with the executive function are complex. Each type of process, as it pertains to the actions of the therapist, is described in the sections that follow. As the reader will see, these actions take place both within and outside the group therapy sessions. To provide the reader with a reasonably vivid image of these activities, we consider the situation of a therapist organizing a group in a large community mental health center. The therapist has to undertake the following executive or control activities (summarized in Table 5.1) more or less sequentially.

Group Design, Context Cultivation, and Member Recruitment

Before beginning the group, the therapist must assess a variety of factors, including the needs of the potential group members, the likely time frame available, and all other components of the patient's treatment package. For example, if a high percentage of members were to be recruited from a pool of individual therapy patients, it would be important to ascertain what treatment needs were being addressed by the individual therapy. Having established an appropriate target area of change and goals within that area (Chapter 2), the therapist must identify the potential resources in the group that could be cultivated in the service of these goals (Chapters 3 and 4) and the interventions leading to the mobilization of these resources. All of these

Table 5.1   Therapist Function: Executive Activity

Definition	Actions that structure the group through the reinforcement of internal and external boundaries and the direction of members to engage in activities that will move them toward their goals.

Therapist Behaviors	■ Designing the group, cultivating the context's support of the group and recruiting candidates
	
	■ Screening and preparing members
	
	■ Maintaining the therapeutic frame
	    Observing time boundaries
	    Observing membership boundaries
	    Enforcing rules
	
	■ Directive activities
	    Modeling and reinforcement
	    Agendas
	    Exercises
	    Homework
	    Use of treatment manual

elements constitute the *group design*. Research has shown that to the extent that the therapist creates a sensible plan or design for the group, the experience is more coherent to group members and they will thereby derive more from group participation (Dies, 1994).

Beyond the creation of a group design, however, the therapist must develop a strategy for both obtaining referrals and for promoting the group in the broader treatment environment. Perhaps the therapist decides to give a presentation on the plan for the group to all staff members in the outpatient center. Or the therapist may decide to meet with key staff members individually. The smooth operation of any group and its ultimate survival and success depend on identifying and executing an effective strategy to obtain support. A group that is not supported by the broader environment faces constant challenges and encroachments. The therapist may arrive to the group room and find that it has been reassigned for some other organizational purpose. Or the therapist may discover that a staff member within the organization recommended to a group member to drop out of the group when the member expressed some mild dissatisfaction about a particular session. These impediments will be rare in an environment in which the therapist has cultivated an awareness of the compatibility of the group's goals with the organization's mission.

This set of executive functions, particularly the nurturing of contextual support, is one that tends to be neglected. Perhaps more than other modality, groups require compatibility and support from the setting. Too often the therapist sees his or her efforts in isolation from those of others and gives the setting short shrift. However, any time the therapist invests in the planning stage of the group is likely to benefit the group throughout its existence.

Screening and Preparation of Members

Presumably, if the therapist designs a group appropriate for one of the populations treated at the center and cultivates the context's receptivity to the group, he or she should enjoy a flow of referrals that would enable the group to begin. An essential task of the therapist is to screen members to ensure that the group is appropriate for each member—and that the prospective member is appropriate for the group. This distinction is an important one. There may be members who could make a contribution to the other members and the group as a whole but who may be more likely to benefit from another type of group. In this case, the prospective member may be appropriate for the group; the group may be inappropriate for the prospective member.

In a setting such as a community mental health center, the therapist will often have considerable responsibility for, and control of, the screening process. In other settings, such as inpatient facilities, patients need to be placed in treatment very quickly. In such settings, the therapist and the group's members are deprived of the luxury of an extensive screening process. Other staff members may refer persons to the group with the expectation that they will be placed in it. Nonetheless, the therapist cannot ethically abdicate responsibility for the screening process (Weiner, 1993). Group therapists must ensure that members accepted into the group will neither pose a danger to other members nor be at risk themselves of being damaged by a particular group.

If a candidate is not accepted for a given group, the therapist's obligations to that person do not end. The therapist must ensure that the individual has support in coping with any distress from being turned away from the group. The therapist does not have to provide the support; indeed, as the source of the rejection, the therapist may be in a compromised position in doing so. Rather, the obligation merely requires that the therapist take steps to guarantee that such a forum exists for the person. Furthermore, the therapist should share any knowledge of other groups that may be appropriate.

The preparation of the member for the group may follow the selection process or may occur simultaneously with it. The former is likely to occur in a longer term group situation in which there is not the pressure of placing the individual immediately. The latter is typical in a setting in which the brevity of treatment requires immediate placement. Too often, this circumstance leads the group to abandon preparation altogether. Chapter 8 discusses both selection and preparation more extensively and describes the research literature on preparation. However, at present let it suffice to note that to optimize group participation, especially early in a member's involvement, preparation is extremely useful. Therefore, even if a group member must be placed quickly, the therapist must find the means to prepare the member for entry into the group.

In preparing the new member for group participation, the therapist must educate that individual about the goals of the group and how those goals are accomplished. Additionally, the therapist must develop the member's understanding of, and willingness to abide by, the rules of the group. These rules mandate behaviors that guarantee the safety of members and facilitate the progress of the group toward its goals. Because goals vary from group to group, rules can vary. Decisions about rules are a major step in the group design.

By performing the executive function of describing the rules in detail and explaining the basis for the rules and any consequences for their violation, the therapist is laying the foundation for the group's moving to maturity. Admittedly, in a short-term group the therapist may have to assert and enforce the rules throughout its life. In a long-term group the therapist's providing this structure early on may enable the group to assume this executive activity.

Maintaining the Frame of the Group

During the group sessions themselves, a critical executive function of the therapist is to maintain the therapeutic frame. Perhaps the clearest grasp of what the therapeutic frame is can be achieved by illustrating its disruption. Imagine you are a member of the following outpatient group:

> *Members sat waiting for the tardy group therapist to arrive for the eighth session. The therapist entered the room 10 minutes late, offering no explanation. After the group began, there was a knock on the door. The therapist went to the door and the secretary of the center said, "I have to get the VCR. Dr. Bird wants to show a film to the interns." The secretary, who was known to all of the group members as the person who collects fees, joked with the group members as she unplugged the television. She said that this was her only means of finding out their secrets. She and the therapist then struggled to get the cart out of the room.*
>
> *Upon the therapist's return, members made several comments about wanting to join the interns to see the movie, comments that the therapist found quite amusing. Then tentatively, one member said she had something difficult to say. She said all week she had been brooding over another member's reporting in the prior session that he had shared something she said with his wife. She turned to the therapist and said, "Isn't that a violation of confidentiality? Weren't we told in the beginning that we had to keep what we hear in the group to ourselves?" The therapist shrugged and muttered, "Well, if he didn't mention your last name . . . I suppose it's a gray area."*
>
> *Before the group could discuss the issue further, another member of the group walked in with a great flourish. He was carrying several large bags of clothing and stood in the middle of the room. With no particular efficiency, he removed his raincoat. The group members asked why he had the bags. He launched into a narrative about his conflicts with his girlfriend that led him to move out of her apartment. His delivery was comedic, and group members, including the therapist, were obviously entertained—all except for the woman who expressed the concern about confidentiality. The session ended, and as members left, the therapist and the late member ambled out of the room together still chatting about the romantic difficulties of the member.*

In this vignette, the therapist failed to establish a consistent therapeutic frame. The *therapeutic frame* consists of those elements of regularity and predictability that allow members to see the group as a place of order. Contributing to the therapeutic frame are consistencies of time, place, membership, and enforcement of rules. The responsibility for building and maintaining the therapeutic frame falls largely on the shoulders of the therapist. Our analysis of this session will show that the members of the group would likely see this therapist as a bad manager. While the therapist's managerial weaknesses fall under the first category of executive function, they also have negative ramifications for other functions, particularly caring. A therapist who neglects managerial responsibilities will ultimately be seen as having insufficient caring for the group's well-being.

Temporal Boundaries: Chapter 3 introduced the notion of group boundaries. The beginning and ending times in the group constitute an external boundary that defines the group in temporal reality. When temporal boundaries are violated, members have an understandable confusion about what belongs to the group and what does not. In the vignette, the therapist neglected this critical executive function in a variety of ways. The therapist did not begin the group on time. Further, was the conversation between the therapist and group member after the session ended about the member's relationship part of the group session or a private exchange? To the extent that the group begins and ends on time, a clear demarcation exists between the group's work mode in pursuit of therapeutic goals and activities directed toward other goals. As Agazarian (1997) noted, "Time boundaries are among the most important boundaries and yet they tend to be neglected. The group that starts and stops on time has a working quality that is never present in a group whose starting and stopping times are blurred" (p. 67). When time boundaries are violated, the key means of reinstating the boundary is to acknowledge the violation and to stay alert to any reactions to the violation.

Membership Boundaries: A second boundary that was unstable in this session was the membership boundary, which demarcates those inside and outside the group. This boundary, more than any other, is likely to define the group in the eyes of its members. When the therapist began the session, he provided no acknowledgment that a member was missing. Perhaps his own lateness hindered him from calling attention to another's lapse in punctuality. Furthermore, he permitted an intrusion into the group by the secretary, who at least briefly became part of the group's transactions. What the therapist conveyed by not attending to these circumstances is that who enters and leaves the group is of no consequence. The type of violation that occurred with the entrance of the secretary is characteristic of settings in which the staff lack a sufficient understanding of the mission and methods of the group. The therapist may have attended inadequately to the task described earlier of creating a *pro-group climate* (Rice & Rutan, 1981), an environment that actively supports the goals and processes of the group.

Rule Enforcement: A third executive function unfulfilled was the enforcement of the group rules; hence, the boundary between the acceptable and unacceptable was blurred. The therapist failed to clarify whether confidentiality had been broken. While it may be appropriate in a mature group to encourage discussion about possible gray areas, certainly no group should be left uncertain as to whether a violation occurred. Because the therapist did not identify a violation, he was also unable to impose consequences consistent with the group contract. Such indifference toward the group rules inevitably creates a lack of safety in the group. Individuals enter the group wary of the dangers of revealing themselves to others, and unaddressed violations confirm their fears.

As the analysis of the vignette suggests, the therapist is the boundary manager of the group, regulating its defining features such as its membership and its location in time and space. This activity is crucial early in the life of the group. When the therapist fails to perform these executive functions minimally early on, the group is likely to have difficulty achieving the cohesion it needs to activate key psychological processes such as interpersonal learning and self-disclosure. While executive activity may be especially great early in a group's development, the therapist will have opportunities to perform executive functions throughout the life of the group (Lieberman, Yalom, & Miles, 1973).

Directive Activities within the Sessions

The therapist engages in executive action whenever he or she directs the group members to engage in particular behaviors either within or outside the sessions. A variety of activities are available to the therapist, the usefulness of any one being determined by its compatibility with the group goals. While this section will not provide an exhaustive account, it features a sampling of directive interventions that are used across many approaches. The interventions that will be covered are modeling and reinforcement, agendas, exercises, homework and its review, and the broader topic of treatment manuals. The reader should note that other categories legitimately contain some of these activities. For example, "agenda" is a technique that both structures the group's activities and also lends meaning to events. Hence, this technique could be placed under "meaning attribution."

Modeling and Reinforcement: In considering the therapist as a model and reinforcer of behavior, we will be helped by drawing our attention back to the case of the tardy therapist. What behaviors did the therapist model? The therapist modeled being late, turning away from difficult issues, focusing on concerns lying outside the group, and assuming a cavalier stance toward violations of the temporal and spatial boundaries of the group. The therapist also differentially reinforced or rewarded certain behaviors through laughter and attention, chortling when members expressed a desire to watch a movie and holding a semiprivate conversation with a group member about romantic difficulties.

The research has resoundingly shown (see Dies, 1983, 1994) that these behaviors play a powerful role in shaping group members' behaviors. Whether consciously or not, the therapist teaches the members how to be in the group. For didactic purposes, the vignette depicted extreme behaviors on the part of the therapist. However, far more subtle behaviors, such as leaning forward, looks at a watch, or nodding in response to a certain topic or speaker, are detected by the group members, especially early in the life of the group. Therefore, it behooves the therapist to be extremely aware of how he or she is behaving in the group. This awareness will do more than prevent the therapist from engaging in, and promoting behaviors at odds with, the group goals; it will enable the therapist to support in an active way the group's movement toward his or her goals. For example, Liberman (1970) demonstrated that therapists can be trained to reinforce members for behaviors that promote cohesiveness. The members of a group in which the therapist used social reinforcements to promote cohesion exhibited greater symptomatic relief than the members of a control group in which the therapist did not use social reinforcement techniques.

In the vignette the therapist's recognition that safety is a primary condition for work in the group might have led to behavior quite opposite to that which occurred in relation to the member's stated worry over confidentiality. When the obviously anxious member began her tentative discussion of the topic, the therapist might have leaned forward. After she made her comments, the therapist might have remarked on the criticality of the topic and of the group's coming to an understanding of whether a rule had been violated. Finally, the therapist would not have permitted the dilatory member to derail the group's focus on confidentiality. Such behavior on the part of the therapist would not only have discouraged behaviors antithetical to the group's purposes but would have actively fostered the group's growth.

Modeling and reinforcement may be important not only in fostering behaviors that already exist in members' repertoires but in teaching members new behaviors. For example, Chapter 4 described the extremely important process of feedback. As noted, feedback is a complicated mechanism with such factors as the time and valence of feedback playing important roles in the benefit members are likely to derive from the feedback. Early in the life of the group, therapists play an important role in teaching members how to be effective feedback providers.

In one study, data was collected from nine six-week personal growth groups in which leaders and members engaged in a structured feedback exercise (Morran, Robison, & Stockton, 1985). Each member was given feedback by each member and by the leader during various group sessions, and the members rated each piece of feedback for its helpfulness. Observers also rated the quality of the feedback along a variety of dimensions. The investigators found that leaders' feedback tended to be more useful in that it was more specific, more tied to observable events, and less directive. Early in the life of the group members rated leaders' feedback as more helpful. However, as the group progressed, the difference between the perceived helpfulness of leader and member feedback disappeared and members' feedback to one another took on some of the characteristics of leader feedback. For example, member feedback became less directive over time.

What these results suggest is that there are skills that members must acquire to help each other to take advantage of all that a group has to offer. In the Morran et al. (1985) study, the members' feedback became more similar to that of the therapists, and once it did, it was seen as being just as helpful, suggesting that having examples of new potentially constructive social behaviors would have an advantage over reliance on trial and error.

Agendas: One directive activity therapists use to focus the group's work is individual member agendas. An *agenda* is a problem that is a focus of the member's work during a given session. The essential idea behind agendas is that a member can work more effectively if the intended work is planned (Kivlighan & Jacquet, 1990). Agendas are often used in brief group therapy, when limited time requires that work be highly circumscribed to what can be realistically managed.

An example of the use of agendas is found in Yalom's agenda group model. This model, designed for inpatients who may be participating in group therapy for only a single session, requires that each member develop an agenda that can be formulated in interpersonal terms and can be fulfilled within the session—for example, that the person will take initiative in her relationship with another member by resolving to ask the member a question sometime during the session. The agenda then determines the therapist's activity in that the therapist makes an effort to have each member make some progress on his or her agenda during that session. To the extent possible, the therapist endeavors to orchestrate agendas, that is, to have multiple agendas fulfilled within the same interaction:

> Tara indicated in the beginning of the session that she wanted to work on being more open in expressing her feelings. Delores wanted to work on having a greater sensitivity to others' reactions. The therapist encouraged Delores to "tune in" to Tara's nonverbal behavior to ascertain whether she was having a feeling that she might attempt to describe to the group.

A benefit of the agenda approach is that even in a single session, members can see improvement. For inpatients, this sense of progression contributes to a view that therapy works, thereby encouraging them to pursue therapy after discharge (Yalom, 1983).

The catalyzing effect of agendas has been demonstrated in the research literature. For example, group members who were interviewed after completing a group experience identified the agenda as one of the most helpful aspects of their experience (Leszcz, Yalom, & Norden, 1985). Members who recorded two problems on an index card and read one problem to the group increased their participation during the session (Flowers & Schwartz, 1980).

What type of agendas are likely to be most effective? The reader may recall the general finding from outcome research described in Chapter 1 that approaches that capitalize upon group process produce more positive results. This principle applies to many specific techniques used in group design, including the agenda. To the extent that the agenda focuses upon the here-and-now, it is likely to be helpful to members. If a member says, "I want to learn to control my rage toward my husband," the therapist would recast it as, "I want to work on expressing my irritation toward members when my irritation is still mild." Yalom identified other features of serviceable agendas, such as that they be concrete and amenable to fulfillment within a given session. Therefore, the preceding agenda may be transformed into, "In this session today, I will express my irritation the first time I notice its presence."

The characteristics of agendas that increase their usefulness may depend on such other moderating factors as the developmental phase of the group. One study found that agendas that are focused on the here-and-now (rather than the there-and-then) are particularly helpful in the middle and later phases of a group in promoting engagement and discouraging avoidance of important issues (Kivlighan & Jacquet, 1990). However, more research needs to be done to help group therapists use the potential of the agenda-structuring technique.

Certainly the agenda technique has its limitations. Some members may feel that the pressure to create an agenda early in the session adds to the threatening quality of the group experience. The process of having each member formulate an agenda is time-consuming. In a group of 8 to 10 patients, the demand to have each formulate an individualized agenda may significantly limit the time available for other activities such as agenda fulfillment. One solution to this problem is to limit the number of people who formulate agendas in any one session (Froberg & Slife, 1987). This strategy is especially feasible when members are likely to be present in the group for multiple sessions. Finally, agendas can limit spontaneity. The guiding effect of agendas may join with members' defensive efforts to avoid the emergence of impulses, affects, and other psychological contents whose exploration may be critical to the realization of the group's goals.

Initially, it was noted that agendas focus the member's work. However, the agenda has an impact not only on the member's behavior during the session but also on the therapist's. The therapist focuses the member's work in the area delineated by the agenda. Some of the effect of the agenda may be its impact on the therapist. A recent study (Barlow, Burlingame, Harding, & Behrman, 1997) demonstrated that to the extent that therapists in a short-term group home in on a particular core treatment aim, a concept called *therapist focality*, members derive more from the group experience. They also showed that professional therapists show a greater engagement in such focusing than "natural helper" nonprofessionals. Future research might distinguish between the differential effects of the member's use of agendas versus that of the therapist to enable the group to obtain maximum benefit from their use.

Exercises: The therapist may organize structured experiences such as exercises and games to train the group members in particular skills. Such training may occur at the beginning of the group as a prelude to a less structured segment. For example, the therapist may introduce exercises to train members in giving feedback to one another or to practice their listening skills. Strengthening these skills presumably enhances the effectiveness of members' relating to one another in later sessions.

Some evidence suggests that such training early in the life of the group is beneficial. In one investigation (McGuire, Taylor, Broome, Blau, & Abbott, 1986), researchers examined techniques early in the course of the group to see if they would favorably affect members once they had an opportunity to interact spontaneously. The experimental group proceeded through three phases. In Phase 1, each member was paired with another group member. The pair of members met to discuss their goals and agendas for the session. The experimental group was divided into two subgroups, with one member from each pair included in a different subgroup. Each subgroup met in a fishbowl format and was observed by the other subgroup. Then, the pairs met again and each member gave his or her partner feedback on the partner's behavior in the group and the extent to which the partner progressed toward his or her goals. In Phase 2, all eight members met together for a session, but members were again paired. Before the group experience the pairs met to plan for the group, and they met after the group session to discuss one another's behavior during the session. In Phase 3, members met without any structuring techniques. The control group met for the same span of sessions as the experimental group without the advantage of any structuring techniques.

Trained observers rated members' behaviors on three dimensions: frequency and type of self-disclosure behavior, feedback behavior, and depth of processing. Members in the experimental and control groups did not differ in depth of processing. However, the members of the experimental group did exhibit greater self-disclosure in the first phase of the group. The members of the experimental group also showed fewer verbalizations incidental to the group task than members of the control group. Amount of feedback was unaffected by structure. Hence, this study shows that structuring techniques can have specific positive effects such as increasing on-task behaviors, but some changes may take place in the natural course of the group's development and are not dependent on the therapist's executive activities.

While structuring techniques can be used in the early phase of the group to prepare members for more effective functioning in less structured phases, they can also be used throughout a group's life. Structuring techniques also figure prominently in groups emphasizing skill development. An excellent example of a technique-oriented approach is the social-skills training model, used primarily but by no means exclusively with low-functioning patients. This model teaches microlevel social skills such as initiating contact, listing, appropriate self-disclosure, terminating contact, and so on (see Brabender & Fallon, 1993, pp. 46, 89 for further description of this model). The members would take part in role plays in which skills would be practiced. During the role play, members would be coached by the therapist and would give one another ongoing feedback, carefully orchestrated by the therapist to be at all times constructive. Members would also learn to perform their own self-evaluation of success in executing these skills. Modeling of the skills by the therapist and the verbal reinforcement of members would also accompany these techniques as members made progress in approximating the skills. The therapist also frequently assigns homework to practice the skills acquired in the group. The following section describes the technique of homework.

Homework: Chapter 4 briefly discussed the use of homework under the mechanism of guidance. Homework is assigned most commonly in those approaches that have skill acquisition as a goal. However, any group therapy approach could incorporate some homework feature.[1] Homework carries many potential benefits. It provides additional opportunities to practice a skill or apply a new awareness about the self. This feature is extremely important in group therapy in a managed care environment. The therapist and members may lack the luxury of a long period of time. Thus, the therapist would want to make in the time available as intensive an experience as possible to enable members to progress toward their goals. Homework enhances the likelihood that gains in therapy will be transferred to life outside the group by requiring the application of learning in the group to more real-life situations. Through homework, members can identify obstacles to their use of skills or insights acquired in the group. The group, then, can help the member find ways to remove the obstacles or lessen their effects. Finally, as MacKenzie (1990) noted, "Therapeutic homework not only maintains the continuity of therapy, it carries an implicit message that the patient must shoulder a portion of the therapeutic responsibility" (p. 202).

Homework requires many structuring activities on the part of the therapist. During the preparation for group involvement the therapist must inform the member that it is an element in the group treatment and explain its relevance to the goals of the group (Kazantzis & Deane, 1999). During the sessions themselves the therapist must make sure that the homework assignment is appropriate to each member's ability and to the work that the member has done in the group. Suppose a member of a group designed to teach basic

---

[1]Homework has least commonly been used in psychodynamic approaches. Although homework is certain a possibility within a psychodynamic orientation (Spitz, 1997), in many instances it may fundamentally change the therapy because the nondirective nature of the treatment gives rise to certain reactions on the part of group members that constitute the therapeutic grist for the work. Homework adds direction, and this direction is likely to alter the perceptions of members of the therapist and the group. How substantial this alteration would be is a matter of future investigation. See Halligan (1995) for a discussion of the types of homework assignments that have been used in individual dynamic therapy that might be extended to group therapy. Examples include dream recording and writing a letter to someone who has a conflictual relationship. These assignments seem to involve a greater emphasis upon reflection than action relative to the types of assignments typically used in group therapy.

social skills and has practiced making positive statements to others. The homework assignment should be limited to this skill rather than extended to other activities such as asking the other to engage in a further social interaction such as taking a walk. The therapist must assist each member in considering when, with whom, and where to carry out the assignment. The therapist must also help the member to anticipate any obstacles or difficulties in executing the assignment. If the member is in a broader therapeutic context such as a hospital, the therapist will need to work with other staff to ensure that conditions facilitate rather than hinder homework completion. For example, staff may need to be reminded to provide the member with time to perform the homework and with verbal prompts to do so.

In the post-homework session, the therapist must check on the assignment to discover whether it was completed and if the member encountered any difficulties. If the homework was not completed, the therapist must determine why and formulate an intervention consistent with this determination. In a very low functioning group, the lapse may be the result of members' difficulty keeping the group in mind outside of the session. In that case the therapist may simply have the member complete the assignment in the session. However, the therapist may ascertain that failure to complete homework is a behavioral expression, conscious or unconscious, of a reaction to the therapist or some aspect of the group. While the individual member may be expressing the reaction only for himself or herself, the reaction may also be on behalf of a larger unit such as a subgroup or the group as a whole. For example, the group may reach the developmental stage of challenging the therapist's authority. Homework neglect may be the group's means of mounting the challenge. The therapist may wish to respond interpretively to members' expressions. That is, the therapist may say something such as, "I think that not doing the homework is your way of letting me know that you're angry that you are not progressing more quickly." In so doing the therapist is departing from the executive realm and entering the meaning attribution realm, to be discussed subsequently.

If the member did perform the homework, it would be important to explore the member's perception of his or her success. At this point the therapist may wish to deploy some of the techniques described earlier in this chapter. For example, particularly in a low-functioning patient, the therapist may use verbal and other types of reinforcement to support members' homework attempts. If the member reports difficulties in carrying out the homework (for example, "I tried to walk up to her and say 'hello' but I became paralyzed by fear"), the therapist can initiate a role play in which the member can experience some success in performing the skill.

As the reader can see, incorporating homework into the group design must involve a high level of commitment on the part of the therapist to engage in activity inside and outside of the sessions to support its effectiveness. Because homework can have a positive effect only if it becomes a major focus of the group, the therapist must carefully weigh its expected contribution to members' progress in relation to other activities and processes against its potential disadvantages.

There are several possible disadvantages of homework. It heightens the executive role of the therapist. While it increases members' responsibility for their progress outside of the group, it may lessen their capacities to take control and initiative within the group. Furthermore, homework adds a high level of structure that is likely to interfere with more spontaneous interactions among members. Such spontaneity is essential to realizing the potential of the group to function as a microcosm, where members' characteristic difficulties in relating emerge clearly enough to enable members to address them. Moreover, because reporting on homework involves a focus on the there-and-then, it may significantly detract from the group's ability to delve into more typically affect-arousing here-and-now phenomena. In summary, as with any technique, whether homework is appropriate in a given group design depends on the goals of the group and the other processes deployed in relation to these goals.

As noted in Chapter 4, although homework is a central component of a number of approaches to group therapy, research on this technique is relatively sparse. This neglect within the literature reflects a broader inattention to the topic of homework across modalities (Kazantzis & Deane, 1999). Future research could be helpful in clarifying the specific benefits of homework as well as the technological features of homework that are likely to increase its positive effects.

Manualized Group Therapy: Group therapy takes place in an era of great concern that treatment be both effective and efficient. Third-party payers, particularly under managed care systems, reimburse only for services that are needed and that produce the desired results. One way of ensuring that any intervention has these features is to use a treatment manual outlining in detail an approach with demonstrated efficacy. The clinician essentially replicates interventions that were shown in a study—or even better, a series of studies—to have produced the intended outcomes. Under these circumstances the approach that the therapist uses can reasonably be classified as empirically supported.

Treatment manuals for group therapy have been created primarily for short-term groups lasting typically up to a half-year, often less. A cardinal characteristic of these models is specificity in the statement of group goals and methods to achieve them. They also specify all of the organizational elements, such as the rules of the group that exist to support its design. Finally, they specifically describe the activities of the therapist. Often on a session-by-session basis, they give instructions on the sequence of activities. Many of the techniques described earlier in this chapter, such as reinforcement, role play, agenda setting, and homework, are incorporated in an orchestrated way. The therapist whose actions and observations are highly prescribed is placed in an extremely directive role.

Treatment manuals have a number of potential benefits for group therapy. First, they increase the usefulness and comprehensibility of research on group therapy. I have had the experience of reviewing many outcome articles in some area of group therapy. Even current articles describe a positive pattern of results as a consequence of group intervention but specify in the vaguest terms possible what the intervention actually was. For example, an author might write, "The therapist used a combination of insight and analysis of members' interactions." With such a lack of specificity, no practitioner would be able to replicate the therapist's approach or even understand why the researcher obtained the results he or she did. The detailed presentation of methods characteristic of treatment manuals enables more ample communication between researcher and practitioner. Such communication enhances the extent to which research can guide practice.

A second potential benefit of treatment manuals is that the process of generating the manual facilitates the development of a solid group design. Dies (1994) reviewed 30 treatment manuals for various types of therapy groups and reported the following:

Generally, investigators attempt to furnish a coherent framework for thera-
peutic change. The basic rationale for treatment, ground rules for interaction
(e.g., confidentiality, attendance), clarification of patient and therapist roles,
and similar issues are reviewed early in treatment. Goal-setting and evalua-
tion of expectations also occur early in therapy, and sessions are planned to
insure meaningful progress toward individually defined goals. (p. 124)

As Dies also points out, in the 1960s and 1970s many studies examining the effectiveness of therapy groups produced disappointing
results. Only until carefully developed approaches emerged could the
potential usefulness of this modality be demonstrated. Treatment
manuals encourage the creation of well-thought-out approaches that
are likely to compare favorably to their more haphazard predecessors.

Another benefit of manuals is that the coherence of their group
plans can be conveyed to prospective members. We have discussed
that when a plan makes sense to members, when they understand
why they are doing what they are doing, their motivation to immerse themselves in the group process increases. Along the same
lines, treatment manuals may make group therapy more available to
persons with psychological difficulties. The therapist using a clear,
coherent framework can present that framework to a third-party
payer. The latter, seeing the evident link between goals and methods, is far more likely to approve reimbursement for group therapy
sessions than when the link is obscure. This point assumes that
third-party payers are willing to reimburse for psychological services. This assumption is not always valid.

Yet, treatment manuals carry with them potential risks and disadvantages. The first is that because no two settings are identical,
manuals are typically used in settings that differ from those in
which they were developed. The usefulness of an approach outlined
in any given manual is likely to be diminished by the therapist's failure to consider context fully. That is, the therapist may not identify
all the characteristics of his or her setting and how the approach may
need to be adapted to fit into the context harmoniously. Authors of
manuals contribute to therapists' practice of applying manuals literally when they fail to make clear that they are providing a set of
guidelines rather than an exact blueprint. Writers of manuals might
also describe ways in which the approach at hand might be altered
in other treatment contexts.

Second, treatment manuals devote great attention to technique, sometimes to the neglect of a focus on the quality of the therapeutic relationship (Addis, Wade, & Hatgis, 1999). Writers of manuals may assume that group therapists will naturally apply their skills in fostering group cohesion and an atmosphere of acceptance. Yet readers of manuals may infer that it is only the technique that is important. As is discussed later in this chapter, the quality of the relationships in the group and the overall group climate are crucial to the realization of goals. This point should be made clear in any presentation of a particular approach.

Third, while an approach presented in a treatment manual may be supported by well-designed research studies, the clinician cannot make this assumption. Group treatment manuals exist on every point along the continuum from no research support at all to considerable research support. However, even if research support is substantial, rarely is data sufficient show whether all elements described in a manual contribute to the positive outcome. An example from earlier in the chapter is homework, whose touted benefits greatly outstrip the empirical support for its importance. The group therapist must be a local scientist (Peterson, Peterson, Abrams, & Stricker, 1997) who investigates whether members seem to be making the positive changes that were expected through application of a model or approach. Simple before-and-after measures often reveal a great deal about the usefulness of treatment. The goal of such investigative efforts is not necessarily to produce the data for a publication in a refereed journal. Rather, the major goal of such efforts should be providing information or feedback to enable practitioners to refine or redirect their efforts (Dies & Dies, 1993).

Evaluation of the Executive Function

The effects of executive activity are multiple. The executive activities outlined early in this section regarding boundary establishment and norm regulation enhance members' perception of the group as predictable. This predictability fosters a sense of safety that is critical for the group's successful functioning. Without a moderate level of this type of executive therapist activity, members focus necessarily on self-protection to the neglect of advancement. Because a sense of safety on the part of members is so vital to all of the group's efforts, this kind of structural contribution is required of therapists of all theoretical orientations. However, a high level of executive activity related to boundary maintenance and rule enforcement can have adverse reactions. For example, the therapist may appear despotically concerned about order over members' individual needs. The negative effect of high and low levels of executive activity was seen in the earlier-cited study by Lieberman, Yalom, and Miles (1973). Their participants in encounter groups showed no positive change when the leader was extreme, that is, high or low, in the expression of executive functions.

The second type of executive activity pertains to specific techniques used to move members toward the goals of the group. Because the goals vary, the extent to which any one technique is used varies. Moreover, some goals may not be relevant to many of the techniques described. For example, a highly structured technique-oriented format is generally at odds with the goal of intrapsychic conflict resolution, which requires a relatively unstructured process in which the various elements of a conflict can emerge with reasonable clarity. While some evidence shows that developmental conflicts do emerge in highly structured groups (Schopler & Galinsky, 1990), it is doubtful whether a highly technique-based approach would be conducive to their full expression or exploration. For this reason the psychodynamic approaches having some variety of intrapsychic change as a goal have minimally used the kinds of structuring techniques described in this section.

Caring

Caring is the therapist's conveyance of regard and affection for group members, acceptance of each group member in the fullness of his or her person, and the conviction that each member has a capacity for change. Caring is related to the therapist characteristics of genuineness, empathy, and warmth studied by the famous research team Traux and Carkhuff (1967), who found that when these qualities are absent in the therapist, patients can actually get worse as a result of therapy. High levels of caring are associated with a deeper level of self-exploration. Lieberman, Yalom, and Miles (1973) found that in groups whose leaders were low in caring, members had poor outcomes relative to groups with leaders high in caring. MacKenzie, Dies, Coché, Rutan, and Stone (1987) investigated 54 training groups at the annual meeting of the American Group Psychotherapy Association (APGA). Participants rated the group leaders on a list of adjectives. These ratings were then examined in relation to the members' ratings of the benefit of the group experience. They found that the dimension most closely associated with positive perceptions of the group experience was the caring exhibited by the leader.

How does the therapist show caring? As Table 5.2 shows, the specific therapist behaviors associated with caring are many and varied. For example, caring is shown when the therapist conveys an accurate grasp of members' experience. Caring is seen in the therapist's honesty even at the expense of his or her comfort, such as when members accuse the therapist of being distracted in a given session and the therapist affirms the accuracy of this observation. Caring is shown in the therapist's reliability in performing certain executive functions such as starting the session on time and giving members' adequate notice of cancelations. Caring is conveyed by the therapist's ability to remember key events for the member or to detect subtle changes. Caring is communicated when the therapist

Table 5.2   **Therapist Function: Caring**

Definition	Behaviors that demonstrate the therapist's warmth, respect, interest, and acceptance in his or her interactions with group members.
Therapist activities	■ Exhibiting accurate empathy
	■ Being honest with members
	■ Being dependable
	■ Being attuned to individual member's subtle manifestations of growth
	■ Opening him or herself up to members' expressions of a range of feelings toward him or her, particularly negative reactions
	■ Showing acceptance for all elements within the psychological lives of the members

recognizes when a member is in a position of vulnerability, even when the member is attempting to conceal it. Caring is manifested by the therapist's willingness to be the object of members' negative feelings and show acceptance as members express what they perceive as the most objectionable parts of themselves.

The caring of the therapist cannot be captured by a snapshot of members' reactions to the therapist at a moment of group life. Caring reflects the perception of the therapist that members develop over time. In the moment, the members may see the therapist in a way that may appear at odds with caring, for example, when the therapist explores a rule violation, does not directly answer a question, or fails to provide concrete solutions to problems. The therapist may be seen as indifferent, depriving, withholding— anything but caring. However, over the long run the therapist's consistent engagement in the kinds of behaviors listed earlier will lead members to recognize and appreciate the therapist's caring for the group.

To authentically demonstrate caring, the therapist must feel a sense of caring. The therapist who has a generally positive stance toward other persons, borne out of his or her own history of healthy relationships, is likely to bring this orientation to relationships within the group. As part of this orientation, the therapist will convey to members the expectation that outcomes of interactions among human beings tend to be more positive than negative.

Yet, the therapist with a positive bearing toward others may fail, at times, to show it. This failure can be the result of feelings and impulses that arise in the sessions and defenses that may be raised against them. For example, individuals who are new to the activity of leading a therapy group commonly feel great anxiety (Frost & Alonso, 1993). The group situation exposes not only the members but the neophyte therapist. Understandably, the developing therapist worries that his or her lack of knowledge and skill will be evident to members. This worry often adversely affects manifestations of caring. Over my many years of doing cotherapy with psychology interns, I observed that the interns were often very timorous and tentative, particularly in their early weeks of leading the group. During this period the interns would have some difficulty exhibiting warmth to members and would give a rather uptight, constricted presentation. As the interns gained in confidence and know-how, they would invariably convey much greater empathy and concern for members.[2]

More experienced group therapists may confront more specific factors that impair their ability to experience and express caring toward members. For example, a group therapist may find jealousy to be an unacceptable feeling. In everyday life this stance will lead the therapist to be self-critical about jealous feelings. In the group the therapist will also have difficulty tolerating jealousy expressed by a group member. Because jealousy is common during the stage of group development following the group's resolution of authority issues (see Chapter 3), the therapist may pull back from not merely an individual member but the group as a whole. Such recoiling conveys to members that this aspect of their own psychological lives is unsafe. They thereby follow the therapist in the withdrawal from the new, "objectionable" material.

At each developmental stage, members are likely to express a range of affects and impulses. The therapist must have a capacity to welcome all of them to facilitate the group in continuing its work. Therapists in all modalities must devote considerable attention to developing an acceptance of all elements within their own psychological lives and those of others. For group therapists the demand may be especially great because the group setting provides a more powerful stimulus for the activation of feelings within the sessions. Therapists certainly differ in their comfort levels with their own psychological lives. However, probably every therapist needs to engage in personal work, typically in therapy, to address aspects of his or her own person perceived to be unacceptable. By coming to accept them, the therapist is able to have a more tolerant attitude toward members and show greater caring in a sustained way.

---

[2] This example raises the issue of how the group therapist-in-training should be introduced to the group. Should the members be told that one member of the cotherapy team has student status and the other, senior/supervisory status? This type of arrangement is called a *Nequipos* team and is very common in training sites such as teaching hospitals (Roller & Nelson, 1991). The advantage of identifying each person's role is that it gives the person in training freedom to be exactly that. The junior person feels less pressure to appear to be a full-fledged group therapist and can devote more energy to learning rather than acting. The group members are also helped to make a correct attribution about any possible reticence on the part of the student-therapist. Rather than mistaking the lesser participation for coldness or indifference, they will recognize that this individual is learning the ropes" of the group.

Even when the therapist has a healthy stance toward others and is unfettered by personal issues that may hinder responsiveness to group members, there still may be circumstances in which the therapist fails to show adequate caring. Sometimes the therapist's way of showing caring is different from members' assumptions about how a caring individual appears. This discrepancy between the therapist's style and the members' assumptions may occur when the therapist's cultural background differs from that of the members. Group members from a highly expressive culture may find a therapist from a culture characterized by greater emotional restraint to be far more unfeeling than the therapist actually is. Reciprocally, members from a culture of restraint may find the therapist from an expressive culture too encroaching. For example, the latter may use affect terms that connote more intensity than group members can tolerate. The therapist may accurately say "You were enraged" when "You were angry" is as much intensity as members can acknowledge. Therapists attuned to such cultural differences can be sensitive to the effects of his or her behaviors and make adjustments.

Beyond these barriers to the therapist's demonstration of caring are simply any behaviors that convey feelings and attitudes other than those the therapist wishes to express, or even actually feels. As such, these behaviors constitute miscommunications. Perhaps the therapist frowns when attempting to figure out some elusive aspect of the group. While the frown may be the therapist's idiosyncratic response to mental activity, the members may construe it as disapproval, at least at the moment.

Without feedback to the therapist on this behavior and how members interpret it, the therapist is likely to be unable to bring it under control. In a group atmosphere of openness where feedback is given and received routinely, the therapist will eventually hear about the focusing from the members. However, such information may be obtained at an earlier point in a group's life from a cotherapist, if one is present, in the processing period following the group session. Videotaping is also a way of garnering feedback about one's self-presentation. Finally, group therapists can obtain invaluable information about their interpersonal behaviors through their own participation in therapy groups and in experiential groups such as those featured by the American Group Psychotherapy Association at its annual meeting.

In summary, the expression of caring is critical to the successful functioning of the group. To show caring in a way that members will regard as genuine, the therapist must have a basic sense of trust in others and expect that relationships with others will have primarily positive outcomes. The therapist must have a tolerance of the gamut of human experience that leads to an acceptance of self and others. The therapist must possess a repertoire of caring behaviors comprehensible to the population from which the group members are drawn.

The conveyance of caring by the therapist involves both didactic and personal exploration. The didactic element requires an investigation of how affective stimulation is processed and how affect is expressed among the group members. The personal exploration entails the therapist's achievement of his or her own healthy interpersonal relations, typically through his or her own therapy and the removal of blocks to the demonstration of caring. Some individuals may enter the enterprise of conducting therapy groups with a great capacity to show caring; for others, intensive work may be necessary. However, it is likely that all new group therapists require personal work in some realm of their own psychological functioning.

Meaning Attribution

The third basic function of the group therapist is to assist members in cognitively framing their experiences and behaviors. That is, the therapist helps members to find meaning in their diverse reactions in the group. This therapist activity is critical to the success of the group, as Lieberman, Yalom, and Miles (1973) demonstrated in their study of encounter groups. These investigators found that groups whose leaders were high on meaning attribution had more successful outcomes than those whose leaders were low on this function.

Why is meaning attribution important? Members may realize a variety of benefits from finding meaning in their group experiences. One was identified in Chapter 4 in the discussion on interpersonal learning. The first step of interpersonal learning, the reader may recall, is activation of affect. While this step is essential to engage members fully in the group process, affect in the absence of understanding is likely to be extremely threatening to members. Understanding is a vehicle by which members can harness and channel feelings in a way that enhances a sense of safety in their presence:

Bert came to the group session angry with everyone and he expressed his anger intensively. Although initially members could not identify any precipitant to Bert's anger, eventually it became clear that Bert was angry with the therapist for raising her fee: Her action stimulated in him a fear that he would no longer be able to continue with the group. Once this connection was made, Bert remained vexed at the therapist, but his expressions were focused on the money issues rather than on a number of disparate concerns. He was also able to find solace in learning that other members shared his worries about the ramifications of the fee increase.

Bert's lack of understanding of the source of his anger made him vulnerable to an affective experience that was especially uncomfortable in its diffuseness. Once Bert understood his anger, it become more delimited and less consuming. This development liberated more positive, enjoyable feelings toward those who were not truly the object of his irritation.

This example suggests several other benefits of meaning attribution. Through enhanced understanding, members learn that their experiences are not as chaotic as they may seem but rather have some reasonableness in relation to the issue at hand. This notion in no way assumes that a member's reaction may not be in fact an overreaction. Rather, the point is only that there is a fit between the stimulus and the response. Recognition that their reactions do not occur randomly diminishes the strength of their perceptions of themselves as strange, bizarre, weird, or out of the mainstream, perceptions that adversely affect their self-regard. Moreover, having the incoherent become coherent can increase members' curiosity about themselves and enhance their therapeutic persistence as they learn that explorations can have valuable yields.

Another benefit is that a cognitive framing of members' experience can increase their empathy for one another. Members learn to look deeper and withhold negative judgments. Bert's group members probably felt a reciprocal annoyance in response to his seemingly unprovoked lashing out. However, once they recognized the actual source of his distress, they had the basis for kinder feelings toward him.

Finally, the use of a cognitive frame can help members with the transfer of their learning in the group to the world outside. I had the opportunity to lead a short-term inpatient group whose members, after a hiatus, joined a long-term outpatient group that I was also leading. On entering the long-term group, a member would typically recount the challenges of leaving the hospital and describe how he or she dealt with the return of old interpersonal stressors, such as a critical boss or an intrusive neighbor. Often the member would summon a particular formulation acquired in the inpatient group that would in the member's perception bolster his or her ability to cope with circumstances that had been unmanageable prior to hospitalization. For example, a member might say, "When I felt myself getting hostile toward him, I reminded myself 'You tend to get hostile when you feel really insecure.' Then I would ask myself if I had good reason to feel insecure and when I realized I didn't, I calmed right down." We might suspect that for this member, both the incisive formulation and the positive emotional experience with which it was associated contributed to its positive effect.

Selection of a Meaning System

If meaning attribution is a critical function for the therapist, how does the therapist accomplish this task? To help members find meaning in the events of the group, the therapist must also possess a system of meaning attribution. Such a system must define what types of events in a group are important, how these events are interrelated, and how members' understanding of their interrelationships supports the goals of the group. Each of the major theoretical approaches and models that have been developed from these orientations provide the therapist with a system of meaning attribution with these features.

For example, the cognitive-behavioral approach identifies individual member's affective experiences as important events. These affective experiences are then examined in terms of members' cognitions. Members' grasp of the interrelationships between cognition and affect is presumed to be a component of their greater control over their affective lives. Such an increase in control is a typical goal of a cognitive-behavioral group.

The therapist has no obligation to use one of the dominant theoretical orientations available. However, it is critical to achieve clarity about the cognitive framework that is part of the group's design. This clarity enables the therapist to use the framework in a consistent way that makes this framework evident to members. To the extent that members recognize the operative framework, they can use it in pursuit of the group goals.

Types of Interventions

The therapist can make a variety of interventions in helping members find meaning in the events of the group (see Table 5.3). At the simplest level, anytime the therapist labels what is occurring in the group, he or she is providing some cognitive framework. The following vignette demonstrates the power of labeling in transforming the events of a group:

> *Toni had been in the group for two months. She exhibited an unusual capacity to identify with other members' experience, even those that seemed remote or strange to other members. Another more long-standing member, Vicki, appeared threatened by Toni's sensitivity. Prior to Toni's arrival, she was the member with the greatest readiness to resonate to others' feelings. Yet relative to Toni, Vicki was both more selective and superficial in her identifications. Vicki's contributions, though, had been invaluable in getting the group off the ground, and her warmth was a much-appreciated commodity in the group.*
>
> *Recently, Toni had been achieving greater closeness with Kent, a painfully reticent member. With Toni's deft encouragement, Kent had ventured revealing to the group his shame over his obesity. While other members felt a gratitude to Toni for assisting Kent in entering the conversation, Vicki manifested a peevishness that was extremely off-putting to others. During Kent's fledgling efforts to describe his comfort with bodily self, she posed ill-timed and intrusive questions. When other members attempted to*

Table 5.3 **Meaning Attribution**

Definition	Assist members in finding meaning in, and cognitively framing, their reactions.
Therapist behavior	▪ The didactic presentation of a system of meaning
	▪ Labeling members' affects, impulses, fantasies, and behaviors
	▪ Identifying patterns in group events
	▪ Summarizing broad units of behavior (e.g., session wrap-up)
	▪ Interpretations of unconscious motives, feelings, urges, and so on as they affect the members' behaviors and experiences in the group

find similarities between their own experiences and Kent's, Vicki attempted to accentuate differences.

The therapist perceived that Vicki's behavior was increasingly arousing hostility. The therapist noted Vicki's long-recognized enthusiasm for, and skill in, forming connections with other members and observed that very recently, she had been interacting with other members in a different way than ever before. The therapist speculated that perhaps Vicki acted a different way because she felt *differently during the sessions. Vicki became tearful and admitted that she felt "off" in the group lately and didn't know why.*

The therapist queried, "Might it have to do with envy? Envy can be a feeling that's difficult to acknowledge to oneself and others. Yet most people do feel it from time to time." As the therapist uttered these words, the expression on Vicki's face was one of recognition, as if she instantly grasped the accuracy of this label. Other members rather quickly assumed a more patient posture toward Vicki, as if now they saw the coherence in all of her disparate puzzling behaviors. Using their new awareness, members proceeded to support Vicki by talking about their own envy toward people in their lives. One member revealed that in fact Vicki had aroused her envy by the ease with which she could interact with others. This revelation seemed to fortify Vicki, who then discussed rather directly her feelings of envy toward Toni.

Highlighted in this vignette is the labeling function. The mere act of putting nonverbal reactions into words is a cognitive act. Had the therapist allowed the group to continue on a nonverbal affective plane, Vicki may have been a scapegoat, with little or no recognition of why she was driven to engage in the behaviors that so adversely affected her relations with others. The group may have been no more than a recapitulation of the interpersonal struggles Vicki had outside the group. The label provided Vicki and the other members with the necessary information to move in a more productive direction.

At a higher level of complexity are interventions in which a pattern of group events is described. Such patterns may concern verbal and nonverbal behaviors, feelings, impulses, cognitions, and any physical stimuli that impinge upon the group. The following statements are descriptions of patterns:

- "In last week's session, I announced the group session would be canceled in two weeks, and this week, three members are absent." [verbal behavior–nonverbal behavior]

- "Early in the session, several members expressed annoyance that a new member will be arriving, and since that time, there have been many long silences in the session." [feeling–nonverbal behavior]

- "This week, we had to move our session to a new room. Somehow this new setting has inspired the group to talk about what a dangerous place the world seems to be." [physical stimulus–verbal]

While these statements vary from one another in terms of the type of group event on which they focus, they are similar in that they are descriptive. They concern events that are directly observable. These statements are useful in that they reveal the connections among psychological events that deepen members' understanding of such events. For example, if Vicki learns that the experience of envy leads her to respond in certain acrimonious ways toward others that create distance, she may learn to respond to the envy in an alternate way that has a different interpersonal outcome. More specifically, rather than seeking to ward off her envy, she might subject her feeling to a test of its reality base: Was she less envious because another member had various interpersonal strengths? This reality-testing process was what the therapist had effected in assisting the member in labeling her feeling. Upon acquiring her ability to provide the label herself, Vicki could also take greater charge of both the reality-testing process and the way she expressed envy to others.

At still another level of complexity is an intervention in which the therapist summarizes for members broader units of behavior. A therapist, for instance, may summarize at its end an entire session. Such a cognitive technique can be especially useful when a session has been wrought with intense affects. What the therapist conveys is an anxiety-lessening message: "No matter how chaotic events may seem, there is an order here that can be understood." For members who may have memory impairments, the summary provides an opportunity for the rehearsal of information and can thereby enhance retention. This cognitive step can also involve an affective element. For example, Smead (1995) advocates the use of a type of summary in sessions with children, where children are thanked for their various contributions to the group. Such a step would involve a blending of the caring and meaning attribution therapeutic functions.

The preceding interventions involve the cognitive framing of experiences that are relatively accessible to members. For instance, although Vicki did not label her own reaction as one of envy, when the therapist did so, it was immediately recognizable to her. This reaction was in the periphery of her consciousness; it was preconscious. Sometimes, the therapist will draw attention to psychological contents that are not in members' awareness even peripherally. For example, the therapist might call attention to a motive operative in the group that, while undergirding members' behavior, was wholly unknown to them:

> *The group members had been focusing on Joey's difficulties for these sessions and were getting nowhere. Joey would describe his ineffectual behaviors at work and in his dating life, and the negative outcomes of these behaviors. Members would urge him to relate to others in a more assertive and self-respecting way. Joey, after initially appearing mildly interested in the other members' ideas, would lapse into a posture of helpfulness while he exasperated the other members. Despite their frustration, they could not seem to transfer their attention to any other topic, person, or concern. At the same time, they increasingly deprecated Joey for what they called his "Milquetoast" behavior.*
>
> *The group therapist mused aloud that the group, like the moth to a flame, could not resist returning to assist Joey even though members strongly felt that their efforts were futile.*
>
> *Joey noted, "Yea, in fact, it's making me tired . . . like I'm supposed to be doing something I can't do but I have to keep trying."*
>
> *The therapist continued, "Well, I wonder if it's sort of like this: By focusing on Joey's difficulty in being strongly independent, members can pretend that it is his problem alone. In fact, the more the group advises Joey, the more beaten down he feels. The more beaten down he feels, the more he acts in that way that members feel is so objectionable. Perhaps the group has persisted in doing what appears to benefit neither Joey or the group because by so doing, we can pretend that it is only Joey who is more passive than he would like to be."*

In this vignette, the therapist made an interpretation that raised a connection between a puzzling piece of group behavior—members' persistence in engaging in behavior that was not effective—and an unconscious motive that may underpin this behavior, the wish to deny dependency longings. If the therapist's interpretation were sensitively timed and accurate, it would effect a shift in the group. Members' increased awareness of their dependent longings as well as their efforts to reject them would diminish their collective need to select one member to be the repository or container (Bion, 1959) for such needs (the projective identification process described in Chapter 3). Through their lessened defensiveness, they thereby would proceed to activity that would be more productive and less frustrating. Once the group no longer needed Joey to be the dependent member, there would be room for him to grow into other roles.

From these examples, it may seem that cognitive structuring is exclusively the province of the therapist. By no means is this the case. Rather, group therapists benefit their groups by finding ways for members to participate in the cognitive structuring of members' reactions. Therapists set the conditions for member participation by being consistent in the meaning attribution system that serves as the basis for cognitive restructuring interventions. Therapists who shift from one system to another will hinder members from learning how to organize cognitively their feelings. The therapist may pose questions to the group such as, "How do we understand what has been happening here?" When members do offer their own interpretations, the therapist should receive these efforts thoughtfully and respectfully. Yet members may accept certain types of interpretive statements only from the therapist. For example, group-level interpretations are frequently perceived as the therapist's domain (Cohen, Ettin, & Fidler, 1998). Members who attempt to make such interventions are often seen as striving to be junior therapists in order to curry favor with the therapist or avoid identifying with the other group members.

Emotional Stimulation

In Lieberman, Yalom, and Miles's (1973) original study, this category referred to rather provocative facilitator activity that intensified the pitch of feelings in the session. There are two major types of such activity. The first is the facilitator's own expression of feeling. The facilitator might make comments such as, "I feel enraged at you for making that comment" or "I was really moved by your words."

Earlier in this chapter "modeling" was described as a means of influencing members' behaviors. When the facilitator or leader of a group engages in any behavior, particularly early in the life of the group when members are looking for signs of appropriate group activity, such modeling is likely to be a powerful stimulus. Members think, "If the leader is expressing these strong feelings, it must be what one should do here." This aspect of the emotional stimulation function is discussed in the next chapter.

Another aspect of the facilitator's activity is confrontation in which the leader challenges the members' views and assumptions about themselves. The therapist might say, for example, "You think of yourself as such a tolerant person, but you subtly reject anyone who isn't in your race or your social class or doesn't have your highbrow and elitist interests."

Lieberman, Yalom, and Miles (1973) found that a moderate level of emotional stimulation produces more favorable outcomes than either low or high stimulation. This discovery is an extremely noteworthy and potentially reassuring one to persons who wonder if they have the right personality to be a group therapist. Individuals who are high on the dimension of emotional stimulation are often seen by members as charismatic leaders. This finding suggests that not only is it not necessary to be charismatic, it may not be especially helpful. This conclusion should be reassuring to those who worry that some absence of a magnetic quality in their interpersonal style will hinder their effectiveness as a group therapist. As noted in the beginning of the chapter, there is no single personality profile for the effective group therapist.

Yet, a low level of emotional stimulation is also not beneficial to a group's work. As discussed in Chapter 4, feelings must be activated or stimulated. Otherwise, group transactions boil down to little more than hollow intellectual discourse. The therapist's expressions of feelings or confrontations of members are means of stimulating emotion. However, both of these types of intervention carry the risk of arousing extreme levels of anxiety in members. Excessive or ill-timed confrontations can evoke humiliation in a member who is the target of the intervention, as well as a precipitous loss in self-esteem. While therapist self-disclosures (see Chapter 6) and confrontations have their place, there are other types of intervention that stimulate emotion (see Table 5.4). For instance, the

Table 5.4 **Therapist Function: Emotional Stimulation**

Definition	Behaviors that intensify members' experience and expression of affect in the group.
Therapist activities	▪ Modeling—the therapist expressing his or her own feeling
	▪ Confronting challenging members' views or assumptions about themselves
	▪ Being attuned to and reflecting members' feelings
	▪ Encouraging members to attune themselves to one another
	▪ Identifying blocks to members' expression of feelings (such as fears of the consequences of such expressions)

therapist can maintain a sensitivity to feelings members may be having and facilitate their expression:

> *While members were speaking with animation, Jonah sat looking dejected. The therapist invited Jonah to talk about his feelings. As Jonah slowly and hesitantly spoke, the therapist made reflective comments to convey an understanding of what Jonah was communicating.*

The therapist may also foster a group climate wherein members are sensitive to one another's feelings. Instead of the prior intervention, the therapist might have said:

> *There seem to be two emotional strains in our group tonight, one of which is upbeat and is expressed by the liveliness of the discussion. The other strain shows itself in Jonah's downcast appearance.*

Such an intervention encourages members to attune themselves to their own and other members' feelings. It may lead members to be curious about Jonah's emotional state and support him in expressing his reactions. Over time the therapist's consistent use of such interventions will enhance members' levels of emotional sensitivity so they rely less on the therapist's prompts. Another benefit of such an intervention is that it does not assume that a member has exclusive ownership of a given feeling. Jonah, for example, may be expressing his melancholy not only for himself but for others as well. It is useful, therefore, to phrase an intervention in such a way that all members can consider its applicability to themselves.

Orchestration of the Four Leadership Functions

Each of the four leadership functions should have its place in the repertoire of the group therapist. They play a role in activating the various mechanisms of change outlined in Chapter 4. For example, consider the mechanism of group cohesion. Executive activity is extremely important in fostering cohesion in that through establishing consistency of place, time, and membership, a palpable sense of groupness is possible. Caring is crucial because as the therapist conveys a sense of value of each group member, members emulate this stance. Furthermore, the therapist's empathy is likely to help members demonstrate empathy for other members. As each member experiences being understood and accepted, he or she is likely to place a greater premium on the group experience. Meaning attribution also plays a role in that when the therapist finds a unifying theme in seemingly varied contributions, members feel a greater connection to one another. Emotional stimulation assists in helping members to be interested in the group and attuned to one another, both essential commodities for cohesion to develop.

Because the four functions are critical to the activation of the mechanisms of change, the therapist is likely to perform activities related to each of them within each session. Yet among groups, and among sessions of the same group, variation is likely and even appropriate. The model the therapist uses will dictate the relative emphasis given to the four functions. For example, skill-building models have historically placed great emphasis upon executive activities, whereas models whose target is intrapsychic change stress meaning attribution. The patient population is also a factor. For example, if members are organized at the psychotic level, they lack the internal structure to effectively organize their expressiveness. Moreover, even a moderate level of stimulation can evoke a sense of fragmentation. Hence, in such groups, there should be a relatively high emphasis upon emotional stimulation.

Furthermore, the developmental stage of the group will have a bearing on the therapist's relative engagement in different activities. Kivlighan (1997) followed the life of a personal growth group composed of undergraduate students led by graduate students participating in a group process course. Group members rated the leaders on the extent to which they were task oriented (roughly similar to executive activities) and relationship oriented. Whereas high task orientation early in the group's life was associated with positive outcomes (reduction in complaints), a high relationship orientation late in the group's life also was associated with positive change. This finding—that different activities have varying levels of importance over the course of the group—is consistent with the Situational Leadership Theory, which holds that the most effective leadership takes into account the needs of the group (Hersey & Blanchard, 1977). Because needs vary, leadership activities should vary.

The Kivlighan (1997) study had another finding relevant to the topic of the emphasis on different leadership activities. Kivlighan found that leaders are relatively consistent. While some appear to adjust their behaviors to the developmental stage of the group, the majority do not. The latter seem to have a particular style of leadership that remains constant through the group. While it may be important for any therapist to learn flexibility, as noted in the beginning of the chapter, the personality of the therapist is always likely to be a force in how the group is led.

Summary

This chapter examined four types of functions performed by the therapist: executive activity, caring, meaning attribution, and emotional stimulation.

Executive activity includes designing the group, developing a receptivity to the group in the clinical context, and recruiting members. The recruitment of members entails selecting members and preparing them for the group experience. Once the group is under way, a major executive activity is maintaining the therapeutic frame of the group, or the features of predictability and regularity that create safety necessary for work to be performed. During the course of the group the therapist engages in a variety of directive activities to move the group toward its goals. The therapist *models* desirable behaviors, encourages other members to model these behaviors, and reinforces these behaviors when they occur. The therapist encourages the members to craft *agendas* for sessions to direct each member's work to an area of therapeutic relevance. *Exercises* are introduced to enable members to practice skills during sessions, and *homework* enables the strengthening of skills in between sessions. *Treatment manuals* coordinate different activities across the life of the group.

Caring refers to the therapist's communication of warmth, interest in, and respect for the members of the group. The caring group therapist manifests appreciation of the value of each member and commitment to each member's growth. The caring therapist conveys authenticity in the expression of his or her thoughts or feelings in the group. Caring also involves accurate empathy for the members' expressions. A variety of obstacles may block the therapist's ability to show caring, such as the therapist's own lack of tolerance for any of his or her own feelings or impulses, lack of cultural competence with respect to the group population, or particular behaviors that members see as incompatible with caring on the part of the therapist. The acquisition of knowledge about the population being tested, personal therapy, participation in experiential groups, and supervision all can contribute to the therapist's capacity to show caring.

The *meaning attribution* function involves the therapist's assisting members in understanding their experiences in the group. Through this understanding members can harness and channel feelings in a way that (a) bolsters members' tolerance of these feelings, (b) strengthens their recognition that their feelings have some reasonableness given the situation at hand, (c) increases their capacities to empathize with one another, and (d) facilitates the transfer of learning to life outside of the group. The insertion of the meaning attribution function requires that the therapist possess a clear framework that can be used to decide the significance of group events and member communications. In making meaning attributions, the therapist can use various interventions such as labeling, identifying linkages between behaviors and feelings, summarizing patterns of behavior, and making interpretations of behaviors and experiences and the unconscious elements underpinning them.

Emotional stimulation, the fourth function, entails increase in the intensity of emotions in the group. Historically, emotional stimulation has been achieved through the therapist's self-disclosure and confrontations of members. However, both of these types of intervention carry the risk of increasing the level of stimulation beyond what members can manage. Other interventions, such as encouraging members' sensitivity to one another's manifestation of feelings and facilitating members' identifications with the feelings of other members, enable the therapist to keep the group adequately but not excessively stimulated.

The extent to which the therapist performs each of these four functions should depend on a variety of factors, including the model according to which the group is seen, the group's developmental status, and characteristics of the patient population. In general, however, group therapists should strive for high levels of caring and meaning attribution and more moderate levels of executive activity and emotional stimulation.

Advanced Leadership Issues

While the scheme presented in the previous chapter outlines major functions to be performed by the group therapist, additional questions remain as the therapist determines what style of leadership would be appropriate for a given group. This chapter addresses three issues that must inevitably be faced as the therapist specifies his or her group design: the structure of leadership, the therapist's treatment of his or her own reactions that emerge in the course of the group sessions, and the therapist's level of transparency or self-disclosure. Some therapists may merely lapse into a given approach to each of these areas. However, the effectiveness of the group in furthering the well-being of its members is likely to be enhanced if the therapist gives each leadership question careful analysis in the context of the overall group design.

The Structure of Leadership

Therapy groups may be conducted by a single therapist or a team of therapists, typically two. When the group sessions are facilitated by multiple therapists, the leadership format is referred to as cotherapy. The group therapy literature identifies both advantages and disadvantages to both forms. While some writers have seen solo therapy as preferable to cotherapy (MacLennan, 1965; Rabin, 1967; Rutan & Stone, 2001), others express opposite sentiments (Andrew, 1995). However, writers identifying one or the other formats often do so within the framework of a particular theoretical orientation and set of goals. Either solo therapy or cotherapy may be preferable depending upon the nature of the group. To create a coherent group design with an optimal leadership format, it is important that the therapist recognize what each has to offer.

In some contexts, it is not possible to select a leadership format. For example, some organizations may not have enough staff for cotherapy. In other settings cotherapy may be needed to train developing group therapists (Rutan & Stone, 2001). Even when the therapist does not have the luxury of being able to make a selection, it is still useful to know about the unique features of each so that the therapist can comprehend the various forces bearing upon the group.

Cotherapy

A first advantage of cotherapy is that it enables a division of labor. Circumstances arise in a group in which the therapist is called on to perform various activities that are difficult to do in combination. For example, suppose a group member is angry at a therapist. It is often more effective for the therapist who is not the target of the anger to facilitate the expression of group member's feelings toward the one who is. Otherwise, the anger can become blunted as the member perceives the therapist as too kindly and encouraging to be the object of anger. In a skills-oriented group, the array of tasks to be performed may overwhelm the solo therapist. With a cotherapy structure, one therapist can, for instance, write on the blackboard and structure a role play while the other participates in the role play and monitors the dynamics of the group. Cotherapy is regarded by many as of particular advantage in working with an extremely difficult population (Concannon, 1995; Geczy & Sultenfuss, 1995). Cotherapy adds an element of safety to any group where members are at risk for such behaviors as leaving the group in distress or exhibiting hostility in a way that is physically threatening to the members. With cotherapy, one therapist can continue the session while the other can attend to any special needs of a member experiencing difficulty responding constructively to the group situation.

Cotherapy allows for multiple perspectives on the process of the group. Given that events are constantly occurring in a group on the levels of the individual, dyad, subgroup, and group as a whole, the amount of information that any therapist can register is inevitably only part of what is available. Having two therapists typically increases the fund of information on which interventions are based. The author routinely did cotherapy in an inpatient setting for many years. In the processing session that occurred after the group session, my cotherapist would often make comments such as, "Did you notice that Tom looked dejected while Sue and Carmella were speaking to each other with such animation?" "Did you see Mack looking at his watch during the last fifteen minutes of the group?" "Were you aware that when you made your comment about some members feeling fearful about the group's coming to an end, Aster rolled her eyes and Genevieve smiled?" These observations would enrich my perception of the group, expanding my knowledge of the range of forces at play at any time.

Cotherapists can also provide feedback on one another's verbal and nonverbal behavior in the group. Some aspects of any therapist's reactions lie outside of awareness, yet it is important to recognize them in order to comprehend fully all the interactions among members:

After a group session the cotherapists of a group discussed the curiously melancholy tone the group had taken. On the one hand, the topics members raised seemed rather mundane and lacked any clear depressive themes. On the other hand, the tone in the group was exceedingly downcast. However, the cotherapists' efforts to get the group to address the negative feelings were unsuccessful.

One cotherapist said to the other, "You know, when you first raised the issue about the group's mood, I thought you stated it in an unusually strong way. . . . Your typical way is to begin slowly. And I wondered if . . . well . . . you thought you should talk about this sadness that seems to be taking hold of the group but maybe not having your heart in it."

"Something about what you're saying rings a bell for me. I know I did find myself having a difficult time discovering the right words, almost as if I was caught up in what had overtaken the group," the other cotherapist responded.

The cotherapists began to explore the possibility that they, too, shared the members' reluctance to explore the dominant feeling in the group. They realized that perhaps by understanding their own reluctance better, they could elucidate the group's reaction. What emerged eventually was that the group members and the therapists were having an anticipatory reaction to the ending of the group. Both therapists were facing the ending of their training year as psychology interns. Their supervisors had suggested that they terminate the group because the next year's class of interns might not be interested in running this elective group. The intern therapists recognized that they had not yet announced the ending of the group to the members, believing that they had plenty of time to do so. Yet, the members were well aware of the calendar of the clinic because it was a long-standing one and several members had individual therapists who had broached the topic of termination with them.

Both therapists came to see that the group's lack of interest in exploring feelings of sadness paralleled their own reluctance to explore termination. Both felt guilty about members' being affected by their own career paths. They also came to recognize that they felt at a loss to handle the group's inevitable question as to why the group could not be continued by next year's interns. Furthermore, they realized that they felt anger toward their supervisor for somehow not being able to guarantee the group's continuation. Because of the desire to avoid a full reckoning with all these feelings, the cotherapists had addressed the affective climate in a way that was ambivalent and ineffectual. However, with the benefit of this discussion, the cotherapy team was able to enter the group the following week with a stance that was less protective of their own feelings and hence more productive for the group.

The realization of the therapists emerging out of their discussion might have been more difficult for a solo therapist to achieve. However, the benefit can be had only if the therapists have a commitment to reviewing carefully the developments of a group and discovering together what may have eluded them in the session.

Just as cotherapists may see the group in different ways, so, too, can group members see the cotherapists differently. For example, at one point one therapist may be seen as more caring than the other, one more controlling than the other. One factor contributing to differential perception is that the therapy team does present real differences to the group member. For example, one therapist may indeed by more intuitive or more able to convey warmth than the other. However, the differences group members see may also be based on the needs of the members:

For weeks, the new group treated the two members of the cotherapy team similarly. However, the male therapist was increasingly seen as cold and intrusive and received a good dose of anger for exhibiting these qualities. The female therapist was seen more benignly. In the review sessions the cotherapists puzzled over this change and could point to no behavioral differences that gave rise to the differential perceptions.

For many people, the expression of anger toward an authority figure is a highly threatening event that stimulates the worry, conscious or unconscious, that the authority figure may retaliate or abandon the angered person. In group, the presence of a cotherapy team gives members the opportunity to express anger toward one member while retaining the positive tie with the other. The preservation of a nonhostile connection with one therapist diminishes members' fears about the consequences of expressing hostility. Hence, the therapists may be seen in polar terms even when they do not differ much from one another. Certainly, the groups' splitting the therapists in this way has a defensive aspect insofar as members are defending against the enormity of their fearfulness about expressing negative feelings toward the therapists as a unit. Nonetheless, doing so allows members to safely express anger, which serves as a forerunner to expressing negative feelings toward therapists who are seen in more integrated, less distorted ways.

Rutan and Stone (2001), rather than seeing cotherapy as creating conditions in which members can express negative feelings toward authority figures, see it as eliciting the opposite reaction. They write, "Many patients find it harder to confront or disagree with two therapists presenting a united front" (pp. 199–200). Such a therapy team might exhibit a style of collaboration and intervention where such potential could be realized easily. For example, therapists may piggyback on one another's comments and thereby overpower the members. This "united front" presentation, making the team an indomitable force, is likely to be rooted in some emotional element that is unduly influencing the therapists' behavior. For example, the therapists may exhibit exaggerated solidarity out of fear of the group's anger or as a reaction formation against competitiveness with one another.

Still another benefit of cotherapy is that it enables greater continuity. When a solo therapist cannot be present for a given session, that session must be canceled.[1] This greater continuity is likely to be an advantage to all groups but particularly to groups having

---

[1] There was an era in which leaderless groups were a fairly common practice. Groups would meet in the absence of the therapist not so much because the therapist could not attend but because the sessions were seen as having distinctive therapeutic value. In today's practice climate, leaderless sessions are not a common phenomenon. A consensus seems to have emerged that the dangers of such a format far outweigh their potential benefits to members.

extremely low functioning members. For such members, a hiatus of even one week could make a difference in their ability to maintain a sense of connection with the group. A life circumstances such as illness or maternity leave may require the therapist to be absent for a number of sessions, placing the survival of the group in jeopardy. This author had the opportunity to interview group therapists who took maternity leaves of varying lengths (Anderson, Fallon, Brabender, & Maier, 2000; Fallon & Brabender, 2002). Solo therapists reported feeling great apprehension over whether their groups would hold together during their maternity leaves. This worry occurred even for those women who had a substitute therapist run the group. In contrast, those therapists whose cotherapists ran the groups reported no anxiety over the continued viability of their groups.

Solo Therapy

With all of the advantages of cotherapy, the reader might wonder what might compel a therapist to do otherwise if cotherapy is a possibility. In fact, solo therapy benefits the group in a variety of ways. First, the solo therapist may evoke stronger transference reactions from members. Depending on the purpose of a group, these reactions may be an essential resource. For example, in a psychodynamic group directed toward intrapsychic change, members' responses to the therapists, often reflecting reactions to authority, are of great importance. As noted earlier, in cotherapy members' dependency upon the therapists is distributed. While this may make it easier for members to express their reactions, it may also mute such reactions, rendering them less available for expression. In solo therapy the interpersonal stimulus is more concentrated and, hence, potentially more potent. For group therapy approaches that do not emphasize the exploration of transference, this potency may be a disadvantage. Members may have intense reactions to the therapist that distract them from the work they have set out to do.

The second advantage of solo therapy is that it may make more palpable to the therapist his or her reactions to the group. As is discussed in the next section, the therapist's reactions are a gold mine of information about the group. However, having a partner in the session may dull these reactions. For example, if members complain about the group's being "a miserable waste of time," the therapist's sense that the complaint is being directed toward the team rather than toward him or herself may lessen the sting of members' dissatisfaction. Furthermore, in cotherapy the processing of the group outside the session may diminish the intensity of both therapists' reactions. For example, cotherapists may commiserate with one another over the vexing behavior of a particular member. When negative feelings are quelled through such sharing, they may be less available for the kind of exploration that would ultimately illuminate a hidden aspect of the group.

In the example given earlier of the cotherapists' discussion of the emotional flatness in the group, the interaction between the cotherapists led to a greater awareness of their own feelings, an awareness that could ultimately enable the group to grapple with avoided issues. Whether the cotherapists' review and analysis of the session leads to the use or dissipation of the therapists' reactions depends entirely on the tenor of the team itself.

A third advantage of solo therapy over cotherapy is that it is simpler. While a duality of perspectives is a potential strength of cotherapy, it is also a weakness, especially if the therapists have not reached accord on fundamental aspects of the group design such as the goals of the group and the processes by which goals will be reached. Achieving such agreement requires typically a considerable investment of time. While cotherapists may not need to iron out all of their differences (provided they are not basic design features), they must at least recognize and accept them before embarking upon the group. Then, once the group has begun the therapists must meet to review each session. Even for senior therapists, as the cotherapy relationship is getting launched, supervision is highly desirable (Dugo & Beck, 1997). While the solo therapist also has an obligation to review each session, this process is less complicated than when there are two perspectives.

Beyond the complexity created by each therapist's point of view is the complexity of the logistical arrangement. As noted in earlier chapters, many tasks must be performed to run a successful therapy group. Cotherapists must decide upon a division of labor that seems fair and equitable to both parties. Moreover, the initial arrangement should be renegotiated as circumstances change. For example, both therapists may intend to be involved in the recruitment of members for the group. Suppose that one therapist no longer has resources for recruitment. Should that therapist have additional duties in another area of the administration of the group? Remuneration for services is another factor. Suppose, for example, that initially cotherapists agree that the senior therapist will receive 75 percent of the group income, the junior therapist 25 percent, based on the fact that the former is supervising the latter. As the junior therapist gains experience, the therapists might develop more of a peer relationship. This team would need to renegotiate the financial arrangement even though within this culture discussing money is difficult for many people (Stone, 1995). Failure to do so might engender resentment in one party and perhaps guilt in the other. Both feelings could adversely affect the therapists' collaboration.

Still another source of complexity in cotherapy is the potential for personal elements of the relationship to affect professional elements. Socialization in therapy groups is typically outlawed because interactions outside of the group could affect members' work within. Yet cotherapists do not hold themselves to this standard, even though just like group members, changes in the relationship outside the group could affect their behavior in the sessions or in the management of the group. If, for example, one therapist rejected the other romantically, both parties might naturally be tempted to cut short postsession reviews to the detriment of the group. Solo therapy is free of such a potential complication.

To remove this possibility, some restrictions could be added to the cotherapy relationship. For example, perhaps cotherapists could impose more stringent requirements upon themselves for the range of their interactions outside the group (Wetcher, 2000). However, the fundamental reality would still remain that the cotherapy relationship is more than a business arrangement: It is a profoundly personal one. Given that the qualities of the therapist have been amply shown to affect the quality of the group (see Chapter 5 and Wheelan, 1997), how could the quality of the cotherapy relationship not affect group outcome? Cotherapists' achievement of a mature working relationship with each member, exhibiting respect for the other's views, a capacity to communicate his or her ideas clearly, and an ability to resolve conflicts and solve problems effectively would provide a favorable context for members' making similar accomplishments.

How does a mature cotherapy relationship come into being? Some theorists, particularly Dugo and Beck (1997), have observed that cotherapy relationships evolve over time. Based upon their observations, they posit a sequence of stages through which the relationship develops that parallels the developmental stages of the group. For example, in Phase 1 cotherapists forge an initial contract and "establish a foundation by creating formal norms for the critical aspects of their relationship and for the conduct of the group" (p. 296). In Phase 2, they form an identity as a group. In Phase 3, they "move into the information gathering that can set up a collaborative working relationship. They begin to learn about the range and depth of each other's intuitions, conceptual orientation, and intervention skills" (p. 297). Dugo and Beck go on to posit six additional stages. They hold that until the cotherapy team moves to Phase 3, they cannot achieve an effective collaboration within the group regardless of the type of group. Furthermore, they assert that the group cannot progress further in its developmental than has the cotherapy team itself.

The relationship between the maturity of the cotherapy team and the development of the group must be studied further. However, to the extent that cotherapy teams must reach a certain level of maturity for groups to prosper, the cotherapy enterprise becomes more difficult. Where circumstances may not provide sufficient stability or time for cotherapists to become a true team (e.g., an institution that does not allow the cotherapists to budget the necessary time for pre- and postsession meetings), then solo leadership would probably be more beneficial to the group.

Theoretical Considerations in Implementing a Leadership Format

Once a particular format has been chosen, either the solo therapist or cotherapy team should create the conditions in which the selected format can be used optimally. A danger for the solo therapist is that his or her perspective on the group may become hardened. Simply because any one human being's perspective is limited, the solo therapist may be unaware of certain patterns and dynamics within the group whose recognition may be critical to the group's progress. All group therapists—those operating solo or within a team—would benefit their groups by nurturing within themselves the humility and skepticism that enable them to view their groups in fresh ways.

Beyond this effort solo therapists support the group's work by allowing knowledgeable others to challenge their formulations and having their reactions to the group probed and illuminated.

Solo therapists also should recognize the group's total dependence on their presence. Solo therapists who have reason to believe that some personal factor such as a sudden worsening of a chronic health problem will force them to miss sessions should make contingency plans for the group's at least temporary continuation so that members' reactions to any sudden event and changes in the treatment can be expressed and explored. Such an issue is likely to figure more prominently in private practice than in organizations in which contingency mechanisms may be in place.

Cotherapy, a more complicated leadership format than solo therapy, requires the consideration of a number of factors. A major factor is whether the therapists can develop a unified vision of what the group will be. Dugo and Beck (1997) speak of the importance of the cotherapists' forging a group contract. In negotiating such a contract the therapists come to an agreement about the goals of the group and the mechanisms of change that will be deployed to pursue these goals. As part of the processes the therapists have to agree on what their roles in the group will be. In the process of developing a contract, some differences between the therapists' perspectives are likely to emerge. Yet as Dublin (1995, p. 84) noted, "The issue is not that there are differences, even glaring differences, but rather how they are dealt with by the cotherapy team." Supporting Dublin's point is a study by McNary and Dies (1993) in which 20 therapy groups were studied, each led by a cotherapy team. Group members were asked to give their reactions to the cotherapists' exchanges. The investigators found that these exchanges tended to be regarded as unhelpful when the cotherapy team acknowledged conflicts they were unable to resolve.

Cotherapy is frequently used to train group therapists. An experienced group therapist will perform cotherapy with a less experienced therapist. In this senior-junior arrangement, each party may not have equal say in the design of the group (Dublin, 1995). The junior person may be present specifically to learn the senior therapist's approach.[2] Nonetheless, the contractual period prior to

---

[2] Some argue that this common configuration is not true cotherapy, which is seen by the writers as a relationship between equals (Roller & Nelson, 1991). However, to eliminate these pairings from the population of cotherapists is to circumscribe the population

the commencement of the group should not be neglected. Even if the goals, processes, and leader roles are not a matter of negotiation, discussion should occur about the compatibility of the approach with the junior therapist's notions about how change proceeds. To omit such a step is to invite two negative consequences. The junior therapist is neither likely to apply the model or approach in an effective way nor to have a successful learning experience. Murphy and colleagues noted that "Trainees who worked with experts described feelings of lack of ownership and passivity" (Murphy, Leszcz, Collings, & Salvendy, 1996, p. 551).[3] Perhaps these experts might have benefited their supervisors more by greater attention to developing an alliance with their junior cotherapist prior to his or her group participation.

As part of the contract cotherapists should develop some mechanism for meeting between sessions to review them. Ideally, cotherapists should meet immediately before and after the session. Particularly but not exclusively in the case of a junior-junior combination, a plan for supervision should also be negotiated during the development of the contract. During both supervision and the review sessions, the cotherapists should attend not only to the events of the group and therapist reactions but also to their reactions to one another both inside and outside the session:

> *A senior and junior therapist had been working together for several months. The senior therapist noticed that the junior therapist had become increasingly less vocal in the group. Moreover, she, the senior therapist, had begun to confine his comments to reflections rather than interpretations. In a post-session review, the senior therapist shared her observation with the junior therapist. Haltingly, the junior therapist revealed that he felt the senior therapist disapproved of his interpretive comments. He noted that shortly after he would make a statement, the senior therapist would seem to nullify it. She would, he observed, either make his comments more specific or phrase them in a way that changed their meaning. He also reported that the senior*

---

radically. Many cotherapy pairs have differences in status, experience, and so on. Moreover, the junior member can achieve great salience as a stimulus to members' reactions precisely because of his or her junior status. Rather than limiting the definition of cotherapy, it is perhaps more useful to recognize that it has different forms.

[3] In contrast, Rice (1995) found that when members of a junior-junior team (both members were trainees within 1 year of experience of each other) were surveyed, 80 percent indicated that they would like to work with the same cotherapist again. Eighty-six percent described the learning value of cotherapy as very high.

therapist had responded in a similar critical way to him in a group seminar that she ran with other trainees.

The senior therapist was surprised by the junior therapist's comments. She had done cotherapy with a succession of junior therapists for many years. She saw this cotherapist as especially perceptive and skilled. She realized that she had been treating him as a colleague rather than as a student. She explained this to the surprised junior therapist and articulated her realization that she had probably not given him the support he needed.

The senior therapist in this example was appropriately attuned to the behavior of her cotherapist and willing to broach the implications of the behaviors for the tenor of the relationship. She was also open to assuming some responsibility for the reactions of her cotherapist and being forthright with him about her contribution to his sense of insecurity about his performance. Postreview sessions that have this type of reflection on the whole will do more to enhance the group than sessions that ignore cotherapist issues and dynamics. In this vignette, for example, the discussion between the senior and junior therapist would have the likely effect of renewing the junior therapist's willingness to participate fully in the group.

Cotherapists must also be keenly aware of any acting out outside the group of conflicts emerging within the group. As noted previously, cotherapists are not limited in the way members are in their extragroup behaviors. This relative freedom of the cotherapists makes them vulnerable to expressing through their interactions whatever material the group cannot address directly:

The outpatient group had recently proceeded through an intensive phase of challenging the cotherapists' authority. Both members of this junior-junior team felt that they had worked together effectively to assist members in challenging their fears about expressing negative feelings toward them.

In one of their postsession reviews, one therapist revealed to the other an intense attraction and a wish to pursue the relationship on a more social basis. The other cotherapist expressed similar feelings.

Following the phase in which members address authority issues, they move into a phase in which there is a heightened sense of intimacy. Group members often experience an urge to challenge all boundaries between and among members. The unconscious wish is to achieve a kind of perfect union with one another and obliterate differences. The rules of the group typically play a useful role in restraining members from engaging in behaviors that might undermine the integrity of the group. It is possible that in their attraction to one another and consideration of moving their relationship to the social realm, these therapists were acting out the unconscious wish of the group.

As the preceding example might suggest, it behooves any cotherapy pair to consider how changes or wishes for changes in the relationship may be a response to conscious and unconscious aspects of the group's current life. When this type of exploration is done, the cotherapy relationship can serve as one diagnostic indicator of the status of the group.

The Group Therapist's Reactions

What is likely to be evident to any new practitioner of group therapy is that one's own reactions can be a powerful force with which to contend while leading a therapy group. Some writers (e.g., Goodman, Marks, & Rockberger, 1964) have argued that in group therapy, there are many more pulls for strong therapist reactions than in individual therapy. Whether this is true or not, the beginning group therapist will find that at any moment in the life of the group, he or she is likely to have a variety of emotional and cognitive responses, and as the group progresses, these reactions are likely to change. However, what also changes is the therapist's capacity to make sense of these reactions. As they develop, group therapists typically moves from being overwhelmed by their emotional responses to the group to an appreciation of these responses as valuable tools to learn about the group and about themselves.

Among the theoretical approaches available to the group therapist, the approach that gives greatest attention to the therapist's reactions is the psychodynamic/psychoanalytic approach. Freud (1910) noted that in an analytic session, the patient will have a reaction to the analyst that derives from, and properly belongs to, early figures in the patient's life. Such reactions he referred to as transference reactions. In like manner the analyst may have reactions to the patient rooted not truly in present reactions but in the analyst's own early history. These therapist reactions Freud labeled countertransference.

Freud saw countertransference as an impediment to treatment, for it challenged the neutrality and objectivity in the analyst that was required for analysis to proceed fruitfully. When operating under the sway of countertransference, the therapist, Freud believed, is likely to view the patient in a distorted way and the interventions proceeding from such distortions are less likely to be helpful than those flowing from a more accurate perception. For this reason Freud exhorted the therapist to "recognize this counter-transference in himself and overcome it" (1910, p. 145).

This classical view of countertransference was embraced by psychodynamic therapists for many years. Group therapists who used a psychodynamic approach would make an effort to be alert to any elements of their response that might be countertransferential. They would seek to better understand these elements and their origin in their personal histories so that the influence of these elements would be lessened. Frequently, therapy and supervision were vehicles by which the group therapist might explore their countertransference responses.

In recent years group therapists have continued the critically important task of discerning what personal issues may be activated by events within the group. However, in all modalities there has been a shift away from a one-person psychology in which one person (the therapist) functions as the neutral observer, while another (the patient) provides the fund of experiences for exploration toward a more relational perspective. Within this new perspective mutuality is a feature of all interactions. As Wright (2000) wrote, "Mutuality refers to the fact that all parties in the therapy setting are undergoing experiences and reactions, and that each influences and is being influenced by the other or others in an ongoing fashion, i.e., the therapeutic process is reciprocal" (p. 183). The experiences that both patient and therapist have are co-constructed, with each party affecting and being affected by the other. Neither can the patient's experiences be construed without reference to the therapist, nor can the therapist's experiences be construed without reference to the patient.

This more relational view of therapist reactions has implications for how the therapist treats them during the group process. Therapist reactions are only in part, as the classical view of countertansferences requires, aspects of the therapist's responses to the group to be discarded or diminished through the therapist's own personal work. Ormont (1991) referred to these aspects that are idiosyncratic or unique to the group therapist as *subjective counter-transference*. He distinguished this type of countertransference from *objective countertransference*, which is responses that are more universal. These latter therapist responses provide information about the group's concerns, conflicts, processes, and other psychological elements, information that might not be easily accessible otherwise. As Rutan and Alonso (1994) noted, listening to one's affective reactions in a diagnostic way is especially useful when the therapist is experiencing some uncertainty about what is happening in the group because these reactions can be highly elucidating. Chapter 11 explores the issue of countertransference further in the context of the model that has made a major contribution to the elucidation of objective countertransference, the object-relations approach.

Transparency

In the example of the imminently departing cotherapists, perhaps it occurred to the reader that the therapists might have shared with members something of their reactions to the group's upcoming termination. For example, one might have said, "I feel distressed that group members must suffer this loss when you are making so much progress" or "I feel sad over disrupting the group." In making such comments, a therapist is being transparent, that is, allowing members to recognize what is occurring in his or her internal life. In its greater specificity, the second comment involves more transparency than the first. Even more disclosing would be a revelation to the group that the therapists felt guilty over subordinating members' needs to their own career plans. Hence, the transparency of the therapist is on a continuum ranging from no disclosure (or opaqueness) at all to an extremely high level.

What might be the benefits and costs of such communications? There are a number of potential benefits of some level of transparency on the part of the therapist. In this instance, the therapists' conveyance of some feelings of concern about the ending would show empathy for members' understandable disappointment and sorrow that they were losing something of great importance to them. In fact, "judicious self-disclosure" can often be one route to establishing empathy (Rachman, 1990). A second potential benefit is that members might become aware of a connection between their behaviors and the reactions of authority figures. For example, a member may learn that her attunement to the therapist for any trace of negative reaction engenders in the therapist a wish to withdraw.

Despite the potential benefits, the cost of certain communications may be considerable. If the cotherapists were to reveal a high level of guilt over the group's ending, members might see them as quite fragile and wonder whether they are too vulnerable to be of any assistance to them. They may also feel some sense of responsibility for the therapists' discomfort and experience some guilt. Not only would they question whether the therapists could act as caretakers for them, but also they may be led to see themselves as caretakers of the therapists. Several studies support the notion that the therapist's disclosure of personal problems or negative feelings may lead the members to question the therapist's mental health (Weigel & Warnath, 1968; Weigel, Dinges, Dyer, & Straumfjord, 1972) and, hence, capacity to lead the group effectively.

Factors Affecting Reactions to the Therapist's Self-Disclosures

In weighing the costs and benefits of making self-disclosing statements to the group members, the therapist might consider other factors that have been shown to influence their impact. In an excellent review article written over two decades ago that still comprehends most of the important research on transparency, Dies (1977) cites three factors that bear on the effects of therapist transparency: developmental status, type of group, and type of disclosure. These dimensions are discussed and related to the example of the vacationing therapist.

Developmental Status: One factor is the developmental status of the group. The more the group has developed and the longer members have been in the group, the more tolerant members are of the therapist's self-disclosures (Dies, 1973; Dies & Cohen, 1976). This finding is consistent with the developmental stages presented in Chapter 3. Over the course of a group's life most group members move toward a greater reliance upon one another and less dependency on the therapist for protection and help. They are likely to tolerate evidence of the therapist's humanity once they have stopped idealizing the therapist.

Precipitous demonstrations of fallibility on the part of the caretaking authority figures are likely to jeopardize group cohesion (Cohen et al., 1998) and lead members to withdraw investment in the relationship with the therapist and also possibly the group as a whole.

Despite this developmental trend, there are probably some self-disclosures that group members will forever find to be either unhelpful or even harmful. Dies and Cohen (1976) had undergraduates rate different types of potential therapist disclosures from the vantage point of having been in a therapy group for 1, 7, or 15 sessions. The ratings were on a scale from 1 to 7, with 7 corresponding to the category of "harmful." Although the investigators found that as the session number increased, members said that an increasing number of therapist disclosures were helpful, a number of disclosures were seen as harmful over the three ratings. Examples of statements receiving a 4 or higher across the three-session length conditions are the following: "questions about his own emotional stability"; "feelings of sexual attraction toward a member of the group"; "the fact that he is currently in therapy"; "his distrust of a group member"; and "the feeling that he is being manipulated by a group member." The obvious limitation of this study, however, is that it is based on the ratings not of therapy patients but of individuals imagining how they would respond as therapy patients.

Type of Group: A second variable is the type of group. A comparison of findings of studies on personal growth groups versus those on therapy groups suggests that the more the individual perceives himself or herself as having psychological needs to be met by the group experience, the less tolerant he or she is of the therapist's transparency. Generally, members of personal growth groups perceive a high level of therapist transparency in positive terms. For example, in one study on personal growth groups in a college setting, there was a strong positive relationship between the group leaders' level of self-disclosure and the leaders' level of perceived mental health (May & Thompson, 1973). While some studies on personal growth groups show that leader transparency is associated with gains by members in the group (Hurley & Force, 1973), others do not (Bolman, 1973). In contrast, therapy group members tend to see high-disclosing therapists as less psychologically healthy (Dies, 1973) even if they like these therapists better (Weigel et al., 1972). This difference between personal growth and therapy groups may be the result of expectations and goals. As Dies

(1977) noted, members of personal growth groups see themselves as, like the leader, a part of the general population. They do not expect that the concerns of the leader would be so very different from those of group members. Therapy group members, on the other hand, define themselves as persons with problems. The notion of the therapist also having problems may lead to questions of whether the therapist is truly in a position to help them.

Content of the Disclosure: A third variable is the type of self-disclosure made by the therapist. In the Dies and Cohen study (1976) described previously, disclosures of emotional reactions of the therapist that were perceived as helpful had two characteristics. First, they were reactions that would generally be deemed to occur in most people's normal range of experiences. For example, the therapist's acknowledgment of past experiences of loneliness was generally perceived positively. Second, disclosure should relate to reactions having their origin outside the group (i.e., "then-and-there" reactions). An example of a disclosure involving both of these features would be the therapist's admitting to sadness in relation to a loss that was familiar to group members, such as the death of a parent. In contrast, members found negative therapist reactions directed toward individual members to be unhelpful and disturbing. This fact is consistent with a study on individual therapy patients showing that members found reassuring therapist disclosures more helpful than challenging disclosures (Hill, Mahalik, & Thompson, 1989). Furthermore, it seems that group therapists instinctively make the type of self-disclosures that members find to be more useful. In a study of 20 outpatient groups (McNary & Dies, 1993), it was found that therapists far more frequently make positively toned disclosures that group members regard as helpful.

The Uses of Self-Disclosure

The discussion of the factors affecting members' reactions to a particular therapist disclosure or to a general level of transparency adopted by the therapist makes clear one key point: Many contextual factors must be considered in the therapist's decision making about disclosures. The list that is offered is probably only a partial one. Such factors as the level of functioning and dynamic issues of the group members are examples of insufficiently investigated variables that probably should figure into the therapist's deliberations on this matter. Level of transparency is a fundamental feature of group design. It is a dimension that the therapist should consider in planning the group while recognizing that the group's likely response to different levels of maturity will likely change as the group matures. In the group design the therapist should have a conception of the kinds of situations in which he or she would make a disclosure. To explore this matter fully, the therapist or cotherapy team should begin with a recognition of the possible uses of the therapist's disclosures and consider these uses in light of the goals of the group.

A first potential use of therapist self-disclosure is to affirm the member's perception of the interpersonal world. Opportunities for self-disclosure occur when one or more group members have discerned a particular affect state in the therapist. For example, consider the following situation:

> *A group member came into the group late. Another member was sobbing and describing how her husband had been transferred to another branch of his company, requiring her to leave the group. The tardy member was habitually so. Sometime during the middle of the session, the tardy member said to the therapist, "You seemed quite irritated by my lateness today." The therapist knew that in fact she had been annoyed by the lateness because it had punctured the spellbinding effect of the departing member's narrative. She was taken aback because this member was typically oblivious to others' reactions. She considered whether she should own up to her annoyance.*

In some individuals who enter group therapy, a major aspect of their difficulties is an imperceptiveness to others' reactions (Rutan & Stone, 2001). For these persons, a goal of the group experience is to foster a greater sensitivity to others. The therapist's denial that she was annoyed would be inconsistent with the cultivation in this member of greater awareness of others. While the therapist's reaction to this member involves the communication of negative feelings, such feelings are within the scope of everyday experience, both in terms of intensity and cause. That is, most people become at least slightly vexed when an absorbing activity is interrupted. Given these features of the therapist self-disclosure, it is unlikely that the member would construe the therapist's reaction as conveying dislike of her. Nonetheless, the therapist should attend carefully not only to the reaction of the recipient of the communication but to the reactions of all members.

Particularly when authority issues are dominating the group's inter-actions, a therapist's expression of negative feelings can easily be ex-aggerated and evoke primitive fears of retaliation or abandonment.

A second use of self-disclosure is the conveyance of empathy with the group members' reactions. Particularly important is the therapist's acknowledgment of behaviors that may have in some way adversely affected group members. The therapist may unwittingly engage in behavior that for a given group member activates feelings associated with early trauma (Rachman, 1990). In the original trau-matic situation, there may not have been any soothing presence within the interpersonal surroundings to lessen the feelings associ-ated with the trauma. In the group circumstance disclosing that in-deed a mistake has been made and that the member's response is an understandable reaction to the therapist's action can have a soothing effect that was absent in the original traumatic situation:

A group member, Katisha, said almost incidentally that after the prior session, Davida's car had blocked her from exiting the therapist's parking lot. Davida had made a delayed departure from the group session because she had been asking the therapist about an insurance form she (the member) was submit-ting. Davida said, "Oh, I forgot I was blocking your car." Katisha shrugged, "Oh, I just listened to my radio." The therapist made no comment. Later in the session, Katisha talked about her sisters' planning events to which she was not invited. When she had made some efforts to express her feelings of being excluded, she was dismissed as being hypersensitive. The therapist noticed that although Katisha was speaking of these matters, she had a very disengaged manner. She was not looking at members as she spoke, and for their part, they seemed to be not truly paying attention. The therapist realized that she had felt a kind of impatience with Katisha's narrative and had hoped Katisha's comments would be interrupted by another member. Upon further reflection, she realized that she had been disturbed by the description of the delayed exit last week and felt responsible for it.

The therapist said, "Katisha, you know I was thinking about what you shared very early in the session. I can imagine that it must have been quite annoying to have to sit in the car while another member was carrying on her business. Certainly the logistics of the parking lot fall under my do-main of responsibility and I made a mistake in having an individual inter-action before I was sure that everyone had left. Furthermore, when you brought up this issue, I didn't really own up to my responsibility in having inconvenienced you and I wonder if that was a further source of distress."

Katisha said, "It's a strange thing to hear someone like you apologize. I wasn't really angry at you, but still, it makes me feel better to hear you say that."

In this example, the therapist had reactivated an old hurt, one of being neglected by family members, by responding indifferently to the member's ambivalently expressed complaint. The member's distancing from the group was a repetition of past responses to the trauma. However, the therapist's response, uncharacteristic of early figures, was a healing moment for the member who felt valued enough by the therapist to be treated with respect.

As is true with all types of therapist disclosure, when contemplating this type of disclosure, the therapist must attempt to discern his or her motives for the intervention, including ones that may not be apparent initially. For example, is the acknowledgment of a mistake an effort at self-flagellation? The therapist should attempt to ensure that the objective of the intervention is to meet the needs of the members rather than those of the therapist. Occasionally, a given intervention may meet both the neurotic needs of the therapist and the legitimate needs of group members. For example, in apologizing, the therapist may both soothe a member who has been the object of the therapist's insensitivity and appease his or her own conscience. By carefully sorting out the motives for the intervention, the therapist will find it easier to deliver the intervention in the best possible way. The therapist's recognition of an urgency to have his or her guilt lessened will enable that therapist to express a sense of regret that is in proportion to, rather than in excess of, the magnitude of the transgression.

A third use of self-disclosure cited in the literature (e.g., Truax & Carkhuff, 1965) is the therapist's modeling of behaviors that are likely to contribute to members' progress in the group or that represent positive outcomes in their own right. For example, by self-disclosing his or her thoughts and feelings, the therapist is modeling openness. When acknowledging a mistake, the therapist is modeling taking responsibility for one's behavior and treating others respectfully. The notion is that when members witness the therapist engaging in these behaviors, they themselves are more likely to engage in the behaviors. In fact, high levels of therapist self-disclosure have been demonstrated to be associated with high levels of member self-disclosure (Kangas, 1971). Certainly the therapist can encourage desirable behaviors in ways other than through self-disclosures. For example, by engaging in a line of questioning supporting one member's self-disclosure, the therapist can increase the openness of all members of the group. However, as Allen (1973) points out, one difference is that the therapist may be more skilled in regulating his or her level of self-disclosure based upon some of the factors that have been cited, such as the developmental status of the group. Some group members may be vulnerable to engaging a degree of self-disclosure that exceeds the group's readiness for that level of sharing.

In summary, the therapist's disclosures may benefit the group in a variety of ways. The therapist's level of transparency should be established as a component of the group design. However, from moment to moment in the life of the group, some variation in the level of therapist transparency will occur. In thinking about any particular disclosure, the therapist should clearly identify the purpose the disclosure is serving, its appropriateness given the developmental status of the group, the possible costs of the disclosure, and any underlying motives that may be driving the therapist's interest in disclosing.

Summary

This chapter extended our discussion of the role of the therapist through an examination of three issues. First, the structure of leadership was addressed. The two common formats of solo therapy and cotherapy were described including the advantages and disadvantages of each. Cotherapy enables therapists to share their different points of view on the group and on one another. It affords members greater continuity in the group and greater safety when members express negative feelings toward the therapists. Solo therapy offers an environment conducive to the emergence of strong transference and countertransference reactions and a greater measure of simplicity. Second, the therapist's use of his or her own reactions was discussed, a topic that is pursued further in Chapter 11. Finally, the topic of therapist transparency was considered. We considered the factors that should inform the therapist's decision about whether and when to disclose. These include the maturity of the group, the type of group, and the content of the disclosure.

Supporting Features of the Group Design

The therapist has made considerable progress in developing the *group design* by establishing goals and identifying processes by which the group can progress toward those goals. The therapist has determined which processes will be important during the various stages of the group's life. Specific leadership activities have been identified that will activate those mechanisms that are important to the group's progress during each of these stages. Now the therapist must decide how to create a group environment that nurtures the group's work. Features such as group size, length, location, and a variety of other factors can be neutral stimuli, deterrents to the group's progress, or catalysts.

Three classes of supporting features will be considered. The first is structural in that the features pertain to the format of the group. The second class is behavioral: How should members comport themselves to ensure that goals are met? The third is financial: How is payment handled within the group?

Structural Features of the Group

When thinking of the important issues of group goals and processes, the therapist may be inclined to view issues such as chair arrangement as mundane. Yet, very concrete aspects as to whether the therapist sits in the same or different chair each week can influence the group's work. In building a group environment, the therapist should consider all of the features that define the group. Very frequently, the therapist may not have control over all of them. For example, in a hospital setting, a group may be allocated a duration that is less than optimal.

What is important is that the therapist be aware of the likely effects of whatever features define the group. This awareness will enable the therapist to be more closely attuned to members' reactions. Whenever possible, however, the therapist should summon any control he or she has in designing the group to ensure that as many features as possible will operate in the service of members' work. To do so, each feature requires its own careful study.

The Size of the Group

How large or small should a group be? What is its optimal size? In determining size the therapist should consider two questions. The reader will see that for size, as for all other supporting features, the optimal size is crucially related to the goals and processes specified by the group design.

The first question is, *What member resources are necessary in order for a group to do its work?* For example, interpersonal groups depend on the presence of different styles and points of view. As the size of the group increases, the variability among members in these important areas increases. There could be a size so small that it limits unduly what members can derive from their interaction. Such a limitation might either affect the pace at which a group could move toward its goals or its ultimate success in reaching them. Groups with four or fewer members may become preoccupied with the survival of the group to the neglect of other issues (Rutan & Stone, 2001). Typically, an interpersonal group will need at least five members to afford the group the needed range of interpersonal behaviors and points of view. Otherwise, consensual validation is hindered (Yalom, 1995). However, highly structured groups such as problem-solving groups have been observed to do effective work with as few as four members (Coche & Flick, 1975). The key for the therapist planning the lower limit is to consider what each member might add to the resources of the group in relation to the total fund of resources needed.

The second question is, *What demand does each member place upon the resources of the group?* The goals of an interpersonal group, for instance, demand that members have the opportunity to obtain feedback on their interpersonal styles. Feedback is a process that occurs in time. The larger the group, the less time is available for members to receive individual feedback. Hence, larger groups require longer sessions (Yalom, 1995).

The resources of the therapist or cotherapy team are also at issue in this decision. Some models require an exceptionally high level of activity on the part of the therapists. In a social-skills training group therapists have an especially large array of activities to perform. As Brabender and Fallon (1993) wrote, "While the therapist is busily directing the format and flow of the session, the cotherapist assists in watching the other members, writing homework assignments, keeping track of goals, and participating in role plays" (p. 594). While cotherapy can aid immeasurably when there are multiple and simultaneous tasks to perform, even with two therapists it may not be possible to do justice to the demands of leading the group if the membership exceeds a certain number.

Temporal Features

The therapist must make a number of decisions related to time. How long should each session last and how frequently should the group meet? How long should the duration of each member's participation be? Should members begin and end the group at the same time or at different times? While the therapist may need to make other decisions in relation to time, the aforementioned are probably the most critical and will therefore be considered in this section.

Length and Frequency of the Sessions: Group sessions typically vary in length between 45 minutes and 2 hours. This variation is accounted for by a number of factors, but among the most important is the level of functioning. Generally speaking, the lower the level of ego functioning, the briefer the sessions must be. Members at the lower level of ego functioning (particularly the psychotic level as defined in Chapter 2) readily experience great fearfulness in relating to others. Keeping the session relatively short helps such members to manage their anxieties both in anticipation of and during each session. Another factor is age (M. S. Corey & Corey, 1997). Younger children may lack the attention span to participate in a longer session. Contextual factors may also bear upon session length. For example, in some inpatient settings, a fixed interval for all activities may be 60 minutes.

Frequency of sessions is a variable that is likely to affect the group's capacity to achieve cohesion. All other factors being equal, the more frequent the meetings, the more cohesion a group can achieve. Cohesion becomes an important consideration in group work with populations that have difficulty in moving toward this achievement. The anxieties of low-functioning members discussed in relation to length of session often interfere with their ability to identify with others' experiences. Their lack of object constancy—the ability to maintain an awareness of the existence of an object in its absence—hinders them from maintaining their grasp upon the group as a force within their lives. For members at this level of ego functioning, it is preferable for sessions to occur more frequently than the weekly meetings of the typical long-tem outpatient group. As Yalom (1995) notes, twice weekly groups provide greater intensity and sense of continuity. In inpatient settings it is not uncommon for groups to meet daily. In fact, one positive influence of managed care has been to encourage inpatient facilities to extend their therapeutic activities throughout the weekend by making the availability of such offerings a condition of reimbursement. Consequently, in some institutions groups meet seven times a week. This situation is a salubrious one for group members whose tie to the group is tenuous.

The Length of the Group: There are two types of membership configuration. In a close-ended group, all members begin the group in the same session and terminate from the group at the same time. Typically in a close-ended group, the number of sessions is a key part of the group design. Most close-ended groups tend to be brief or short term. In open-ended groups, the members enter the group at different times and also have varying dates of termination. While most long-term groups are open-ended, brief and short-term groups may also be. For example, in inpatient units in which there is a need to place individuals in groups immediately, groups are frequently open-ended.

Even if a group is open-ended, the clinician should have a conceptualization of how long the group experience is expected to last. Such a determination would in large part be based upon the therapist's answer to the following four questions:

In what target area lies the intended change? In general, symptomatic change can be obtained relatively quickly. Many of the studies done on cognitive-behavioral group therapy have demonstrated that the common presenting symptoms of anxiety and depression can be substantially lessened after 12 to 20 sessions (e.g., Free, Oei, & Sanders, 1991; Zerhusen et al.,—20 weeks). Groups devoted to skill development can also effect positive change in as few as 8 sessions. For example, a number of studies show that improved problem solving (e.g., greater ability to generate multiple solutions to problems, enhanced capacity to evaluate potential solutions) can occur in as few as 6 sessions (Jones, 1981) but more typically between 8 and 12 sessions (e.g., Pierce, 1980—11 sessions; Intagliata, 1978—10 sessions; Small & Schinke, 1983—12 sessions).

Interpersonal change often takes longer than symptomatic change. For example, Bateman and Fonagy (1999) compared a group of patients organized at the borderline level who participated in an analytically oriented group in a partial hospital setting versus a group that received standard psychiatric care (psychiatric review, visits from a psychiatric nurse, and so on). These fairly disturbed patients showed symptomatic improvement relative to the controls after 9 months of program participation. Interpersonal change did not occur until after 18 months. While some types of interpersonal change may be possible in a time-limited group, others may require a long-term involvement.

Historically, approaches emphasizing intrapsychic change have been conceptualized in the context of long-term group therapy. Such approaches have typically been geared to modify features of the person that developed over the course of many years and, unlike symptoms, that have achieved stability within the individual's personality. Moreover, the nature of the processes used are such that they unfold over time. For example, Chapter 3 discussed universality as a change-producing mechanism that exists at different levels. A relatively superficial level of universality can be achieved in a brief period of time. However, deeper levels require the establishment of a degree of trust that requires a considerable fund of interactions of members with one another.

Nonetheless, because of the pressures of managed care, clinicians using approaches geared to produce intrapsychic change have moved to adapt these approaches to briefer time frames (Rutan & Stone, 1993). This adaptation occurred first in individual therapy. For example, Thomas Mann (1981) proposed a 12-session model in which members would have an opportunity to address the central issues underlying the presenting symptom. The central issue is a feeling about the self that has developed from past experiences and is always present on a preconscious basis. The patient in his or her current situation is presenting with symptoms because features within that situation resemble those of past events in which the feeling about the self originated. What Mann proposes is to use the time-limited character of the treatment to create a condition that will enable the correction of the individual's negative self-image. In facing the time limit, the person experiences in vivo the pain attached to the negative self-image. With the full emergence of the pain in treatment, and the patient's experience of the therapist's empathy in relation to this pain, the patient has the opportunity to reconstruct his or her self-image by recognizing that many elements of the self-image are no longer warranted by present realities.

The notion that is at the center of Mann's treatment method—that the time limit of treatment should be used rather than lamented—has increasingly been applied by group therapists. Chapter 2 described the group therapy format for persons with pathological grief reactions (Piper et al., 1992). This short-term group was similar to Mann's individual approach in that it actively used the time limit of 12 sessions. Particularly during the termination period, the members had heightened access to conflicts related to events of loss in their lives in that they were now losing the group. As noted earlier, members exhibited change on a variety of levels, ranging from the symptomatic to the intrapsychic. Hence, intrapsychic change is possible within a relatively short time frame. However, we know much less about the kinds of intrapsychic goals that are suited to short- versus long-term treatment than about other types of change, especially symptom relief and skill building. This area is one that could benefit from further study.

How focused versus broad is the desired change? The more focused the goals, the briefer the treatment can be. To some extent, a reason groups geared to lessening symptoms and developing skills have been able to show positive change over a relatively brief duration is that the goals to which the groups were directed were relatively circumscribed. For example, the goal of symptom alleviation is typically established in relation to a particular symptom such as anxiety or depression. Not unusually, groups devoted to interpersonal and intrapsychic change are typically far-reaching in their efforts. For example, most long-term interpersonal groups aim to assist each individual with, not a single interpersonal difficulty, but a spectrum of problems.

Interpersonal and intrapsychic changes have been far more amenable to pursuit on a short-term basis as group therapists have restricted the goals in these areas. In the example given earlier of the loss groups (Piper et al., 1992), the conflicts addressed in the time-limited group were only those pertaining to loss. An even more dramatic example of goal delimitation is Kibel's (1981) object-relations model used in inpatient settings. This model has an extremely specific goal—that of helping those members organized at the borderline level to reacquire their premorbid defensive system (particularly the defense of splitting). Through this reacquisition members can achieve a sufficient sense of well-being to be able to leave the hospital. Once discharged, members can pursue longer-term therapy in which more ambitious intrapsychic goals can be pursued. Kibel's approach to inpatient group therapy is designed so that a member can derive benefit even if he or she is in the group for only a few sessions. While no outcome study has yet been done on this model, it is based on the kind of careful goal delimitation process that is likely to lead to positive results.

What kinds of cognitive, emotional, and motivational resources do members bring to group treatment? To the extent that members do not possess resources critical to their pursuit of particular goals, these resources must be developed in the group itself. The cultivation of a needed resource becomes a subgoal, which requires additional time relative to the circumstance in which members already possess the resource. Whether the time is great or little depends upon the resource itself.

For example, in the 12-session loss group (Piper et al., 1992) described earlier, members are selected on the basis of their ability to appreciate the connection between the presenting complaint—such as anxiety or depression—and loss. Such an appreciation reflects the individual's psychological mindedness, some modicum of which is required for members to be accepted into the group. As noted earlier, members of the group generally give evidence of making great progress in addressing loss-related conflicts within the confines of the 12 sessions. However, had the therapists been required to develop in the members the necessary psychological mindedness, the 12-session time frame would have been unrealistic.

What resources does the setting offer in bolstering members' group work? This question is most pertinent when the therapy group is embedded in a larger treatment environment. Some inpatient groups use the same model within the group that is used in the unit to guide interactions between patients and staff. For example, some inpatient units embrace a social-skills training approach. All staff members in the unit are (or are expected to be) well-versed in this approach. In the therapy group members receive instruction in social skills and opportunities for practice. On the unit staff are ready to assist group members with their homework from the sessions and to frame interpersonal difficulties emerging in the social-skills language learned in the group. Relative to the treatment environment that operates independently with the group, the supportive environment allows the group to work more efficiently.

The Spatial Features of the Group

Our physical environment can be a major influence upon the kind of experience we have in that environment. For this reason it is important that the therapist's attitude in establishing the environment be careful rather than casual. Many dimensions characterize the group environment, the most important of which will be discussed in this section.

The Location of the Group Room: In planning the group, the therapist should attend to the relationship between the group room and the broader context. How firm is the boundary between the group and the environment outside? A group room that creates a firm boundary protects members from possible intrusions of the outside environment. For example, if during an inpatient group session members overhear a loud and angry exchange between two staff members outside the group, then that material necessarily becomes part of the session, implicitly or explicitly. A firm boundary also prevents group communications from being transmitted outside the group. For example, a door ajar may provide nonmembers with access to communications members intend to be private. Of course, the boundary separating the group from the outside environment in created and fortified in ways other than the structure of the physical environment. For example, the reader may recall the vignette in Chapter 5 in which the group therapist permitted a secretary to enter the group room to procure a VCR. When such intrusions are permitted, the sanctity of the physical environment becomes irrelevant to the firmness of the boundary between the group and the outside environment.

Therapists in private practice should also consider the location's accessibility. If possible, a location that is accessible by public transportation is preferable to one that is not. The therapist is likely to receive a greater number of referrals when prospective members do not have to depend on a car. Furthermore, members are more likely to attend regularly when there are alternate ways to reach the group.

The Characteristics of the Group Room: The internal boundaries of the group become a consideration in the seating arrangement, the level of illumination, and the furniture. Across most models, the goal of the therapist is to create an environment where the internal boundaries between members are porous. *Porousness* means that there is a free flow of information, verbal and nonverbal, from one member to another. At the same time, boundaries that are too permeable may evoke in members a sense of danger.

Exchange of information is maximized by members' sitting in a circle. Individuals should be seated at a sufficient distance and angle to see easily the members on their left and right. Moreover, too much proximity can violate members' sense of personal space. A variety of factors determine the amount of personal space necessary for members to enjoy a reasonable level of comfort. One is culture. Persons from northern European countries generally prefer greater interpersonal distance that persons from southern European countries. In a culturally mixed group the therapist will have difficulty taking the cultural factor into account. Additionally, it is helpful if the chairs are light enough to be moved. In exploratory groups members' movement of chairs can provide useful information about the group's dynamics (Foulkes, 1986). Other types of groups may involve role plays and other exercises that require the reconfiguration of chairs.

The level of illumination of the group room should be moderate. The lighting should not be so dim as to hinder members from seeing one another. Excessively bright light may contribute to members' sense of being exposed and may thereby create an atmosphere not conductive to emotional expression.

The chairs in the group room should be comfortable given the relatively long period they are occupied. Some group therapists have a table in the middle of the circle of chairs because it creates an ambience of relaxed informality (Foulkes, 1986). However, the table should be low enough to enable members to have visual access to one another's body language. A high table is also unsuitable because it creates the aura of a business meeting.

One decision that the therapist must make is whether there will be designated chairs. As others (e.g., Rutan & Stone, 2001) have noted, assigned seating for therapists may make a contribution to the work of the group, whereas assigned seating for members may detract from its work. The therapist's occupying a consistent seat each week lends stability to the group that is reassuring to members. On the other hand, giving members the opportunity to choose seats provides information about members' wishes, feelings, urges, fantasies, and so on. For example, two members' sitting next to each other over a period of six weeks and placing themselves more remotely from one another in week 7 may reveal a change in their feelings about one another. Where the members place themselves in relation to the therapist can also be revealing.

Relevant to the group room is the issue of where the members will remain until the session begins. If a waiting room is available, this is an obvious choice. Otherwise, the group room must be opened before the group begins. Members' interactions in either of these venues are a rich source of information about currents in the group that might not be evident otherwise. Many of these interactions will not be observed by the therapist. However, the therapist can work to create a climate in which the members report the interactions themselves in an effort to understand their group better.

Building the Group Contract: The Rules of the Group

There are behaviors in which members can engage that help them to move in the direction of the group goals. Examples of such behaviors are the expression of feelings and other types of self-disclosure, the giving and taking of feedback, the demonstration of caring toward other members, and so on. Both in the preparation of members (see Chapter 8) and in the sessions themselves, the therapist cultivates the capacities to use these behaviors. The particular behaviors emphasized in this cultivation process will depend upon the model the therapist is using.

The presence or absence of another set of behaviors is essential at the outset of the group in order for the group to have any potential to be productive, for members' rights to be protected, or both. Because of the criticalness of members' behavior in certain areas to group and member well-being, rules are established that identify the acceptable parameters of member conduct. In general, the number of rules should be few. A long list of rules reduces the salience of each rule and inevitably mingles the less with the more important, thereby trivializing the latter.

Across types of groups and theoretical approaches, there is some consistency in the rules established. The reason for this consistency is that there are particular behaviors whose presence or absence would preclude any effective group work regardless of type of group. At the same time, the consistency is not absolute. Certain types of groups may require rules that are fairly specific to that group. For example, the contract for a group of substance abusers may include a rule outlawing drinking before group sessions. While most group therapists may see drinking before sessions on the part of members as a detriment to themselves and the group, they may not expect the base rate of such behavior as high enough in the population being treated to warrant a rule outlawing pregroup drinking as a standard component of the group contract. Because the number of behaviors that could adversely affect the group is limitless, the therapist cannot possibly incorporate all of them in the group contract.

The remainder of this section discusses the rules that are common to many groups. One rule, which should be present in all groups, is that of confidentiality. However, because the topic of confidentiality has major legal and ethical dimensions, this discussion is reserved for Chapter 9, which presents a framework for understanding particular ethical dilemmas.

Attendance and Promptness

Across most types of groups, members' regular attendance is critical to the group's success. Missed sessions interrupt the continuity of the group's work. For example, suppose at the end of a session one member gathers his courage after a long period of silence to confront another member. Suppose further that the latter member is absent for the next session. This sequence is likely to give support to the confronting member's perception that engagement in this new experimental activity is dangerous. Missed sessions also prevent members from keeping pace with the group. For example, within some theoretical approaches, instruction about concepts and techniques occurs within certain sessions. Missed sessions for members organized at the psychotic level can undermine their sense of connection to the group as a whole and lead to premature withdrawal from the group altogether.

For these reasons it is incumbent upon the therapist to work toward developing in the group the norm of rare absenteeism. While the therapist may use a range of interventions to establish this norm, a crucial intervention is to incorporate it as part of the group contract. During preparation the member should be helped to understand why consistent attendance is essential (presumably any major impediment to the member's consistent attendance, such as frequent business traveling, would have been identified during selection and taken into account in the selection decision). If members' lapses in regular attendance are likely to be taken up in the sessions themselves, then the prospective member should be apprised of this fact during the presentation of the contract.

Promptness in members' attendance of sessions is also an important norm to establish. When the session begins and one or more members are missing, the group will typically delay beginning its work in earnest. Moreover, tardiness, like absences, can be members' way of expressing in action any fear they cannot express in words. To the extent that members abandon these ready means to discharge feelings and urges, they are more able to grapple with them within the group.

In connection with the absence and lateness policy, members should be strongly encouraged to inform the group, when possible, when they expect to be late or absent. The member should also be encouraged to contact the therapist before the session when emergencies arise. Valuable session time can be wasted by members wondering whether a member will appear. For example, if a member has announced several weeks before that she will be absent for a given session, members are less likely to make false attributions to events in the preceding session to explain her absence.

Socialization Outside of the Group

Many group therapists prohibit members from socializing outside of the group sessions. In an inpatient situation, this prohibition is typically not possible. Members typically encounter one another in other therapeutic activities and in leisure periods. Some hospital day programs (e.g. Piper et al., 1996) permit participants to interact during program hours but not outside of the program. The no-socialization rule is applied most commonly in outpatient groups.

Socialization among members outside of the sessions is outlawed for a variety of reasons. First, members' interactions outside the group may diffuse the productive tension that fuels a group's motivation to address problems that arise in the group:

Carline has been extremely agitated by her confrontation of Madeline in the last session. In that session Madeline appeared wounded but said nothing. Carline found herself thinking about it repeatedly and felt apprehensive about the session to come. She called Madeline and apologized, saying that she was in a somewhat bad mood and had overstated her case. Madeline received the news with relief, responding, "I'm glad I'm not as bad as all that." In the next week's session, neither Madeline nor Carline broached the latter's confrontation of the former. The other group members also seemed to have forgotten about the event.

That members want to rid themselves of the tension associated with a conflict is understandable. However, in achieving quick closure members deprive themselves of learning opportunities. Perhaps Carline did overstate her case. If so, it would be important for her to learn what interpersonal circumstances prompt this response, which she later regrets. On the other hand, Carline's statement may have been on target and might have been validated or specified further by other members. Both of these possibilities would require that members come to the group ready to explore these issues. Interim contacts can reduce members' sense of urgency to do so.

A second disadvantage is that extragroup contacts prevent all of the members from participating in the conflict-resolution process. Suppose Carline and Madeline had a more in-depth exchange. Carline may have provided Madeline with additional details about those behaviors of Madeline to which she responds negatively. If Madeline had been able to assimilate this information in a constructive way, the group would not have been privy to this sequence. Moreover, when members express their reactions, they do so not only for themselves but also for other members. In taking the issue away from the group, members such as Carline and Madeline silence voices for the group as a whole.

Some group therapists who permit extrasession socialization argue that these disadvantages can be avoided by stipulating that members must talk about any interactions outside the group inside the group. This less restrictive rule still creates the condition for the emergence of the two problems described previously. While it is true that Madeline and Carline would be required to share their interaction, preventing it from going underground altogether, their interest in it would in all likelihood be reduced substantially, as interest always is for yesterday's news. Moreover, while members might receive a report about the members' problem solving, they would not have witnessed it. It would be a there-and-then summary rather than a here-and-now immersion. As such, it would be less likely to engage and therefore benefit members.

A third reason for the socialization prohibition is that role conflicts may develop that endanger the socializing member's group work. In some cases individuals who enter group therapy do so specifically because they have a poverty of relationships outside the group. A friendship with a group member outside the group may acquire more importance to a member than his or her relationship with the person in the group. A likely consequence is that the parties may avoid confronting each other in the group lest they place the friendship in jeopardy. Moreover, they may withhold information in an effort to protect one another's privacy and perhaps to hold on to a sense of intimacy during the group sessions.

A fourth reason to prohibit extragroup socialization concerns risk management. Historically, the focus of risk management and professional ethics has been the client-therapist interaction only. Increasingly, in part because of litigation, risk-management thinking has shifted toward the inclusion of the client's interactions with other parties (including other clients). This shift has implications for how contact among members would be viewed from a risk-management perspective. Any group therapist who actively endorses contact among members most likely does so in the expectation that such contact will benefit members. Yet the possibility of a negative outcome exists, particularly given that the therapist is not present to monitor and guide members' interactions. The most conservative strategy from a risk-management perspective, therefore, is to require members to refrain from socialization, though outlawing socialization does not absolutely protect the therapist from being seen as responsible for any negative outcomes resulting from member interactions outside the group. The least conservative strategy is the active endorsement of such interactions, because with therapist endorsement, the extra-session interactions can more plausibly be seen as an extension of the therapy. Intermediate between these points is the therapist's silence or neutral stance on the issue of socialization.

Eating and Other Oral Activities in the Group

Particularly for groups with members organized at the borderline- and neurotic-levels, a rule is often established that members must refrain from certain oral activities during the group sessions. Typically, these include smoking, eating, drinking, and chewing gum. The rationale for this abstinence is that all of these activities can dampen the intensity of feelings and urges in the sessions, making these reactions less available for communication and exploration. Occasionally it may be appropriate to relax this rule of oral abstinence. A member with a cough may be able to participate more fully by being permitted to take a cough drop.

The group therapist may also require members to refrain from drinking alcohol prior to the session in order to prevent the diminishment of the strength of a member's reactions. In a high-functioning population, members may see this restriction as obvious and may experience the therapist's articulating it as patronizing. The therapist may therefore address this issue only if it emerges as a problem.

When working with members functioning at the psychotic level, the therapist must be concerned that members' anxiety levels may reach unmanageable proportions. For the same reason that the therapist would not want borderline- and neurotic-level members to refrain from utilizing oral substances, the therapist may wish to make certain oral items available to psychotic members. By serving, say, juice and cookies, the therapist may reduce members' anxiety to a level that may be more tolerable. In groups with children and adolescents, food may be a means of providing nurturance to members and at the same time be a powerful stimulus for exploration (Mishna, Muskat, & Schamess, 2002).

Terminating from the Group

Optimally, members leave the group when they have accomplished their goals. There may be many obstacles to the member's doing so. While some obstacles are external (such as a member being discharged from the hospital), others are internal. The member may be frightened by the group's entrance into some new area of exploration. The member may leave early to express anger toward other members, the therapist, or the group as a whole. The member may precipitously depart as a self-protective response in relation to some hurt.

Whatever factor propels the member to leave the group, the member can be helped to avoid basing a long-term decision on a momentary reaction by taking sufficient time to make the decision. Members can be assisted in making a considered rather than impulsive decision by agreeing as part of the contract their willingness to remain in the group for a prescribed period of time after announcing an intent to depart. The interval should be long enough to permit sufficient processing of a group dynamic but not be so long as to risk the member's compliance with this contractual feature. For many groups, several weeks' notice may be an interval that balances these considerations.

Having established this stipulation about termination, the therapist can do very little to enforce it. Nonetheless, this stipulation helps create a group climate conducive to members' assuming the same reflective attitude toward the issue of termination that they have for all other group phenomena. Moreover, it encourages members to work collaboratively rather than alone in reaching their decision about termination.

In presenting this termination requirement, the therapist should clearly convey that the interval represents the minimum of time the member should remain in the group after announcing the wish to leave. Especially for members who have been in the group on a long-term basis, a much more extended termination period is desirable. The termination process itself represents a tremendous therapeutic opportunity. The specter of the loss of the group invites the emergence of new conflicts and issues. There also is the possibility of consolidating earlier learning and understanding. For these reasons, the termination should not be short-changed.

Payment for the Group

In some types of groups, payment may not be an area of concern for group members. For example, in an inpatient setting the group may be part of the per diem charge covered by the patient's insurance policy. In groups of children and many adolescents, the group members may have no direct cognizance of the payment plan because payment is handled by the parents. When the group member is financially responsible for the group experience, the therapist must consider two topics in formulating the group contract. The first is how payment is rendered. The second concerns the handling of problems related to payment during the course of the work.

The Structure of Payment

To establish a fee, the therapist must know for what the member is paying. The two major alternatives are that the member pays either for individual sessions or for his or her seat in the group. The former alternative is more consistent with the payment plan typically used in a medical model system in which the patient goes to the practitioner for a particular professional service and pays when the service is delivered. The second format is more compatible with an educational framework in which the individual reserves a place in some instructional situation such as a course or workshop. Within the duration of a course the student who misses individual classes is obligated to pay the same tuition as if he or she was present for all classes. In group therapy the seat-based policy recognizes not only the fact that the member has made a commitment to be consistently present but also that when the member is physically absent, he or she continues to have a psychological presence in the group. During such sessions members who are present will continue to do work that will benefit the absent member.

In the session-based payment system, typically the member would pay either at the end of each session or at the end of some period of time such as a month. If a member misses, he or she would not be required to pay for the session. However, some stipulations may be placed upon freedom from payment. For example, the therapist might require that the absence be the result of a planned vacation, a work obligation, or an illness that is sufficiently severe to prevent the member from engaging in other activities. In the seat-based system, the member pays regardless of the reasons for missing the session. Within this system the member may be billed prior to some unit of time such as a month and payment rendered before all sessions have taken place.

The seat-based payment system, which may be relatively unfamiliar to therapists who are accustomed to working in other modalities such as individual therapy, has a variety of advantages. This system discourages absences and thereby protects the stability and continuity of the group. In most cases it is more expensive to the member to be absent because insurance companies do not provide reimbursement for missed sessions (a fact of which members should be apprised before group participation). This system also encourages group work in that it makes an otherwise convenient acting-out route decidedly less attractive. In groups in which the therapist permits some absences and not others, considerable group time can be devoted to deliberations on each absence. While an argument could be made legitimately that such deliberations are valuable, after a certain point they can bog the group down and detract from the group's here-and-now explorations.

A final advantage is that a seat-based policy protects the group therapist's income. Particularly for professionals who derive a large portion of their income from group work, this protection can have a significant role of reducing the therapist's level of stress. Without such protection the therapist may have a level of worry that can distract him or her from full attendance to group phenomena.

The alternate system, the session-based method, has the advantage of compatibility with the prevailing medical model of insurance reimbursement. Most insurance companies or managed care plans will not find a monthly fee reconcilable with their service-based reimbursement plan. Some managed care plans very specifically stipulate that the therapist cannot charge the full fee for a missed session. A second advantage of the session-based system is that it affords the therapist more flexibility. Suppose, for instance, a member had a serious illness requiring her to be away from the group for four weeks. Suppose further that the therapist knew that the member had significant financial difficulties. It may be the therapist's wish to provide the member some relief from stress by removing the obligation to pay for the missed session. This accommodation can be made more straightforwardly in the session-based than seat-based method.

Regardless of which payment method the therapist uses, it is crucial that prior to the beginning of the member's participation the therapist communicate which method is in operation. Particularly important is anticipating how absenteeism will be handled. Some (e.g., Tuttman, 1992) have argued that such specificity at the outset is encumbering and therefore such matters should be dealt with only when the situation arises (for example, when the first absence occurs). I would argue that such policies must be described up front because imposition of unanticipated fees can undermine the member's trust in the therapist. Moreover, it is more likely that the therapist will offer a detailed rationale for such a practice during the preparation phase by providing an explanation of the coherence of goals, processes, rules, and other policies.

A second issue regarding payment is whether fees will be the same for all members or variable, that is, on a sliding scale. There are advantages to each policy. The sliding scale allows the therapist to accommodate persons from a diverse socioeconomic range. This accommodation has a humane dimension in that it makes group therapy available to persons with relatively limited financial resources. Such flexibility allows the therapist to use other factors that may be more important in the selection process. Also, a sliding scale may enhance the stability of the group. In some instances members may commit to the group without being able to sustain their commitment economically. Others may experience a drastic change in their financial situation and be forced to leave the group. With a sliding scale, the therapist can set the most appropriate fee at the outset and make an adjustment if necessary.

With the standard fee policy, the therapist has the advantage of simplicity. The group therapist does not have the challenging task of determining where on the sliding scale each member's appropriate fee lies. Moreover, the therapist need not stay attuned to the specifics of each member's financial condition to know if a given fee remains appropriate. For example, if a member low on the sliding scale announces an anticipated absence due to a Hawaiian vacation, the therapist is freed up to contemplate aspects other than the possibility that the member may be paying an inappropriately low fee. A second advantage is that the standard fee safeguards the therapist's income. With the sliding scale, the therapist's group-related income can be quite variable as composition changes (unless the therapist limits the number of members at the low end of the scale).

One advantage that is sometimes cited for the standard method is that it avoids members' becoming resentful when they feel other members pay less. I have never found this factor to be a compelling one. Members can be resentful either because the fees are different or because they pay the same despite different resources among members. When the issue emerges prominently (whether directly or not), it most likely does so because it is related to an area of dynamic concern and as such is worthy of exploration. Likewise worthy of exploration is any member's belief that because he or she is paying a reduced fee, the therapist holds him or her in lower esteem than members paying a fee higher on the scale.

Handling of Payment During Sessions

Once the member begins the group, financial issues will inevitably arise. For example, in one long-term group, the following situation developed:

> *Sadie opened the session indicating that she was giving her four-week notice. Her husband had lost his job and there was no way she could afford the fee for weekly therapy. Sadie was aware that the therapist had a sliding scale. Yet she seemed unable to consider the possibility that the therapist could make an adjustment for her. When other members suggested that Sadie might ask for a new fee, she responded with horror mixed with mortification. The therapist noted to herself that Sadie's stance toward this financial issue was similar to her seeming incapacity to ask group members for time and attention when she was in a state of distress. At such moments Sadie declared that she preferred managing her problems on her own.*

As is true in Sadie's case, a member's behavior in relation to money is meaningfully tied to other group behaviors. Given that money-related behaviors are as worthy of exploration as any other manifestations, the therapist must be ready to bring the topic of money into the group. Yet within our culture, the taboo against talking about monetary issues is great (Gans, 1992; Rutan & Stone, 2001). Motherwell (2002) agrues that women are especially subject to this taboo because women are socialized to believe that money is a concern of men. Money is inextricably tied to a person's social and self-worth and can therefore stimulate feelings of shame and embarrassment. The cultural antidote to these feelings is the avoidance of the topic of money altogether. In the group, both members and therapist are likely to operate under the sway of a prohibition against delving into this realm. Once again, the female therapist who operates under "the expectation that women nurture for free" (Motherwell, 2002, p. 52) may feel particularly tempted to remain silent when financial issues arise. Unless the therapist combats the prohibition actively, great opportunities for learning will be lost.

How can the therapist work against this cultural prescription? The therapist should address his or her own reluctance to talk about monetary issues in supervision. For new group therapists, role-playing a conversation about money may be useful in overcoming a sense that raising financial issues is an inappropriately intrusive act.

From the standpoint of the member, this prohibition can be attacked in several ways. First, the therapist should establish in the preparation for the group that concerns related to money such as unpaid bills will be discussed in the group. It is helpful to members if the therapist presents a rationale for doing so, that is, the fact that behavior related to money may have significance. Second, the therapist should distribute bills and receive payment within the meeting rather than through the mail. As Gans notes, "Leaders who only mail out bills may be sending an unconscious and subtle message that bills are not for group discussion" (1992, p. 137). Third, whenever there are financial problems with members or a change in fees, these issues should be discussed directly in the group.

Summary

In this chapter, we continued to refine the group design by considering features that forward the group goals. The first set of factors discussed are structural. One is the *size* of the group, or number of members. Two questions the therapist might pose to help himself or herself address this issue are: What member resources are necessary in order for the group to do its work? What demand does each member place upon the resources of the group?

An array of *temporal features* that define the group was considered. In setting the length of the sessions, the therapist gives attention to characteristics of the members such as level of ego functioning and age. The frequency of sessions was discussed as a variable related to cohesion: The more frequently a group meets, the greater the cohesion level it is likely to achieve. The temporal feature of length of group participation was discussed in some detail. Useful information to consider in setting this feature includes the target area in which change is sought; the breadth of change; the cognitive, emotional, and motivational resources members bring to the group; and the resources within the setting for bolstering members' work.

The *spatial features* of the group design are the location of the group room and its physical characteristics. The latter includes such elements as the furniture, seating arrangement, level of illumination, and the presence of a waiting room. For most types of groups, the therapist's goal in establishing the physical conditions should be to create a firm boundary between the group and the outside world and a relatively permeable boundary between members.

The second set of supporting features discussed were the rules of the group. The rules for any group should regulate those behaviors most critical to members' rights, well-being, and progress. While rules may vary from group to group, groups typically have rules concerning attendance and promptness, confidentiality (which will be discussed further in Chapter 9), socialization outside of group, oral activities in the group, and the termination period.

The third set of features include the therapist's policies concerning payment. Two issues that therapists should establish prior to a member's entrance into the group are whether the member is paying for a seat or a session and whether the fee is standard or variable (i.e., on a sliding scale). The therapist should also specify in the contract that members' behaviors in relation to fees will, at times, be part of the group's focus and exploration.

Composition, Selection, and Preparation

The next several chapters of this book discuss more specifically the mechanics of the group. The progression of activities from the time the therapist organizes a group until the members depart from the group, either individually (as in an open-ended group) or together (as in a close-ended group) are described. This chapter focuses on activities of the therapist prior to the first session entailing the selection of members, their preparation for the group experience, and the preparation of the group for the introduction of a new member. However, because the therapist's selection of individual members should be predicated upon a conception of the overall composition of the group, this topic is our initial focus.

Composition of the Group

All of us have attended social events that were delightful and others that were dreadful. Undoubtedly, many factors have given these events one character or another. However, prominent among them was the mix of people. Most likely, at those events that were especially pleasant, the melding of personalities was just right. Those attending could talk easily with one another and find entertaining common activities. Conversely, when good chemistry is lacking, interactions are laborious and ungratifying.

In getting a group off the ground, the therapist has a great investment in including individuals whose personal attributes are likely to click. To accomplish this aim, the therapist must have a picture of what an optimal combination of individuals would be. In assessing an individual candidate, the therapist consults this picture. However, the prudent therapist constrains his or her thinking by reality. The size of the pool from which the therapist can recruit group members will determine how selective the therapist can be. As Yalom (1995) points out, group therapists are often in a position of merely excluding persons who are clearly inappropriate and including everyone else. But where there is a large cohort (e.g., in a large inpatient facility with a number of different types of groups in operation at any time), the therapist can develop a more articulated view of what a good combination of members might be.

The number of variables that could be considered in determining the optimal combination of individuals is as vast as the variation in the human condition itself. How similar or different should members be in age, level of intellectual functioning, symptom patterns, level of psychological awareness, level of ego functioning, motivation for treatment, cultural background, socioeconomic status, and so on? Should members be of the same gender or not? Should members have the same sexual preference or not? As the number of variables considered increases, the pool of candidates for the group shrinks. To ensure the birth of the group with enough members to allow for a rich set of interactions, the therapist must discern which variables are most crucially related to the success of the group. In making this determination, the therapist should consult the clinical literature on his or her population, including any research on composition, his or her own clinical experience with the population, and the distribution of characteristics in the population available. Each of these areas will be addressed in the context of an extended example.

Suppose a clinician working in a residential treatment center is interested in launching a psycho-educational group for persons with eating disorders. The goals of the group are to increase self-esteem and to support normal eating behaviors. The therapist must investigate what subject variables are most relevant to this population in this setting. As with most populations, the research provides some but not a great deal of direction, primarily because compositional variables are difficult to subject to systematic investigation. Establishing groups differing in their degree of heterogeneity on particular variables while being relatively comparable on other major variables requires a larger subject pool than is normally available. Hence, decisions about composition must be made on other bases.

For example, limiting the group to individuals with eating disorders would be a major decision. An alternate decision would be to run a group with persons of heterogeneous symptomatology, only some of whom have an eating disorder. Although the decision the therapist makes is not rooted in actual studies, it is consistent with a well-established clinical view about individuals with eating disorders. The view advanced by many clinicians working with this population is that eating-disordered individuals are so different from others in their symptoms and approaches to psychological work that they are likely to have difficulty relating to others in a symptomatically heterogeneous group. Because of their relational problems, they are likely to offer themselves as prime candidates for scapegoating (see K. Moreno's excellent review of the research on an eating-disordered population, 1994).

Another major decision is whether to include patients with different types of eating disorders. That is, is some symptom heterogeneity beneficial to the group's work? Opinions differ on this score (Moreno, 1994). Some view a group that is symptomatically homogeneous—for example, either all anorexics or all bulimics—as promoting the development of group cohesion, a precious group commodity associated with positive outcomes (see Chapter 4). Others feel that persons with different symptom patterns add to the resources of the group, with the anorexic providing containment and the bulimic, stimulation. This trade-off is a classic one. In general, homogeneity of symptoms or problem areas provides relatively quick bonding of members. It also increases the group's efficiency in working toward its goals when the symptoms or problem areas are the specific focus. On the other hand, symptom or problem heterogeneity provides a relatively greater range of resources for the group's work. While bonding may take longer, members may also achieve greater depth in their interactions.

The research offers the therapist some assistance in resolving this particular dilemma. Studies to date support a heterogeneous composition in that homogeneous anorexic and bulimic groups had higher attrition rates than mixed groups. The clinician may also have some direct observations of how anorexic and bulimics interact. Moreover, practical factors may compel the clinician in one direction or another. For instance, there may not be a critical mass of one subtype to form a group. Alternately, there may be so few in one category that the representatives in it are likely to feel like outliers.

The members' range of ego functioning is a critical variable that the therapist must always consider in the planning stage. As defined in Chapter 2, ego functions are those basic psychological activities an individual uses to adapt to the environment and realize his or her own goals. The observation of clinicians and the results of research agree that persons of different levels of ego functioning have different needs in therapy. Persons operating at a low level of ego functioning (at the psychotic or low borderline level as defined by McWilliams, 1994) require support, warmth, and in many cases individual attention in order to benefit from their group experiences (Leopold, 1977). The high level of anxiety these members bring to group involvement requires a high level of structure that has a containing role, enhancing members' sense of safety. Conversely, individuals operating at a higher level have a capacity to tolerate anxiety and to engage in exploratory work. Many studies have supported such long-held clinical views about these different types of patients. For example, in one study lower-functioning members were more likely than higher-functioning members to rate as helpful supportive therapeutic factors such as receiving advice and instillation of hope (Leszcz et al., 1985).

The upshot of the varied needs that members at different levels of ego functioning have is that when these different levels are represented in the group, the therapist is unable to pitch the group so that it is productive for all. In this psycho-educational group, members' exploration of their body images could play a role in enhancing their levels of self-esteem. However, with members who are relatively low in ego functioning, such lines of investigation could promote disorganization.

In sum, while generalizations about composition are difficult to make, a guideline can be offered for the level-of-functioning dimension. The members of the group should not be greatly heterogeneous in their functioning. In this way the therapist can tailor the group experience to meet the needs of participants and avoid the harm that can occur when members are placed in a group that is too stressful or stimulating to be useful.

Another dimension the therapist must consider is age. Should members of the group be within a narrow or broad age range? Age is almost always an important variable to consider because it covaries with an array of important psychological processes. For example, cognitive capacities vary as a function of age. Twelve-year-olds are generally capable of assuming an abstract attitude that is only in the future of a six-year-old. Also, the developmental tasks that confront persons differ at different ages. The person in her early 30s launching a career faces a set of problems and issues that is distinct from that of a woman experiencing new widowhood after 50-plus years of marriage.

With an eating-disordered population, age can be a major factor. Although eating-disorder diagnoses are most common within a fairly narrow age band, a group composed of persons in their late teens will nonetheless have a different set of themes and issues than groups consisting of individuals in their 20s. The therapist must consider whether combining persons from these different age groups would enrich the group or dilute the concerns that each subgroup might develop. This question is in essence the same one that emerged in relation to heterogeneity and homogeneity of symptoms.

A final feature that is considered is gender. Currently there are all-male, all-female, and mixed-gender groups, although the latter greatly predominate. Same-sex groups have been seen to hold many benefits, including a more relaxed environment where members can be more open, a greater opportunity for identification, and a lessened degree of sexually stereotyped behavior. Mixed-gender groups are seen as providing a more real-world environment for members.

The research has provided partial support for these views. Relative to women in mixed groups, women in all-female groups have been observed to engage in a greater range of social behaviors (Aries, 1976; Carloch & Martin, 1977). However, men in all-male groups appear to have a greater tendency to exhibit sexually stereotypic behaviors than when women are present (Aries, 1976). Supporting the real-world benefit of the mixed-sex group was the finding that men are able to be engaged by a much greater range of themes than in all-male groups (Aries, 1976).

The literature on eating-disorder groups contains some observational reports on the usefulness of having males and females in group therapy together. However, so many more women than men have eating disorders that it is not unusual for very few men to be available. What if there is only a single male candidate? This circumstance is one that most group therapists face in regard to some demographic variable—gender, race, age, and so on. The dilemma is a major one. On the one hand, the candidate should not be denied potentially helpful treatment. On the other hand, the therapist would not want to set the candidate up for an adverse group experience.

Systems-centered therapy's distinction between functional and stereotypic subgrouping is useful in understanding why the inclusion of a member who exclusively represents a demographic category poses a challenge to the group (Agazarian, 1997). Functional subgrouping is a technique explicitly employed by the therapist to forward the developmental goals of the group. By first exploring similarities but eventually differences within the safety of their subgroups, members can come to accept diverse parts of themselves. This step is accompanied by a greater capacity on the part of members to identify with the positions of members in the warded-off subgroup. Once members achieve greater comfort with the psychological forces on both sides of a conflict, they can move onto their integration, the accomplishment of conflict resolution. On a group level, members' identification with the positions of not only members of their subgroup but also those of the alternate subgroup, enables the conflict at hand to be resolved, a prerequisite to the group's moving into the next developmental stage.

Stereotypic subgrouping is not a therapeutic technique but rather a group structure that emerges naturally to enable the group to defend against a threat (Agazarian, 1997). Members subgroup on the basis of a shared stereotype of other members. For example, a single male member of an eating-disorders group might be seen almost exclusively in terms of other members' preconceptions about how men are and are not in terms of their session-by-session experience with this individual man.

While stereotypic subgrouping is not unusual, it always carries the danger of achieving a hold on the group. Because this mode is inherently nonexploratory, it undermines the group's development. For the members being stereotyped, it annihilates their unique identities. Yet, if multiple members are being stereotyped, the annihilation is somewhat easier to bear. The members within the subgroup can dispute the stereotype by recognizing the variation among themselves (unless they, too, are swayed by the stereotype). The discovery of differences within the stereotyped subgroup may ultimately help dissolve the subgrouping structure.

When the subgroup consists of a single member, that member cannot share the burden of being stereotyped. Nor is the member able to explore differences among members of his or her subgroup in a way that would affirm the member's identity and challenge the stereotype itself. Hence, the subgroup of one is in a most vulnerable position to remaining a subgroup. If the subgrouping structure succeeds over time in relieving the group as a whole of some real or fantasized discomfort, the stereotyped person's position becomes a relatively fixed group role, or role-lock, in the language of systems-centered therapy (Agazarian, 1997). Members become so dependent on the stereotyped member to relieve their discomfort that they discourage behaviors at odds with the role.

Does this mean the therapist should steadfastly avoid having a member who is singular in some conspicuous way? Many seasoned group therapists can provide examples of members, unique to a category, who have flourished in their groups. Possibly these therapists, in deciding to include this member, took into account, implicitly or explicitly, a variety of contextual factors concerning the group. What is this particular member's likely response to being the different one or being the target of others' projections? Occasionally, I would conduct an inpatient group in which there would be a single male. Some male members would appear to enjoy being in this special position and would either slough off any stereotyping or find solace in the stereotype. Other males would be disturbed by being the sole representative of their gender. The therapist must give particular attention to the prospective member's level of ego functioning. As discussed in Chapter 2, persons organized at the psychotic level are especially at risk for feeling as if their very fragile sense of self is disintegrating in the face of others' projections.

The length of the group is also a relevant factor. A long-term group has time to work through a stereotyping subgroup structure. However, in a short-term group a particularly tenacious stereotype may last throughout the life of the group. Another related factor is the maturity of the group. This consideration is relevant when the group has been meeting for some time. As a group matures, members acquire the capacity to recognize their own defensive maneuvers as they emerge on the group, subgroup, and individual levels. A mature group that employs stereotypic subgrouping will be likely to recognize much more readily—with or without the assistance of a therapist—the operation of a defensive element. The shift in the nature of the interaction between the group and the stereotyped members from stylized to authentic is likely to affect that member greatly. He or she learns the valuable truth that with work, neither inaccurate perceptions, undesired roles, nor the pain attached to each need be lasting.

The variables that have been examined in relation to composition—symptomatology, level of ego functioning, age, and gender—are only some of the variables that might be evaluated. These particular variables tend to be relatively important ones, but they also illustrate the process by which the therapist goes about making compositional decisions. As the reader can see, the consideration of subject variables should be specific to the target population. For example, heterogeneity of symptoms may play out in a different way among persons with eating disorders than in a population of individuals with affective disorders. The therapist's intimate knowledge of the target population, including an awareness of the relevant research literature, is extremely helpful in developing a viable compositional picture to be used in member selection. Yet, once a group is under way, the therapist should garner information about the consequences of different compositional decisions (see Piper et al., 1992, Chapter 4, for an excellent example of such an analysis). Based upon this information, the therapist can revise the selection criteria to achieve a more satisfactory combination of members.

Selection of Individual Members

Selection of members for a group requires that the clinician possess both clear criteria for determining who is suitable and methods to determine whether a candidate meets the criteria.

Selection Criteria

In selecting members for a group, the therapist should consider a candidate's goals, resources to meet those goals, and capacity and willingness to behave in consistency with the treatment contract. To evaluate these different realms, the therapist should consult the group design, which specifies group goals, therapeutic processes, and group behaviors necessary to realize goals.

Are the treatment goals for the group meaningful for this individual? If, for example, the individual's interest in pursuing group therapy is to obtain immediate relief from anxiety and the goal of the group is to foster interpersonal change, then the group goals and the person's needs may be incompatible. The interview process is exploratory, and many individuals arrive at a different conception of their treatment needs than they had when the interviewing process began. The person could realize that he or she was vulnerable to periods of intense anxiety caused by interpersonal strife. If so, both the interviewer and candidate may come to recognize that the interpersonal focus of the group is indeed useful.

Information about the prospective members' fantasies about the possible benefits of group membership may emerge slowly over the course of an interview or series of interviews. The candidate's initially stated goal may not be his or her real goal. I once interviewed a man whose initial problem formulation seemed very compatible with the interpersonal focus of my group. He spoke of overcoming his loneliness and sense of isolation through freedom from his paralyzing self-consciousness in most social situations. However, as he spoke, it became clear that he expected the group itself to provide the social connections needed to remedy his social needs outside the group. Once he learned that one group rule was refraining from socializing outside of the sessions, his interest in the group diminished markedly. Even though he was given a rationale for this component of the treatment contract, his disappointment that entry to the group would not provide an immediate social network could not be assuaged. Both he and I together determined that this group would not meet his personal goals for involvement.

The group design specifies the therapeutic processes that will be deployed in the group, and these processes have implications for the resources the person must bring to the group. For example, in an interpersonally oriented group, the therapeutic mechanism of universality requires the capacity of each member to see him or herself in others. While the ability to identify can deepen over the course of group participation, the member needs some modicum of this ability to successfully begin in an interpersonal group. In an interpersonal problem-solving group, members learn to generate and evaluate different solutions to social problems. This type of group requires some ability to think synthetically and retain information (Coche, Cooper, & Petermann, 1984). The task of the therapist is to analyze the processes within his or her approach to determine what resources members have to have for therapeutic processes to be deployed. The therapist must also ascertain what resources can be cultivated through group participation.

The therapist should consider each element of the contract to determine the individual's likely ability to meet it. Particular focus should be given to the rules of the group. A most basic rule, typically, is regular attendance. Because the presence of members is so key to the group's effectiveness, absences are expected to be rare events. A member who clearly has a low level of motivation to participate in the group will generally have difficulty disciplining himself or herself to make the sacrifices necessary for regular attendance. Some prospective members may have a relatively high level of commitment but may have other obligations that interfere with consistent attendance, such as a job with unpredictable hours. The therapist must carefully probe the issue of each person's capacity and willingness to attend regularly. The importance of this factor may seem so evident that the therapist may assume incorrectly that if there were an obstacle to regular attendance, the candidate would volunteer this information. However, the candidate at this juncture is merely learning about group therapy. He or she does not yet have an experiential base to appreciate fully the value of all of the features of the treatment contract.

In the same way that the clinician considers attendance, he or she should consider every other group rule to determine whether the prospective member provides evidence of having the capacity to observe it.

Other Factors in Selection: We have considered how the selection criteria must be derived from the group design. Because group designs vary, selection criteria must vary. Yet, are there any selection criteria that run across different types of groups? Are there any characteristics that would make a person unsuitable for any type of group? Today, so many varieties of groups are available that there is a group for almost anyone. However, a few general guidelines can be offered that might disqualify a person from group therapy.

If the person does not want to be in a group, group therapy is probably contraindicated. Because treatment requires informed consent, this issue is generally moot. However, there may be a case in which consent, while being desirable, is not ethically or legally necessary for treatment to proceed. (The issue of informed consent is pursued in the next chapter.) Suppose a parent wants a young adolescent to join a group, but the adolescent makes it very clear that she does not want to do so. Should the group therapist accept her into the group? When a group is heavily populated with those who do not want to be there, this special compositional feature must be taken into account in the group design. In general, however, a person who does not want to be in group treatment is unlikely to derive much good from it and may even interfere with others' benefiting from the group. Generally, people who are unwilling to be in a group expect that group participation will fail to benefit them. Indeed, research has shown that low expectations of the usefulness of group are associated with less constructive activity during the group (Caine & Wijesingle, 1976) and poorer outcomes (e.g., Block, Bond, Qualls, Yalom, & Zimmerman, 1976). Pearson and Girling (1990) found that poorer outcomes were associated with the belief that it was only the therapist who could provide help and the expectation that only symptoms would improve (as opposed to broader personality change). Prospective group members who do not want to change are unlikely to derive benefit from the group. For example, Mussell et al. (2000) found that two significant predictors of success in treating women for the symptoms of bulimia nervosa in a cognitive-behavioral therapy group were the desire to discontinue bulimic behaviors and the expected success from group participation.

This guideline should be applied only after a careful exploration of why the individual does not want to be in group therapy. For example, the person may have some very specific fears that can be productively addressed. However, if after a thorough discussion about the group the person is resolutely against it, his or her wishes not to participate should be respected. When group leaders were asked to explain selections errors they made in their groups, a very commonly cited one was the leader's failure to consider sufficiently the member's motivational level (Riva, Lippert, & Tackett, 2000).

If the individual is in such a state of crisis that he or she cannot tolerate sharing the attention of the group with other members, then the person should not be placed in a group until the crisis abates. The presence of a crisis alone in no way contraindicates group treatment. In fact, many groups are devoted specifically to crisis management (for example, see Dembert & Simmer, 2000, for a discussion of group treatment of members of the community following a disaster). Yet one way a person may respond to a crisis is to require the unbroken and extended focus of another person. This person may experience the withdrawal of attention that occurs as a group shifts its focus from one member's difficulties to another's as a total abandonment. If so, the person may do better in individual treatment.

If the individual is likely to engage in violent activity in the group, he or she should not be placed in group therapy. Members have a right to be safe in the group. When the placement of a candidate in the group compromises the therapist's ability to make this assurance, then alternate treatment should be sought, possibly in a group specifically designed to help individuals to find alternatives to violence in managing aggressive impulses. However, built into such group formats will be resources to ensure members' safety beyond what is found in the typical group.

Methods of Evaluation

The therapist has many ways to obtain information about a prospective group member to determine his or her appropriateness. The information that the therapist garners serves three purposes: (a) learning if the individual is an appropriate candidate for a particular group; (b) developing specific goals for the member; and (c) increasing understanding of the individual to enable the therapist to work more effectively with him or her in the group sessions.

Interviewing: Perhaps the most common means of selecting group members is through one or more interviews. A typical structure for such interviews is the following: The therapist begins with a description of the goals of the group followed by a conversation about the extent to which the goals are relevant to the individuals' needs and reasons for pursuing group therapy. If a reasonable compatibility exists between what the group can offer and what the individual is seeking, then the therapist can move into a presentation of the processes involving in pursuing the group's goals. For instance, the therapist might describe the feedback process as follows:

THERAPIST: We spoke last week about how you feel there is something that you do that offends or irritates other people. You said you believe that this is why you have had difficulty sustaining friendships. One way that you can address this problem in group is to obtain information about how people in the group see you. We call this information feedback. Often it is difficult to get this information on the outside.

INTERVIEWEE: But these people are strangers. They don't really know me.

THERAPIST: Over time they will know you better and better. But in the beginning you will have the opportunity to learn what first impressions people may form about you.

INTERVIEWEE: It kind of scares me . . . hearing about the things people like about me least.

THERAPIST: Most people have some apprehension about the prospect of learning about other people's reactions to them. But they are also pleasantly surprised to discover that much of the feedback they receive in the sessions is positive and that makes the negative far easier to take.

INTERVIEWEE: Well, that makes me feel a little better.

THERAPIST: Good, and it's also important to realize that all members are participating in the process of receiving feedback about themselves. So you will be giving feedback as well as getting it.

INTERVIEWEE: I can't imagine what I'd say to another member!

THERAPIST: As you're in the sessions, you'll get a better idea of it. But say you're in a session and you notice that a member, let's pretend her name is Ariel, always changes the topic when another member talks about something sad. When she does it to you, you realize that it makes you feel like withdrawing. It would be important for you to point out to Ariel the pattern in her behavior and your reaction to it—how her behavior affects you. Ariel might be greatly helped by this information; it may give her something she needs to improve her relationships within the group and outside.

INTERVIEWEE: But might not Ariel become upset if I were to give her this . . . feedback?

THERAPIST: Yes, she might. None of us are happy to hear about negative aspects of our behavior. But keep in mind that Ariel has made a commitment to this process in order to improve her relationships. To Ariel, it's worth the discomfort. Also, giving Ariel this information provides her with the opportunity to experiment with new ways of responding to others' feelings. Ariel can try to hang in there with others when they feel sad. As she makes progress, she's likely to get favorable feedback. We would also try to help Ariel, and perhaps others too, to understand why it can be difficult to sit with others' unhappiness. That understanding can be very helpful in making constructive changes in our ways of interacting with others.

The reader may be struck with the fine line between selection and preparation. The therapist is not only collecting data about the prospective members' reaction to how the group works but also is teaching the person to be a group member. Notice that the therapist has addressed some of the conceptions and misconceptions that the individual has about his or her likely group experience. For example, the therapist affirmed the prospective member's assumption that group interactions could arouse disturbing feelings. The therapist also acquainted the member with a number of the therapeutic processes, such as feedback and its use for the purpose of experimentation. Additionally, the therapist underscored the importance of understanding one's behavior and experience.

Why is it necessary to discuss the processes used by a group to move toward its goals? First, informed consent requires that the individual knows to what he or she is committing. A candidate who is unaware that, for example, a group has an in vivo aspect does not have enough information to make a decision. As stated earlier, group therapy, to be effective, almost always requires voluntary participation. Voluntary participation requires that the person knows clearly what the group entails. Second, the element of surprise could have its own iatrogenic negative effects. Third, the prospective member's responses can be very helpful in evaluating the person's suitability for the group. An individual who is utterly dismayed at the prospect of obtaining feedback may not be a good candidate for a processing group.

For all of these reasons, key elements of the group contract such as the group rules are described. Initially, this description can be cursory, but once the individual has been accepted for the group, an expanded discussion of the rules should take place.

As the interview proceeds, therapists typically attend to what the interviewee says and how the interviewee relates to the therapist. Therapists will make inferences about how the candidate is likely to relate in the group based on the individual's style of relating in the interview. However, the interview is a dyadic or two-person situation, whereas the group has multiple participants. Can one accurately predict from one to the other? According to Piper's (1994) review of the research, dyadic behavior in the interview is not a highly accurate predictor of the benefit the member is likely to derive from group, whether the member is likely to remain in the group, or how the member is likely to behave in the group.

Direct Observation of Group Behavior: An excellent predictor of future behavior is past behavior in the same or similar circumstance. One means by which the therapist can determine candidates' likely response to being in a group is to provide them with a kind of mini-group experience. The candidates can be observed to see whether they engage in behaviors that will enable them to benefit from the group experience.

This technique of direct observation of group behavior was one that I routinely used in selecting members for an inpatient group. The selection was somewhat atypical of inpatient groups in that referrals came from eight different psychiatric units rather than a single unit. I therefore had the luxury to truly consider composition in the selection of members. My procedure was to conduct a small group interview in which I spoke to the group members about the three elements mentioned earlier—goals, processes, and rules. Then, in a brief unstructured segment members were given the task of getting to know one another. Almost invariably the interviewees talked about what brought them into the hospital. However, I was able to observe such important dimensions of group behavior as degree of openness, activity, and connection with others.

This procedure proved to be helpful in various ways. First, it acclimated members to the group experience. Second, members came into the group having familiarity with several other members, putting them at ease (much like walking into a party and seeing several people you know). Because members came from a variety of units, this familiarity was not otherwise guaranteed. Third, I could anticipate the likely character of the group, helped me to respond with greater rapidity to emerging group phenomena—a rapidity that was important given the short-term nature of the group. My ability to quickly make sense of group happenings helped me to work more vigorously to move the group toward its goals. Fourth, the procedure would enable me to identify certain individuals who simply were not suitable candidates for the group, most often because of extreme anxiety about group participation.[1] Once the group formed, the stability of attendance was great during its eight sessions. I attributed this stability in large part to the selection procedure.

Research has supported the usefulness of the direct observation of prospective members' group behavior to forecast their behavior in group sessions and the benefit they are likely to derive from group participation. Piper (1994) reviewed four studies on the issue of direct observation of group behavior as a predictor of group performance. For example, in one study (Connelly & Piper, 1989) two dimensions of group member behavior were examined in pretraining sessions: degree of participation and on-task behavior. The investigators founds that members' pregroup behavior on these dimensions was highly correlated with their performance in these areas in the group sessions themselves. Moreover, the pretraining scores were associated with members' outcomes. For example, a significant relationship was found between leader-rated work (the person's total amount of on-task behavior over his or her total participation) and improvement on symptoms.

The studies reviewed by Piper provide support of group observation as a useful tool in member selection. What group observation does is to enable the use of interpersonal variables in member selection. Recent studies on member dropout also underscore the importance of interpersonal behavior. Oei and Kazmierczak (1997) found that demographic and symptom factors did not distinguish those who prematurely left versus those who completed a cognitive behavioral group. The only factors that did were the amount of participation (as rated by the therapists) and comfort in self-expression (as rated by members). In a cognitive-behavioral group for depression, the only factor discriminating dropouts from completers was capacity to place trust in others. Despite the potential helpfulness of pregroup observation of interpersonal behavior, most therapists use the interview as the primary if not sole means of selecting members, though one

---

[1] Often these patients would begin a one-on-one behavior modification for anxiety management. After completing the program, the patient would enter, often quite successfully, one of the hospital's groups. Of course, in many hospital settings today, there is not sufficient time to take this stepwise approach.

survey suggests that it is the least used method (Riva et al., 2000). There may be several reasons for this bias. Setting up a pregroup experience may be logistically difficult. In an open-ended group in which members are added after a group has begun, not enough candidates may be available at one time. A therapist may also not want candidates to identify one another as prospective group members. While the therapist could require participants to commit to maintaining confidentiality, the strength of the commitment may be affected by whether or not the member actually enters the group. This problem is less of an issue in an inpatient setting in which individuals are likely to encounter one another elsewhere. Finally, therapists may not know what interpersonal behaviors should be considered in selection decisions. As the research based on relevant interpersonal behaviors increases, pregroup observation is likely to become a more popular solution.

Personality Assessment Tools: Group therapy typically involves a focus on a person's interactional style, which is a core aspect of personality. A range of tools provide information about personality. These tools, especially when used in concert with one another in a battery, provide a plethora of information about personality processing, including interpersonal functioning. To what extent is the individual open to others' feedback in developing a conception of self? What is the person's proclivity to be emotionally expressive in interactions with others? Are the emotional expressions highly controlled or relatively unbridled? Does the person experience an ease in the longing to affiliate with others, or does the person experience discomfort with such a longing? All of these are questions that can be answered through personality assessment.

There are major differences between the kinds of information that can be obtained through interviewing versus personality assessment. In an interview the content of responses is more likely to be affected by the person's attempt to present in a certain light, for example, appearing virtuous to the interviewer. In assessment, the inference making is more inscrutable. It is less obvious how the assessor moves from the data to a hypothesis about personality. For those instruments that might be more affected by self-presentation, indicators built into the tools often reflect such an effort. A second factor is that psychological tests are normed, so it is possible to compare an individual's response to the responses of a population of individuals. Through a comparison one can ascertain with some precision the major organizing features of the individual's personality, for example, passivity.

Because psychological batteries are extremely expensive and have to be performed by trained professionals, their use in every case would be prohibited. However, they can be particularly useful when some major issue related to personality bears upon the selection decision. For example, when after one or more interviews I still question whether a candidate's level of ego functioning is appropriate for a particular group, I refer him or her for an assessment. From the assessment I can learn about the individual's reality testing, associative processes, capacity to modulate feelings, ability to reflect upon experience, and a variety of other processes. Moreover, if the individual is selected for the group, I will have much additional material from which to formulate goals and anticipate the likely course of treatment. For some individuals who are referred for group therapy, a personality assessment may already have been conducted. It is worth the therapist's time to procure the report and to read it carefully, gleaning information related to appropriateness, goals, and course of treatment.

In Piper's (1994) review of studies conducted on different selection procedures, he found some evidence of the usefulness of psychological testing. For example, in one study group members' scores on a questionnaire reflecting quality of interpersonal relations were associated with how much the members derived from participation in a short-term group. However, some research finds the connection between psychological test scores and outcomes insignificant (e.g., Steinmetz, Lewinsohn, & Antonuccio, 1983). Unfortunately, the best standardized psychological tests have not been adequately investigated for their usefulness in the selection and planning process. Nonetheless, Piper (1994) concluded that on the whole psychological test findings tend to be more useful than what can be derived from interviews with patients and less helpful than the direct observation of candidates' group behaviors. A recent survey indicated that 27 percent of group leaders use assessment measures focused on individual personality characteristics and 19 percent used measures tapping interpersonal/group behaviors (Riva et al., 2000).

Preparation

When the therapist selects the member, the work is not done. The therapist would want to provide support and information to enable the member to successfully enter the group. Yet it is not only the individual member who must be prepared. If a group has been meeting for a substantial period of time and a new member is introduced, it is an extremely significant event in that group's life. To assist the group in incorporating the new member, the therapist prepares the new member well in advance. The preparation of both the new member and the group will be explored in this section.

Preparing the Member

Preparation for the group experience occurs from the moment an initial conversation occurs between therapist and candidate about the possibility of the latter's joining the group. In all of the exchanges between the two, the candidate obtains information that will be helpful during his or her tenure in the group. Nonetheless, preparation takes on greater intensity once the candidate accepts the therapist's invitation to join the group. Table 8.1 summarizes the elements of preparation for the group.

Table 8.1   **Elements of Preparation**

Basic information about the group:

    Location, time, and length of session

    Size of the group and gender balance

    Tenure of the group

Reinforcing the therapist's contract

Anticipation of other members' reactions

Teaching skills and activating therapeutic processes

Evaluation

Elements of Preparation

Preparation should include a description of the basic features of the group and information to help the entering member to form accurate expectations of his or her early group experiences.

Basic Information about the Group: During the evaluation period, the therapist has shared with the candidate some of the particulars about the group. Some of these (for example, when and where the group meets) might have been shared during an initial telephone conversation to determine whether joining the group was a realistic possibility for the candidate. At this time the therapist provides additional information so that the entering member will have a picture of the group. Knowing how many members are in the group, the gender balance, and the approximate age span can soothe the person's anxieties about entering the group.

The new member might also be told of the length of time the group has been in existence (Agazarian & Peters, 1981). This is a valuable piece of information in that it creates an awareness of the context of members' relationships. For example, in a group that has been meeting for 10 years, new members may realize that some old members may have a backlog of experience with one another. The new member therefore may enter with a respect for the expertise members have about one another.

Reinforcing the Therapeutic Contract: The previous chapter discussed the importance of group rules. At this time, it is essential that the therapist review and explain the rules of the group. Because certain rules are critical to the safety and privacy of the members, the therapist has an ethical obligation to ensure that each group member understands fully the nature of the rules and the consequences for their violation before entering the group.

Anticipating Other Members' Reactions: In the next section, we will talk about ways in which members will respond to the arrival of a new member. As we will see, it is an event that is both major and complicated. Members may not respond in ways that are optimal for the early integration of the new member. In fact, sometimes the group will respond in a way that is utterly at odds with what would put that new member at ease. The new member entering a long-term group might therefore benefit from help in seeing that his or her act of joining the group is an event of great significance for both the group and the new member. A comment such as the following could be helpful:

> *A new member entering the group is in many ways like a baby entering a family. It will be a big adjustment for you getting use to the group, but it will also be adjustment for the members in not only getting used to you but getting used to another person being present.*

A statement such as this serves two purposes. First, it encourages the member to make allowances for others. If others' behaviors are upsetting or provocative, that new member may have greater willingness to "ride out" a difficult period. Second, it sets the stage for the therapist's recommending that the new member give the group a chance by remaining a specified interval before deciding that the group is not right for him or her. Such an interval would enable the new member to experience the group beyond the shakedown period.

The new member might also be helped to anticipate that in the course of his or her participation, there are likely to be periods of various sorts. Some periods, the member might be told, will seem productive and pleasurable, while others may be confusing, irritating, or disturbing in some other way. The fact that this variation is a normal part of group participation should be explained to new members to bolster their forbearance of the difficult times. It might be pointed out that by learning how to derive benefit from stormy or confusing periods, the member will acquire a skill that can be extended to similar periods in life outside the group (see Brabender, 2000, for a discussion of chaos therapy as it relates to coping with stormy periods inside and outside the group).

Activating the Therapeutic Processes: One way to prepare new members for the group experience is by providing them with intensive training in some of the processes that the members will use. The major skills needed for successful group participation must be identified. Then, particular experiences are designed to cultivate these skills. For example, for many types of groups the capacity to give feedback is highly useful. A therapist may decide that the members' group work could be catapulted by skill development in the area of feedback. Prior to entering the group, members might be shown a videotape of a group session. The therapist and the new member could view the tape together. The therapist could point out examples of members' giving feedback to one another. The therapist could advance certain principles such as the importance of giving constructive (negative) feedback *after* positive feedback and of delivering feedback that is behaviorally oriented. The member might identify elements of feedback he or she would have given.

This exercise, at least in design, would not only cultivate feedback skills but also underscore the value of feedback so that this process would be focal. Finally, it may even develop the member's capacity to tolerate constructive feedback by conveying the notion that this type of feedback is part and parcel of the group's process.

So much learning is possible during this type of preparation that it can be legitimately regarded as therapeutic in its own right (Bednar & Kaul, 1993). It is quite possible for individuals to achieve new types of awareness that may be of benefit in their own right. For example, the training exercises described above may help a person recognize the usefulness of feedback in correcting one's behavior, a recognition that could be used independently of group therapy.

Evaluation: Third-party payers, regulatory agencies, and other organizations increasingly call on therapists, including group therapists, to show that their interventions are effective (Dies & Dies, 1993). However, even without these agencies, group therapists have an ethical stake in ensuring that members' well-being is enhanced by participation in groups. How does the therapist know if the group member is improving? An excellent source is group behavior itself. For example, suppose a member, Luba, enters the group to deal with social anxiety. Initially, the member says nary a spontaneous word, speaking only when others initiate interaction. However, after a year of group participation, Luba interacts freely with others, often introducing issues, making queries, soliciting others' observations, and so on. Because Luba consistently shows this new mode of interaction, the therapist can conclude that Luba has improved.

Yet, this therapist's observations about Luba could bear supplementation. Could, for instance, Luba have acquired a comfort in the group that she has not yet achieved outside of the group? While her altered behavior inside the group would nonetheless signify that progress had been made, her unchanged behavior with others might suggest that there is work to be done still.

Therefore, it is helpful to evaluate a group member's movement toward his or her goals using a variety of methods. One method is to introduce questionnaires at various points in the members' participation in the group. Although these questionnaires could be completed by the members themselves, they might also be given to persons in an individual's life. For example, suppose Luba's friends or family indicated that Luba was more active and expressive with them than she had been. Then, even with the discomfort Luba described, the progress she was making in group therapy was evidently transferring beyond the group boundary. With a multimethod approach, the therapist can develop a nuanced portrait of the member's progress.

While individual therapists can always develop their own instruments, a number of published questionnaires, inventories, and other tools that may be useful are available. The American Group Psychotherapy Association has published a CORE Battery (MacKenzie & Dies, 1981), which contains a set of instruments developed specifically for this modality. For example, using the Target Goals/Member form, members are required to state their goals in behavioral terms and rate their level of discomfort and their expectation of success in relation to each behavior. I used this instrument for many years in an inpatient setting and observed that the group members found it easy to complete.

The preparation period is an ideal time to garner the first set of data to be used in evaluation. The process of completing the instruments fosters a reflectiveness about goals and problems that is very compatible with the conversation between therapist and member about goals. By then administering the same instruments at various intervals, the therapist has an opportunity to see what types and degrees of changes occur within different time frames. Certainly, the instruments should be administered at the time of termination and ideally, at an interval after termination.[2]

Preparation, Culture, and Other Member Characteristics: In designing the preparation, it is crucial to consider all features that define the

---

[2] Howard, Moran, Brill, Martinovich, and Lutz (1996) have proposed the establishment of a national database. Data would be input based on standard instruments such as those in the Core Battery. Through the aggregating of this data, the group therapist could see how much change is typical over a given period of time. To know whether his or her group is effective, the therapist could compare the members' degree of progress to national norms for the same time frame.

person, especially the person's cultural background. Organista (2000) provides an excellent example of such sensitivity in his development of a cognitive-behavioral approach in the treatment of Latino clients. He notes the importance of the Latin value of *personalismo*, which he describes as "a valuing of and responsiveness to the personal dimension of relationships, including task-oriented professional relationships, such as psychotherapy" (p. 289). This value is at odds with a preparatory procedure in which members are expected to get down to business and discuss problems without having formed a relationship with each other and the therapist. He discusses a procedure incorporated into the first session in which members and the therapist exchange certain types of information about one another such as personal interests. Having such an opportunity to share this personal data helps Latino members establish the necessary trust to begin to work with one another.

The easing-in step that Organista designed for his group would be less appropriate for Asian American group members, who come from a culture in which personal revelations are made far more slowly (Sue & Sue, 1999). For these members a task focus may increase a sense of safety in entering of the group. Each group therapist must carefully reckon with the particulars of the cultural background of the members. This challenge is especially great when cultural backgrounds vary. Salvendy (1999) recommends apprising prospective members of the fact that the group is or could become racially or ethnically diverse. He writes, "Individuals with strong prejudices that are too cumbersome to work through during those few sessions [referring to the assessment and preparatory sessions] are best not included" (p. 449). Some therapists may prefer making the treatment of the intolerance a therapeutic goal, assuming that the therapist contain the negative effects of the prospective member's intolerance.

Other Features Defining the Prospective Group Member: One factor is socioeconomic status. In a classic study, Heitler (1973) designed a preparation program for inpatients from lower socioeconomic backgrounds. He reasoned that certain aspects of the therapeutic process were likely to be less familiar to persons of that substructure than to middle-class people. An example is the role difference between group member and therapist. He designed a module to educate the experimental group about these features. He found that the members who had the training were more active in the group and forged a working alliance more quickly than the unprepared patients.

Research Findings on Preparation

Two questions arise in relation to the preparation of group members. The first is: Do members provide evidence of benefiting from preparation? Under managed care there is an expectation that practitioners can justify the time they spend with patients, particularly if they bill for this time. In some settings, there may be pressure from other staff to place a patient in a group immediately. Preparing the patient may introduce some delay in the patient's entrance into the group. By providing some justification, the therapist is likely to obtain staff support and understanding for this extra step. The second question is: If preparation does enhance group participation, what types are most effective? Each of these questions will be considered in the light of available research.

Does Preparation Help? The effect of preparation is one of the best-researched topics in group therapy (see Dies, 1993). From the studies that have been done, three conclusions can be drawn:

1. Preparation activities enhance the group process by activating the mechanisms that are key to members' progress. For example, investigators have found that preparation leads to greater interpersonal openness and self-disclosure (Durst, Palmer, Baker, & McGee, 1977; Pastushak, 1978), a higher number of relationship statements (Piper, Debbane, Bienvenu, & Garant, 1982), and a higher level of activity early in group participation (Heitler, 1973).

2. Preparation has been shown to decrease the dropout rate (Heitler, 1973; Piper, Debbane, Garant, & Bienvenu, 1979) and improve members' attendance (Garrison, 1978). Given that members can benefit from group only by remaining in group for some reasonable duration, this is an extremely important finding. Furthermore, we know that on the whole people have negative expectations about group treatment even though the outcomes are at least comparable to individual therapy (Dies, 1993; Slocum, 1987; Subich & Coursol, 1985). Therefore, a

procedure that bolsters members' persistence, perhaps in the face of discomfort, by nurturing their positive expectations makes a very important contribution to treatment.

3. The effects of preparation on outcome are inconsistent as reflected by the inconsistent findings in the literature. Some studies confirm the value of preparation. For example, inmates at a medium-security penitentiary who had been given videotaped presentations and guided performance experience prior to the group made more progress toward individual goals in the group (Hilkey, Wilhelm, & Horne, 1982). Other studies have failed to show the benefits of pretraining. For example, Piper, Debbane, Bienvenu, and Gerant (1982) compared groups in which members had been given highly relevant versus minimally relevant information during the preparation. The investigators found that the nature of the preparatory material did not affect what members derived from the group, although it did affect their verbal behavior in group.

In general, the empirical results concerning the effects of preparation are favorable. The biggest impact may be early on, with preparation easing a member's entrance into the group. It increases positive expectations, decreases unproductive anxiety by helping members to know what group behaviors are useful, and counters catastrophic fears about the group. Once a member has had a lengthy period of immersion in the group, the effects of preparation may diminish. Nonetheless, helping a member to make a good start is of itself adequate justification for preparation. Members who are thrown into a group without explanation or education are at risk for reactions that could discourage them from pursuing therapy altogether.

What Types of Preparation Are Most Beneficial? The practitioner, knowing that preparation can be of benefit, would want to use the optimal method of preparation. Are didactic presentations or experiential opportunities preferable? Is preparation better done in a small group or individually? Bednar and Kaul (1994) divide preparation techniques into those that involve behavioral practice and modeling, cognitive clarifications, and experiential learning. As these reviewers note, the research literature suggests that a number of approaches produce positive results. While no particular approach emerges as superior to any other, there is some evidence (Kivlighan, McGovern, & Corazzini, 1995) that a multiple-method format (e.g., the combination of videotaping and verbal instructions) is superior to a single method.

In view of the lack of direction provided by the research, the clinician should develop a preparation procedure by identifying the information and skills that are most essential. In some instances the preparation can be tailored to the new group member. Suppose a person who has been in a group for a two-year period decided to enter a new group after having had been out of treatment for several years. The new group was similar in all important respects to the old group. Such a person would not need (and probably would not want) the same preparation as an individual who had never participated in a group.

Practical Considerations

In some clinical situations, it may not be possible to do all the preparation that a therapist feels should be done before the member enters the group. In some inpatient settings where lengths of stay are extremely brief, it may be necessary to place the patient in the group shortly after admission to the hospital. The therapist may have time only for a brief meeting with the patient before the first session. In such a circumstance, one can provide the benefits of preparation by incorporating preparation into the sessions themselves.

For example, when new members are being introduced into the group, the therapist can begin the session by reviewing the goals of the group, the processes by which the group pursues its goals, and the group rules. Senior members can assist with this orientation— which is also likely to bolster their self-esteem. During the session the therapist might make a greater number of explanatory comments to "demystify" the treatment process (Yalom, 1993) than may be done in later sessions. Finally, the therapist can provide to the new member written information that will reinforce the critical information about the group.

Another problem that is particularly likely to arise in a private-practice setting is that the member cannot be installed into the group immediately after the preparatory period. The reason for the delay is that the group may not be ready to accept a new member. If the delay would be inordinately long, then the therapist should refer the individual to another therapist. However, if the anticipated delay is reasonably short, the therapist may assist the patient in maintaining the benefits of preparation by having reinforcing sessions during the waiting period.

During preparatory sessions, the therapist can garner more information that can be used to help the member to work more effectively in the group:

An individual was entering a group to develop her capacity to have more satisfying relationships. In the initial set of interviews, the woman presented as an area of difficulty her ability to have constructive peer relationships. However, in subsequent sessions, the therapist learned that there was considerable tension in this woman's relationship with her immediate supervisor at work. Upon investigation, both the therapist and the new member came to recognize that such tension had existed previously in her relationships with other persons who had authority over her in the work environment. The therapist then pointed out to the member that this area of relationships with authority figures was one that could be addressed in the group.

In this example, the therapist put the extra time to good use by broadening the array of themes to which the member could respond. Moreover, the member, seeing the potential of the group to address various of her problems, might have been more motivated to enter the group than when she defined her work in the group more narrowly.

Preparing the Group

Imagine the following situation:

Cecille, a member of a long-term group, enters the session with some trepidation. In the last session, she had confronted Bill on his seductive manner toward her and the discomfort it elicited from her. Because this communication had occurred toward the end of the session, she had not had ample opportunity to obtain feedback from either Bill or the other members. They did have time to say that she had been very brave to reveal what obviously was a long-standing source of distress. However, members did not indicate whether they shared any of her observations. Although she had been very confident of her perceptions before the last session, since that time she worried that perhaps she had imagined the whole thing. The contemplation of this possibility filled her with feelings of shame and mortification. She entered the group session hoping to receive some confirmation of her original perceptions but dreading that she wouldn't. The remembrance of Bill's stony countenance during the end of the session last week only intensified her apprehension.

As she entered the group room, Cecille was stupefied to see a stranger sitting in it. Was it a new group member or perhaps an observer? Another entering member posed this question to the young man. He said he was beginning the group.

Several minutes later, the therapist entered the group. Abashedly, she affirmed that a new member was entering the group. She apologized for not having given the group notice and vaguely alluded to some uncertainties about the new member's work schedule that prevented her from doing so. Members responded by asking the new member, Patrick, about his reasons for entering the group. Patrick gave a fulsome account of the problems he was having in his relationship that led to his decision to enter the group. Bill's visage, initially impregnable as it had been last week, now wore an expression of warm solicitude.

Toward the end of the session, the therapist said, "Perhaps our absorption with Patrick is keeping us from addressing last week's unfinished business." Patrick reddened and muttered an apology about not meaning to "hog the stage." Cecille felt irritated with everyone, especially Patrick and the therapist, but found herself saying in a low, smoldering tone, "It's really important for the group to have a chance to get to know you." Another member asked Cecille about how she was feeling after last week. She choked on her unintelligible words as she yearned for the session to be over.

This vignette has two lessons to teach. The first is the importance of timing when a new member is introduced into the group; the second is to prepare the group for the entrance of a new member. In her heedlessness of both of these basic points, the therapist created a situation that was at best unhelpful to at least one and probably other group members.

The lesson of timing means that the therapist introduces a new member to the group when the group is able to integrate successfully that member. Two conditions may hamper a group from performing this task. The first is if members are in the throes of understanding their reactions to a recent change in the group. If a member who has been with the group for two years departs, the group will need time to address the loss. The length of time will depend upon the complexity of members' reactions as well as the extent to which members engage in defensive activity to avoid becoming aware and expressing different elements in their response.

For instance, if members have some sense of guilt over the departure of a member and wish to defend against an awareness of this painful affect, they may rally around an alternate topic. It may take some work for the group to recognize both the defense and the guilt defended against, and this work requires time. Hence, the therapist may not be able to anticipate what interval a group will require to do justice to their experience of the change.

The second impediment to the group's integrating the member is if the group has been occupied by issues that are particularly anxiety arousing. In our vignette, Cecille's disclosure about her perceptions of, and reactions to, Bill represented an effort to approach the highly threatening topic of members' sexual feelings toward one another and how these feelings are expressed. Generally, a member's foray into such an anxiety-arousing topic suggests some shift in the climate that allows for such risk taking. Hence, Cecille entered this new area of experimentation not simply for herself but for the group as a whole. As she did so, all eyes were upon the success of such an effort. During such a delicate period, the arrival of a new member is likely to have a chilling effect on members' new and difficult work. Cecille and others felt an understandable inhibition in communicating sensitive material in the presence of a stranger around whom they did not feel safe. The retreat of the group is inevitable and in many cases less than temporary. For what the group has learned is that members will be unprotected as they venture into unfamiliar realms.

For the new member, whether it be after an unmetabolized change in the group or in a period of new and difficult work, the activity of getting to know the new member cannot be embraced fully. Not only the new member but the group as a whole can be better served when the group can give the formidable task of integrating the new member its full attention.

The second lesson to be learned from the vignette of Cecille's (and the group's) interrupted work is that the group should be given adequate notice so that it can ready itself for the imminent arrival of a new member. Again, the example of the arrival of a new baby in a family is fitting. It would be unthinkable to bring a newborn home without having given the siblings ample room to anticipate this momentous expansion of the family. Group members also deserve such an opportunity.

When members are deprived of an in-depth exploration of their reactions to the arrival of a new member, they are more likely to act out their reactions in the presence of a new member. If the acting out is sufficiently extreme, the new member may be provoked into leaving the group. Rosenthal (1992) identified four common ways that a group will drive away a member. The group may exclude the member from the discussion. In acting as if the member were not there, the group would be giving direct expression to its wish. The group may intensively and unremittingly focus on the new member. In some groups, members may make the group wholly uninviting by engaging in internecine warfare. Finally, the old members may discourage the new members by impugning the group's efficacy (e.g., "I don't know why I stay here. I'm not getting anywhere").

Although preparing the group for the new member is critical, group members will often show great resistance in this effort. A major intrapsychic reason for this resistance is that the issues activated by a new member are among the earliest encountered in the course of development. Members' identification with the dependency of the new member and any unresolved conflicts that members have in relation to dependency urges have an opportunity to reemerge. Members recoil not only from the psychological pain attached to these conflicts (for example, the pain of experiencing the frustration of dependent longing) but also the awareness of the primitive nature of these conflicts. The resurgence of dependency conflicts challenges any perception members have of themselves as mature beings. The new member also is a stimulus for the arousal of conflicts related to sibling relationships (Leopold, 1961; Shapiro & Ginzberg, 2001). Members readily fantasize that the new member will be capable of achieving a special relationship with the authority figure in the group, the therapist. The feeling of envy of the new member's characteristics (at this point imagined rather than real) is an emotion most human beings will defend against with vigor.

On the interpersonal level, members have an understandable apprehension about how the new member may shake up the social structure of the group. Within the group, at any point, there is a particular type of work to be done. By virtue of their personality characteristics, members will be assigned to certain tasks. When a new member enters the group, these leadership slots are up for grabs. Members acquire approbation in certain roles, approbation that could then be taken away by the usurper. Moreover, members typically feel apprehension at the prospect of taking on themselves a new role. Therefore, anticipating the new member entails reckoning with loss and new threats.

These factors discourage members from examining their reactions to the announcement of a new member. For this reason, some therapeutic persistence is necessary to help members face what they would rather ignore. Support for members' explorations should not take the form of relentlessly reminding them of the imminence of the new member's arrival. More helpful is listening to members' communications on a symbolic level to determine any themes related to the new member:

> A women's group in a college counseling center had been meeting for four months. In the first four weeks of the group's existence, there had been some membership turnover, but in the last three months membership had been stable.
>
> The therapist announced that a woman would be joining the group three weeks later. One member said she had not realized new members would be added to the group. The other members scoffed at this notion, saying that the therapist had made it quite clear that new members would be added on an ongoing basis. The therapist attempted to get the surprised member to elaborate on her reaction, but embarrassment led this member to retreat.
>
> One member proceeded to talk about her suspicion that her boyfriend was seeing someone else, someone she had encountered in one of her classes. When she had expressed this worry earlier in the group, members' attitudes had been dismissive; now the group members took a keener interest in it. While they usually questioned her evidence, this time they alighted on pondering the particular qualities she might have that would be compelling to this young man or men in general. In the context of this analysis, a number of the women preferred characteristics of their own, which would be unappealing to men. Two lesbian members resonated to the idea that qualities they valued in themselves seemed to be liabilities in their relationships. They noted that people with less emotional sensitivity seemed to have more allure. Several of the women talked about the pain of this process of taking stock of oneself.

In listening to the group fragment in the light of the therapist's announcement, the therapist might note that the level of resistance appeared high to pursuing any discussion of the emotional impact of the announcement. The one member who made a foray into this realm was silenced in a manner that served as an effective warning to others contemplating similar attempts. The group then moved to the theme of rivalry. The ostensible stimulus to the lively discussion was the one member's doubts about her boyfriend's fidelity. Yet her worries did not rally members in past sessions in the way they did in the current session. The therapist might hypothesize that the original stimulus was the therapist's announcement about the new member. While new members are capable of evoking a variety of themes, for this group the theme was rivalry. On this hypothesis, the external rivalries were derivatives for the anticipated rivalry in the group.

Why would the group speak so indirectly about their concerns? By talking in code (or derivatives), members are able to accomplish two objectives at once. They are able to hide from themselves their painful apprehensions while providing some airing.

Listening to members' communications as symbolic productions is an activity that has received more emphasis in psychodynamic approaches, which assign a critical role to unconscious determinants of behavior. Yet all theoretical approaches have moved toward a greater recognition of the importance of here-and-now phenomena (Brabender & Fallon, 1993; Scheidlinger, 2000). Such symbolic listening on the part of the therapist can contribute to any therapist's effort to understand the group. However, how the therapist intervenes after developing a hypothesis depends on a variety of factors, including theoretical orientation. For example, whereas the psychodynamic therapist might make a group-level fantasy about what might occur with the arrival of the new member, the cognitive-behavioral therapist might use this material to help members identify their automatic cognitions about competitors. However the therapist uses this information, it should be done with sensitivity toward the often difficult feelings members have in relation to new arrivals.

As noted earlier, a strong group response to the arrival of a new member generally occurs in groups whose membership remains stable. Groups in which there is constant turnover tend to inure themselves to membership changes. Unfortunately, a prime means of doing so is by limiting their degree of connection with one another.

When a group is able to deal effectively with negative feelings in relation to new members, this process often enables them to gain access to positive feelings as well. Members can and do express excitement over the new stimulation a member will provide the group. Some members may hope that the new member will resonate to aspects of their experience that other members cannot. Still, others may see the new member as being a candidate for a group role of which they would like to divest themselves. By having enough time to analyze their reactions to this upcoming event, members can explore how it represents both a challenge and an opportunity.

Summary

In this chapter, we have examined how the therapist builds and sustains a group. In exploring the topic of group composition, a subset of the variables that a therapist typically would consider was discussed: homogeneity/heterogeneity of symptoms, ego functioning, age, gender, and other demographic factors such as race. Particular attention was given to the problem of having a subgroup of a single member. The therapist's use of the research literature and clinical knowledge of the target population was advocated as a basis for determining which variables should be most critical in making composition decisions. The importance of the therapist being reflective about compositional decisions once the group is under way in order to improve his or her clinical decision making in regard to new group candidates was stressed.

After making decisions about composition, the therapist can select members. The therapist should develop specific criteria and methods for determining whether these criteria have been fulfilled. The primary methods are interviewing, direct observation of group behavior, and psychological assessment.

The selection and preparation of the member goes hand-in-hand. During the selection process the member receives much information about the group that prepares the member for participation. However, once a member has made a commitment to join the group, certain points such as the specifics of the group contract should be explored in greater detail. Other important aspects of the preparatory period include helping the new member to anticipate certain aspects of the group experience, particularly difficult periods, fostering the use of therapeutic processes relevant to the group goals, and obtaining pretreatment data.

The rather considerable fund of research has provided inconsistent results on whether preparation positively affects group outcome. However, preparation does seem to increase the use of the processes it is designed to foster and enhance the likelihood that a new member will not terminate precipitously. While the research literature has not established the superiority of any one method of preparation, it does seem to be the case that the use of a preparation package with different components (experiential, video, written materials) is preferable. When circumstances prevent conducting in-depth preparatory sessions, the therapist may incorporate the critical elements into the group sessions themselves.

The necessity of preparing the group (particularly one that has achieved stability) for the arrival of a new member was emphasized. Members should be given time to explore their thoughts and feelings at a time when they are not preoccupied either with other major membership changes or conflictual issues. The therapist can facilitate the group's exploration by an awareness of the variety of themes that the introduction of a new member characteristically provokes.

The Ethical Practice of Group Therapy

In this chapter, we step back and consider how the group therapist can reflect on ethical dilemmas and successfully negotiate them. When an ethical dilemma arises, the practitioner faces a quandary over which course of action to take. It seems impossible to find a course of action that is wholly acceptable (Bricklin, 2001; Kitchener, 1984) and that honors all ethical principles to an equal extent. In encountering such a dilemma, how should the therapist arrive at a resolution that is ethical—and legal?

Ethical Codes and the Law

In resolving ethical dilemmas, the therapist can be aided greatly by consulting the ethical codes of his or her profession. An ethical code provides a set of guidelines for how to navigate professional situations and in some cases aspirational statements, that is, ideals to which practitioners should strive. Among the available ethical guidelines are the Ethical Principles of Psychologists and Code of Conduct (American Psychological Association [APA], 1992), the NASW Code of Ethics (National Association of Social Workers [NASW], 1999), the Code of Ethics and Standards of Practice (American Counseling Association [ACA], 1995), and the Code of Ethics (American Association for Marriage and Family Therapy, 1991).

Additionally, organizations devoted to the advancement of group therapy and related group activities have developed their own guidelines. The American Group Psychotherapy Association [AGPA] (1991) has developed guidelines to handle some of the specific situations that arise in groups that are not covered in all of the discipline-specific codes (see Table 9.1). For example, the AGPA ethical code discusses the situation of members' observing the confidentiality of other members' identities and communications. More specific still are the Ethical Guidelines for Group Counselors of the Association for Specialists in Group Work (ASGW), published in 1989. These guidelines establish standards of conduct for their members in 16 areas, including orientation and providing information, voluntary/involuntary participation, leaving a group, coercion and pressure, and dual relationships. The American Psychological Association (1973) published the "Guidelines for psychologists conducting growth groups."

No matter how specific the ethical guidelines of a professional organization may be, inevitably there will be situations that seem to elude the content of a particular code (Brabender, 2001) or that bring the guidelines in conflict with one another. For this reason, the therapist must have a set of principles that can help him or her navigate whatever situation presents itself. Such a set of principles has been recognized in the philosophical field of ethics and the more specific area of ethics in psychology (Bersoff & Koeppl, 1995; Bricklin, 2001). *Autonomy* is the individual's (or group member's) right to self-direction. *Beneficence* is the obligation to do good for others. *Non-maleficence* is the duty to do no harm (not to be confused with "malfeasance," which is wrongdoing by a public official). *Fidelity* is the placement of the well-being of the client (or in this case, group member) before that of the therapist because of the obligations rooted in the special character of a relationship based on trust. *Justice* is respect for the rights and dignity of all people, including the recipients of one's services. Inevitably, the situations in which the therapist faces a dilemma are ones in which these principles are in conflict.

All ethical codes and guidelines ultimately will be compatible with these four principles. Because of the universality of these principles, they provide a basis for communication between persons across disciplines and professions. As such, they can be of great use to the group therapist who uses a modality that historically and presently is multidisciplinary.

The therapist is also well served by being familiar with federal, state, and local statutes, rules and regulations that clarify or elaborate upon these statutes, and case law that relates to the practice of therapy in general and group therapy specifically. For example, later in the chapter, we see that jurisdictions vary in terms of how they

Table 9.1   AGPA Guidelines for Ethics

Introduction

The American Group Psychotherapy Association is a professional multidisciplinary organization whose purpose is to: "provide a forum for the exchange of ideas among qualified professional persons interested in group psychotherapy and to publish and to make publications available on all subjects relating to group psychotherapy; to encourage the development of sound training programs in group psychotherapy for qualified mental health professionals; to encourage and promote research on group psychotherapy and to establish and maintain high standards of ethical, professional group psychotherapy practice."

Membership in the American Group Psychotherapy Association presumes strict adherence to standards of ethical practice. As a specialty organization, AGPA supports the ethical codes of the primary professional organizations to which our members belong. Providing guidelines for the ethical behavior of group psychotherapists serves to inform both the group psychotherapist and public of the American Group Psychotherapy Association's expectations in the practice of group psychotherapy.

General Guidelines

Ethical complaints about AGPA members will be directed to the primary professional organization of the members. AGPA's response as to sanctions will parallel that of the primary organization. For example, if the primary organization concludes than an individual's membership should be suspended for one year, AGPA will suspend membership for one year. Should an ethical complaint be received regarding a member of AGPA who does not belong to a primary professional organization, the complaint will be directed to the state licensing board and/or the state or federal legal system. If the member is found guilty, AGPA's sanctions will parallel the sanctions of the state licensing board, other governmental agencies or courts of law as to the person's ability to practice; the AGPA cannot parallel such sanctions as fines, penalties or imprisonment.

For those members of the American Group Psychotherapy Association who are psychiatrists, the principles of ethics as applied by the American Psychiatric Association shall govern their behavior; those members who are clinical psychologists shall be expected to comply with the principles of ethics laid down by the American Psychological Association; those members who are clinical social workers shall be expected to comply with the ethical standards established by the National Federation of Societies for Clinical Social Work; those members who are clinical specialists in nursing shall be expected to comply with the principles of ethics of the American Nurses' Association; those members who are pastoral counselors shall be expected to comply with the ethical standards of the American Association of Pastoral Care; and those members of other professional disciplines having published principles of ethics shall follow those principles. Members of the Association who do not belong to one of the above professional groups having a published standard of ethics shall follow the principles of ethics laid down by the American Psychological Association.

(continued)

Table 9.1   (Continued)

Guidelines of Group Psychotherapy Practice

The following guidelines of group psychotherapy practice shall serve as models for group therapists' ethical behavior.

Responsibility to Patient/Client

1. The group psychotherapist provides services with respect for the dignity and uniqueness of each patient/client as well as the rights and autonomy of the individual patient/client.

    1.1   The group psychotherapist shall provide the potential group patient/client with information about the nature of group psychotherapy and apprise them of their risks, rights and obligations as members of a therapy group.

    1.2   The group psychotherapist shall encourage the patient/client's participation in group psychotherapy only so long as it is appropriate to the patient/client's needs.

    1.3   The group psychotherapist shall not practice or condone any form of discrimination on the basis of race, color, sex, sexual orientation, age, religion, national origin or physical handicap, except that this guideline shall not prohibit group therapy practice with population specific or problem specific groups.

2. The group psychotherapist safeguards the patient/client's right to privacy by judiciously protecting information of a confidential nature.

    2.1   The group shall agree that the patient/client as well as the psychotherapist shall protect the identity of its members.

    2.2   The group psychotherapist shall not use identifiable information about the group or its members for teaching purposes, publication or professional presentations unless permission has been obtained and all measures have been taken to preserve patient/client anonymity.

    2.3   Except where required by law, the group psychotherapist shall share information about the group members with others only after obtaining appropriate patient/client consent. Specific permission must be requested to permit conferring with the referring therapist or with the individual therapist where the patient/client is in conjoint therapy.

    2.4   When clinical examination suggests that a patient/client may be dangerous to himself/herself or others, it is the group psychotherapist's ethical and legal obligation to take appropriate steps in order to be responsible to society in general, as well as the patient/client.

3. The group psychotherapist acts to safeguard the patient/client and the public from the incompetent, unethical, illegal practice of any group psychotherapist.

    3.1   The group psychotherapist must be aware of her/his own individual competencies, and when the needs of the patient/client are beyond the competencies of the psychotherapist, consultation must be sought from other qualified professionals or other appropriate sources.

    3.2   The group psychotherapist shall not use her/his professional relationship to advance personal or business interests.

    3.3   Sexual intimacy with patients/clients is unethical.

    3.4   The group psychotherapist shall protect the patient/client and the public from misinformation and misrepresentation. She/he shall not use false or misleading advertising regarding her/his qualifications or skills as a group psychotherapist.

Table 9.1   (Continued)

Professional Standards

The group psychotherapist shall maintain the integrity of the practice of group psychotherapy.

1. It is the personal responsibility of the group psychotherapist to maintain competence in the practice of group psychotherapy through formal educational activities and informal learning experiences.

2. The group psychotherapist has a responsibility to contribute to the ongoing development of the body of knowledge pertaining to group psychotherapy whether involved as an investigator, participant or user of research results.

3. The group psychotherapist shall accept the obligation to attempt to inform and alert other group psychotherapists who are violating ethical principles or to bring those violations to the attention of appropriate professional authorities.

Published with permission from the American Group Psychotherapy Association.

view information sharing among members. To conduct an adequate informed consent, the group therapist should be knowledgeable about the statutes of his or her jurisdiction on this matter.

Model for Ethical Decision Making

With knowledge of the law, specific ethical codes, and general ethical principles, is the therapist adequately equipped to make sound decisions? The one remaining ingredient is a process for evaluating factors relevant to a dilemma. While various models exist for how to resolve a dilemma, we shall consider a model that on the one hand is relatively clear and straightforward but on the other ensures that the practitioner garners the relevant information and asks the key questions. This model, developed by Haas and Malouf (2000), is described by considering its application to a particular dilemma:

> *A group member, Pamela, called the therapist in distress. She had been shocked to discover that she would be crossing professional paths with another group member, Louis, the director of a large organization. Pamela was an organizational consultant whose colleague (not a group member) provided consultation to Louis in his capacity as director. Her colleague at a work team meeting discussed various problems with the organizational leadership, particularly Louis's authoritarian and demeaning administrative*

style. Louis had noted "problem employees" in sessions with no apparent awareness of his contributions to poor organizational morale. Although Pamela was not concerned that she would be interacting with Louis directly, she feared she might obtain additional sensitive information about him through this professional intermediary, who interacted with them both. She felt she could not ask the intermediary to withhold information at team meetings without violating Louis's confidentiality (i.e., being a group member). She assured the therapist that she would be careful not to reveal anything Louis had shared in the group to the consultant.

In thinking about the problem presented by Pamela, the therapist reflected on the original contract with each member. At the time each member entered the group, the rule of no socialization outside of group was presented. One of several rationales given was that the therapist wanted members' observations and impressions of one another to be based on how they acted within the sessions themselves, where everyone could be a witness. Pamela said she did not want to tell Louis about her access to information about him. She insisted that if there was a mutual acknowledgment, both members would feel awkward and inhibited in relation to one another.

The therapist felt disturbed that she and Pamela now shared a secret. On an intuitive level, she felt she was facing an ethical problem that might require a response.

Bricklin (2001) notes that it is often an intuitive or "gut" reaction that something is amiss that launches an ethical inquiry by the practitioner. In the vignette the therapist's sense of disturbance in relation to the secret is such a gut reaction. Bricklin further observes that as the practitioner's fund of experience and knowledge of ethical codes increases, the more trustworthy these gut reactions are likely to be.

Nonetheless, regardless of how much experience the practitioner has, it is important to give explicit attention to whether a problem within the group is a genuine ethical problem. According to Haas and Malouf (2002), this evaluation should precede the activation of a decision-making process (see Figure 9.1). During this evaluation, one must be careful to distinguish an ethical problem from a technical problem. For example, deciding what format of group therapy would most benefit a candidate would be a technical problem. However, the conflict in the vignette is genuinely ethical because it raises the question of whether the conditions under which Louis agreed to be in the group had been substantially changed and if so,

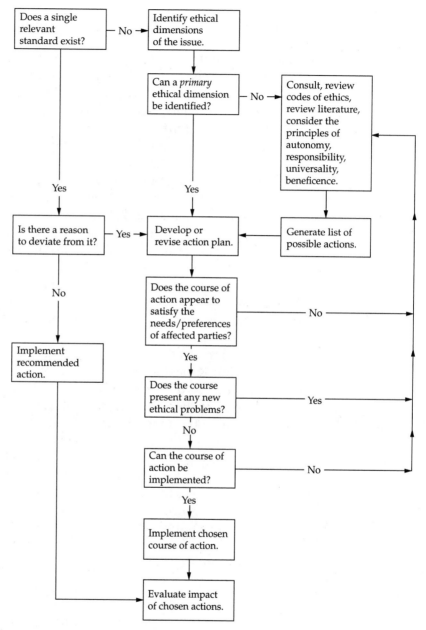

Figure 9.1

The Decision-Making Flow Chart.

From *Keeping Up the Good Work: A Practitioner's Guide to Mental Health Ethics* (3rd ed.)
by L. J. Haas & J. L. Malouf, 2002, Sarasota, FL: Professional Resource Press, p.12.
Copyright 2002 by Professional Resource Exchange, Inc. Reprinted by permission.

whether the therapist had an obligation to inform him of this fact. The ethical conflict is between the one member's right to informed consent (including any departures from the original informed consent) and the other member's right to assume that the therapist will keep certain information private.[1] In fact, many if not most ethical dilemmas practitioners face will involve the two legal rights of informed consent and privacy.

As part of the problem-clarification process, Haas and Malouf (2002) also urge the practitioner to obtain two types of information. First, the therapist should identify the legitimate stakeholders who would be affected by the outcome of the dilemma. In our vignette both group members are stakeholders, but there may be others. For example, the consultant's work may be affected by Pamela's possible reticence in their team meetings if ordinarily the consultant depended upon Pamela's input. Furthermore, to the extent that the consultant's work was affected by changes in Pamela's usual pattern of behavior or degree of neutrality, the recipients of her services may be affected. Second, the therapist should obtain any professional standards that exist in relation to the type of situation at hand.

Having appraised the problem and gathered facts, the therapist is in a position to begin the process of ethical decision making as it has been outlined by Haas and Malouf (2002). The first step is to identify whether there is a single professional, legal, or social standard relevant to the practitioner's situation. Earlier in this chapter, the various professional codes as well as those specific to group work were cited. For example, all relevant codes require the therapist to observe confidentiality about a patient's communication except for disclosures specifically outlined in the informed consent.

If there is a single relevant standard, then the practitioner must consider if there is a reason to deviate from it. As Haas and Malouf (2002) note, one reason the practitioner may deviate is that the standard is too vague to provide direction. Another reason, however, is

---

[1] The assumption here is that as part of the contract the therapist does permit members to share with him or her information that they intend to be kept private. Some therapists do not permit such private communications. By establishing that there will not be private, confidential exchanges between group members and the therapist, the therapist removes the dilemma seen here. However, other problems may arise. For example, there may be a greater pressure to disclose sensitive material to the entire group, and such disclosures could have adverse effects upon the member.

that observance of the standard may have greater negative consequences than deviating from it. For example, suppose member A revealed to member B a plan to commit suicide. Member B then told the therapist of this fact but refused to allow the therapist to discuss it with member A. In this case, keeping member B's confidence may imperil member A. Moreover, member A's self-destructive activity could harm member B if the latter saw him or herself as handcuffing the therapist.

In a more complicated circumstance where no single professional standard applies, Haas and Malouf (2002) direct the therapist to isolate the ethical dimensions of the circumstance. Consider once again the situation in which Pamela may obtain information about Louis through a third party. As noted previously, the conflict is between the need to preserve Pamela's confidentiality and Louis's right to know about a potentially significant alteration in her relationship with another member. Such knowledge might affect what information Louis wished to share inside and outside of group and even his willingness to remain in the group. Louis's right to have the information he needs to make an informed decision is consistent with the principle of autonomy. Recognizing the harm that would result either from the breach of confidentiality or the failure to inform Louis of Pamela's access to intragroup information would evoke the principle of non-maleficence and fidelity.

The next step in the sequence is determining whether a primary ethical dimension can be specified. The principle that supercedes all others is that of "do no harm," or non-maleficence. The principle of autonomy generally has priority over that of beneficence. In this instance the practitioner must weigh the relative degree of harm that is likely to result from either violating confidentiality or keeping the member's confidence. Consultation or supervision with a colleague can be very helpful to ensure that one has identified all relevant dimensions of the circumstance (Schoener & Luepker, 1996).

The next step in the Haas and Malouf framework entails generating a list of possible actions. The therapist should attempt to identify courses of action that would enable him or her to observe those ethical principles that initially seem incompatible. For example, the therapist might decide to make a concerted effort to explain to Pamela the potential that withholding the information has for eroding trust in the group. Within this strategy, the therapist would encourage the line of communication to be member-to-member rather than therapist-to-member. At this time, the therapist would weigh this solution against other alternatives to determine which option optimally resolves potentially conflicting principles. Again, consultation with a trusted colleague may be helpful in identifying solutions that a practitioner may have not recognized or problems arising in relation to a particular conclusion.

Once a particular course of action stands out from other possibilities, it should be subjected to three further tests (Haas & Malouf, 2002). First, does the course of action meet the preferences of the affected parties? Second, does it create any new ethical problems? For example, if the therapist envisioned placing strong pressure on the member to reveal her secret, then the element of coercion would be a new ethical problem. Third, can the course of action be implemented? How viable and practical is the solution? For example, the therapist may not be successful in convincing the member of the potential negative impact of the secret. In some instances, a solution may be too expensive or time-consuming. For example, a member may lose a job and be unable to pay a particular fee. The therapist with a sliding scale may be able to accommodate the member's situation, and in fact may feel an ethical obligation to do so (in consistency with the principle of beneficence). Yet, doing so may have some limitations: Beyond some point, a fee reduction could unduly affect the financial well-being of the therapist. Such practical factors can have a role in ethical decision making.

Once all of these steps have been completed, the practitioner is in a position to implement the solution. As Haas and Malouf note, this step can require a range of skills on the part of the therapist such as "assertiveness, tenacity, the existence of a supportive social network, and the ability to communicate one's chosen action in non-condescending and humane terms" (p. 18). In another decision-making system, that of McCullough and Ashton (1994), the last step of the process is an analysis that is both retrospective and prospective. Based on a study of the situation that created the ethical dilemma, the therapist can contemplate what actions might be taken to diminish the likelihood that ethical principles will collide in a given circumstance in the future. Very often practitioners find that enhancing the informed consent process accomplishes this objective. In our example, including information on how members should handle extragroup contact—whether direct or indirect, intentional or unwitting—might have helped the therapist to avoid his predicament. Finally, Rae and Fournier (1999), in their discussion of ethical issues arising in the treatment of children, discuss the usefulness of re-examining a decision about an ethical dilemma at a later time. After a reasonable interval, the therapist will have information about the consequences of a given decision. This reanalysis, too, will serve McCullough and Ashton's goal of helping the practitioner create conditions in which ethical principles will be unlikely to collide.

Ethical Issues

Armed with ethical principles and a decision-making process, the reader is now equipped to address a sample of the ethical concerns that often arise in the conduct of group therapy. The topics we address are (a) competence, (b) informed consent, (c) confidentiality and privilege, (d) accountability and termination, and (e) the use of technology in group therapy.

Competence

All ethical codes within the human service professions require the practitioner to be competent to provide the services being offered. This is no less the case for group therapy. Underscoring this fundamental point, the AGPA Guidelines for Ethics states, "The group therapist must be aware of her/his own individual competencies, and when the needs of the patient/client are beyond the competencies of the therapist, consultation must be sought from other qualified professionals or other appropriate sources." The ASGW Ethical Guidelines for Group Counselors captures the requirement of competence in Guideline 6, which addresses the need for professional development. In this guideline, group counselors are encouraged and instructed to expand their knowledge base and skill through a range of professional development activities, continuing education, and clinical experiences.

Competence appears in all ethical codes because of its centrality to all the major ethical principles described earlier. For example, to observe beneficence—to do good—the practitioner must be able to mediate the dynamics and power factors inherent in a functioning group. As noted in both Chapters 1 and 2, group therapy has great potential to effect positive change. However, such outcomes are most likely if the therapist has the skill and knowledge (that is, the competence) to activate the processes that are unique to the group. Nonmaleficence is also at issue because groups do have the potential to produce negative outcomes. The competent group practitioner knows how to create conditions that avoid untoward consequences of group participation. For example, the competent practitioner knows how to prevent the kind of coercion that can develop in a group and challenge a member's autonomy or the scapegoating that can precipitously lower a member's self-esteem.

Particular challenges exist with respect to competence in persons conducting therapy groups. Organized training in group therapy has not been prevalent in graduate training programs in the mental health professions. While graduates of psychology programs and psychiatry residency programs will typically have had substantial exposure to theory and research about individual therapy, their exposure to group therapy is often far more limited. Graduate-level programs in social work and counseling are somewhat more variable, and there continue to be programs in which group therapy receive minimal treatment. Yet, in the positions that many graduates assume in organizations, they are often called on to conduct therapy groups. Because of diminishing economic resources in such organizations (e.g., mental health centers), funding is not reliably available for training activities that could compensate for weaknesses in graduate training.

The upshot of the neglect of academic institutions and service organizations to provide adequate training in group therapy is that the burden is placed upon the individual to ensure that he or she is competent. Considerable time and expense is required to fulfill this ethical obligation. Fortunately, professional organizations provide an organized set of training experiences for the new group practitioner. For example, the American Group Psychotherapy Association offers a 12-hour course on the fundamentals of group therapy at its annual meeting and more advanced opportunities in the context of workshops. More local opportunities are offered by the affiliate societies of this organization.

As important as didactic training is, it is not sufficient. To achieve competence the group therapist will require competent supervision. Such supervision can be provided in the context of cotherapy. The advantage is that the supervisor can witness directly the supervisee's behavior. However, in some settings there may be no appropriate supervisor, and even if such a supervisor is present, it may not be possible to work out the logistics for cotherapy. In such circumstances, the supervisee should use process notes, audiotapes, and even videotapes of sessions to provide the supervisor as complete a picture as possible of the supervisee's activity within the group.

Further, Chapter 5 described the strong relationship between the therapist's emotional fitness and effectiveness. To achieve such fitness, many therapists are likely to profit from participation in their own personal therapy. Involvement in a therapy group may be especially helpful to one's work as a group therapist. Furthermore, there may be times in the life of the group therapist when stress may hurt the therapist's work. Competency requires the capacity to monitor oneself to determine the need for therapy or in the instance of impairment, a sabbatical from providing treatment.

To achieve competence, the fledgling group therapist must master the generic aspects of establishing, maintaining, and ending therapy groups that are covered in primers such as this text. However, both for the new and more seasoned practitioner, it is critical to competence that one have an enlightened grasp of the specifics of the environment in which one is working. A thorough understanding of the characteristics of the setting, the population one is treating, and all other factors that would affect the group and determine what group format is likely to be effective should be achieved. This requirement for competence is likely to come into play when a therapist enters a new setting or works with patients with a set of presenting problems other than those with which he or she has dealt in the past.

For example, the reader may recall the discussion of establishing the composition of a group of persons with eating disorders in Chapter 8. To engage in good clinical decision making, the group therapist must become intimately knowledgeable about the characteristics of this patient population, especially as they bear upon the interactions of members in the group. A therapist who intends to lead a group with members of this population and has not done so previously will have to make a considerable investment in training in order to function competently. Therapists attempting to treat individuals within a different age group than they had treated previously must secure training to do so. Soo (1998) notes that too often, practitioners attempt to conduct groups with children or adolescents without having been supervised by a group therapist with expertise in this area.

Practitioners act unethically when they attempt to fall back on generic knowledge when more specialized training is in order. As Salvendy (1999) noted, given that our society is becoming multiethnic, therapists are often in the position of needing to enhance their cultural competence by educating themselves on the cultures of group members. They can do so, he writes, "by acquainting themselves with the available literature, including sociological, anthropological, counseling, and therapy studies. . . . It is also necessary for therapists to be aware of any mythological, religious, historical, or geopolitical reasons for ethnic and cultural beliefs and attitudes for the group to function effectively "(p. 447). Yet, Salvendy stresses that such knowledge is not sufficient: The therapist must also know modes of communication and intervention strategies that are most likely to be effective with a given cultural group. Sue and Sue (1999) emphasize the importance of grasping the values of an individual's culture in order to provide effective treatment. For example, while many forms of treatment entail the use of insight, certain cultures do not value insight. A therapist lacking multicultural competence may mistakenly attribute a person's failure to thrive in insight-oriented therapy to an incapacity to achieve insight rather than valuing insight less than the therapist does.

Competence demands that the group therapists engage in lifelong learning. Most group therapists, over the course of their careers, make changes in their group practice based upon developments in the marketplace. Such changes necessitate the kind of educational involvement described earlier. However, even if the nature of a therapist's practice changes little, continuing education is crucial (Ehly & Garcia-Vazquez, 1998; Ferber, DeMartino, & Prout, 1989). The research base of group therapy is continually increasing in response to the demand for empirically-supported treatments. It is important for the group therapist to be aware of these findings and to apply them to his or her own group efforts. By engaging in this process of renewal that a continuous immersion in the literature brings, the therapist provides an ingredient essential for competence.

Informed Consent

As part of preparation, the group therapist must secure an informed consent. An informed consent is assent to group treatment after receiving accurate information about the essentials of the treatment. Informed consent involves the ethical principle of autonomy. Without informed consent, individuals lack the wherewithal to control their own destinies. However, informed consent is also relevant to the principle of beneficence in that it may render the treatment more effective than when it is absent. Informed consent, if done properly, can enlist the prospective group member as an active agent in his or her own progress in treatment. The foundation for assuming this responsibility is laid with the member's initial agreement to pursue the goals, participate in the processes, and abide by the rules in the group contract. Informed consent also inoculates the treatment against the untoward effects of any surprises that might challenge the group member's trust in the therapist. Chapter 7 gave an example of an event having the potential to erode trust: a group member's being unaware of the requirement to pay for a missed session until a session was actually missed.

This section addresses several aspects of informed consent: what information should be included, how and when the informed consent should be secured, and the informed consent process when treatment is not voluntary.

The Content of Informed Consent: The therapist must give careful thought to what should be presented as part of the informed consent. Included should be the purpose of the group, the therapist's diagnosis of the person or assessment of the prospective member's difficulties, the benefits anticipated, and the methods used. Chapter 8 gave a great deal of attention to the topic of how to talk to the prospective member about the goals and processes of the group to make treatment successful. While all of this material is relevant to informed consent, our emphasis in this chapter is different. Here the question is what information should be provided to enable the individual to have an adequate basis for making a decision about whether or not to join the group, and their level of participation once in the group. For the most part, the information that is provided serves both goals, though occasionally there may be a conflict between the two aims (Widiger & Rorer, 1984). Such a conflict entails a clash between the principles of beneficence and autonomy. That is, withholding certain information might enhance treatment effectiveness while providing it may increase the individual's decision-making power.

For example, we know from our discussion in Chapter 3 of group development that early in the life of a group, members are disposed to exaggerate similarities and deny differences. This developmental phenomenon is important in alleviating members' anxiety about joining the group. Yet, alerting prospective members to this pattern may diminish its intensity and thereby its effectiveness. But would a prospective member require knowledge of this phenomenon to have an adequate basis to make a decision? Would it seem to be the kind of material to lead a person in one direction or another in terms of joining the group? Because withholding this information would not be likely to undermine the individual's autonomy, the therapist could give greater weight to the principle of beneficence. However, if the material is likely to be more relevant to the person's decision making, then the clinician has a greater obligation to share it.[2]

One way to determine whether a particular type of intervention or process within the group should be disclosed is to consider whether it poses any risk to the prospective member. A prime example is self-disclosure. Self-disclosure is risky because whatever information a member discloses in the group could be exported out of the group to the member's detriment. Hence, apprising a member that self-disclosure is an expected part of group activity would be essential to adequate informed consent.

The preceding example points to another element necessary for informed consent. The therapist must disclose the risks and adverse reactions attached to the treatment. While some risks are common to all or most groups, others are particular to a given group format (Roback, 2000). Therefore, the therapist cannot fall back on universals but must do a careful analysis of the specifics of his or her own group as they create risks for the members.

Yet, the potential risks of virtually any activity, including group therapy, are great in number. The task of the therapist is not to share

---

[2] The issue of the potential conflict between treatment effectiveness and informed consent is complex. Within the field of therapy, views differ on how the ethical therapist would resolve this issue (see Graca, 1985; Haas, 1991; and Sombreg, Stone, & Claiborn, 1993 for further exploration of this topic). Within the group therapy literature, this issue has been addressed insufficiently.

every conceivable risk. An attempt to be overly inclusive has its own risk: presenting extremely remote risks alongside relatively significant ones (either in terms of impact or probability). How does the group therapist pick and choose among risks to arrive at those that are explicitly incorporated as part of the informed consent? In other words, how does the therapist establish what is a reasonable risk?

In evaluating any particular risk for inclusion, the clinician may use the decision-making sequence of Haas and Malouf (2002) that we reviewed. Consider, for example, the potential risk that participation might bring physical harm to a member. As members process conflictual aspects of their relationships with one another, intense affects and destructive impulses might be stimulated that could lead to aggression. What is most critical in this evaluation are the steps requiring the practitioner to isolate the ethical dimensions and weigh them—in this case, autonomy and beneficence. By not providing the prospective participant with such information, the practitioner jeopardizes autonomy. On the other hand, providing information about risk can always reduce the individual's motivation to be in the group, thereby denying the benefits of group therapy to the person.

While autonomy generally takes precedence over beneficence, the consequences of violating each principle must nonetheless be weighed for each situation. For example, suppose in a particular group, the practitioner, based on experience with this group or similar groups as well as knowledge of reported findings on this risk factor, knows that the risk of physical harm is negligible. Then, even if physical harm is a remote possibility, not including the risk in informed consent does not significantly challenge the person's right to self-determination. On the other hand, by incorporating it, the practitioner may needlessly alarm the person. If, though, the clinician is conducting a group with a population such as conduct-disordered adolescents where aggression is occasionally acted out, then the challenge to autonomy that attends withholding the mention of this risk becomes much more significant.

As this discussion suggests, an adequate informed consent must be based on the practitioners' knowledge of what the actual risks are and where on a continuum of probability a given risk falls. The empirical study of specific risks in group treatment has been extremely sparse. The major risk that has been investigated, violations of confidentiality (Roback, Moore, Waterhouse, & Martin, 1996), is discussed later. In the absence of a firm empirical base for risk appraisal, the group therapist must rely on a substantial clinical knowledge of his or her group therapy circumstance.

Further, the therapist must rely on the law concerning informed consent within the jurisdiction. As Roback et al. (1996) note, the law is highly variable and in some cases explicitly applies to nonphysician therapists and in some cases does not. When the law does not explicitly cover nonphysician therapists, the law governing physicians is often applied. There are two standards by which the adequacy of an informed consent may be evaluated (Roback et al., 1996). The *professional standard* requires the physician's disclosure of the risks that are generally disclosed or that the physician feels a reasonable person would wish to know. ("Physician" is used because such laws are generally written for physicians.) A *lay standard* mandates the disclosure of all material risks that the reasonable patient would have wanted to know in consenting to treatment. If the lay standard and professional standard conflict, the therapist should apply the standard that would afford the member the greatest motivation.

As noted, every group therapist must assess the risks in his or her own group. However, some risks characterize a broad spectrum of groups. Three in particular will be described: the stimulation of negative reactions during the group, failure to benefit from group treatment, and changes in the group stimulated by changes in membership. A third set of risks associated with confidentiality and privacy is discussed in a separate section.

Negative Feelings during the Course of Group: While therapists are well aware that treatment often arouses upsetting feelings and impulses, individuals entering therapy may not. In a comprehensive, informed consent, the therapist conveys that during the course of the group members may experience a variety of unpleasant reactions. They also may learn of others' perceptions that may be inconsistent with how they see themselves or how they would like to be seen by others. The format of the group determines the extent to which this adverse reaction is emphasized as a risk. For example, in some short-term supportive groups the group design may emphasize processes whereby members are unlikely to receive negative feedback or have unpleasant feelings stimulated. In such groups, negative affects may not be as prominent as they are in exploratory groups. Members nonetheless are likely to have some anxiety stimulation merely by being in group. The reasons for this anxiety were described in Chapter 3. Therefore, for most groups members should be informed of the likelihood of some emotional discomfort.

Failure to Benefit from Treatment: While empirical investigations reveal that group therapy is beneficial, these findings apply to groups. The therapist cannot guarantee that any particular individual will profit from group participation. The fact that progress toward the treatment goals cannot be assured is one of the potential risks of group treatment. The challenge for the therapist is how to describe this risk without discouraging participation or engendering a pessimistic attitude. For some group approaches, the therapist may be able to specify, based upon research findings, the percentage of individuals who improve or fail to improve. Such information helps the entering member to have positive but not unrealistically inflated expectations. Lacking data about the particular approach, the therapist can state generally that while the vast majority of participants benefit, some do not.

Other Possible Risks: Within the literature, other risks have been identified. Lakin (1994) argues that relative to individual therapy, the therapist has less control in the group therapy setting. In the latter, so it is argued, there are multiple agents of change, not simply the therapist or the individual. He notes, "Group therapists can truly anticipate neither the responses of group members in general nor the particular effects of these group members on specific individual participants" (p. 345). Given the lesser degree of control, some might argue that the therapist should acknowledge this unpredictability about what their experiences will be or the likely outcome from group participation. The notion that outcomes are more uncertain in therapy groups relative to individual therapy is not consistent with the empirical findings reported in Chapters 1 and 2.[3] Another risk may be that a member may not be likely to achieve a goal given the structure of a particular group. Consider the following example:

---

[3] Admittedly most studies look at mean differences between groups receiving different treatments. However, until there are a greater number of comparative studies tracking individual's progress through treatment (see MacKenzie & Grabovac, 2001, for an example of a clinical quasi-experimental study tracking individual member's progress), the notion that group treatment is somehow less predictable is speculative.

Roger has been evaluated by a group therapist for possible participation in an eight-session behavior therapy group for the treatment of depression. During the evaluation he mentions that he wants to be in this particular group because his managed care plan will cover all of the sessions. Roger, in the view of the therapist, is clearly depressed and has the potential to obtain significant symptom alleviation from involvement with the group. However, at some point in the interview Roger mentions that he has never been able to sustain a long-term intimate relationship.

The therapist in the vignette would have an obligation as part of the informed consent to tell the prospective member that while the group is appropriate for the treatment of his depressive symptoms, it is not designed to address the significant interpersonal problem he raised. Moreover, he might counsel Roger on the kind of time commitment that may be necessary to pursue his relational difficulty. Armed with this information, Roger's autonomy would be safeguarded. He would have a reasonable basis to determine what treatment goals he wishes to pursue now and the sacrifices, monetary and otherwise, he is willing to make in pursuit of these goals. In general, a part of the informed consent is comparing and contrasting group therapy with other recommended treatments.

Delivery of the Informed Consent: What should be the format by which the member's informed consent is obtained? The formats most commonly used are verbal and written. Each has distinctive strengths, so each has a role in the informed consent process. For consent to be informed, the individual must understand the information. Through a conversation the therapist and the candidate can communicate in a way that is most likely to be comprehensible and meaningful. Moreover, the therapist can obtain substantial evidence of whether the individual grasps the points raised in the informed consent. The strength of the written format is that it creates a level of formality that is appropriate given the importance of the individual's decision. Moreover, it provides evidence that the person has consented. However, a person's mere signature on a consent form does not establish that the person actually understood the conditions of the treatment. It is only through a conversation that the practitioner can know that the person understands the risks and other specifics of the treatment. Therefore, it is crucial that the practitioner document any informed-consent conversations.

A fitting time to conduct the informed consent is prior to the member's entrance into the group. Otherwise, the material in the informed consent is not available for the member's decision about whether to join the group. The practitioner would be well served to include a description of any questions or misconceptions that arise. For example, the therapist in the case mentioned earlier might note, "Roger recognizes that this group is not designed to treat his particular relational difficulty of not forming long-term intimate relationships. He feels he would rather pursue that goal after graduation when he will have more discretionary income to finance his treatment."

When Treatment Is Not Voluntary: Group treatment may occur without the individual's willingness to be treated under a variety of circumstances. Nonetheless, the involuntary character of the individual's membership does not relieve the therapist from the obligation to safeguard the patient's autonomy as much as possible. To this end, the therapist should provide the person with as much information before entering the group as the person who is joining the group voluntarily. The therapist should also make clear any stakes associated with the person's behavior in the group. For example, if the member's behavior is being used as evidence of readiness for parole or parenting skill in a custody dispute, these consequences should be made clear. This communication should also include any special limits on confidentiality regarding the use of information about the member's behavior by sources external to the group. While not able to exercise decision-making capacity about whether to join the group, the individual is empowered to make choices about behavior during the sessions themselves.

Privacy: Confidentiality and Privileged Communication

The right to privacy is a cornerstone of ethical treatment. This right has two components: confidentiality and privileged communication.

Confidentiality: Confidentiality has long been recognized as critical in therapy. Maintaining confidentiality honors many principles. Confidentiality serves autonomy by providing patients with control over information about them. It preserves non-maleficence by avoiding untoward consequences that could ensue from violating confidentiality.

THE RISK OF VIOLATIONS: Within all therapy situations, there are circumstances that necessitate legally-mandated violation of the patient's confidentiality. Among these are threats of physical harm to self or others, child abuse, and in some cases responses to subpoenas concerning a member of the group. The legal and ethical requirements on the therapist to breach confidentiality exist in part because, as noted by Haas and Malouf (2002), other stakeholders in these situations are often likely to be affected by a potential disclosure. Certain disclosures are a legally mandated responsibility of the therapist because to not make them would critically undermine another's well-being. There are also circumstances in which the patient will permit the therapist to share information with external parties, for example, an insurance company to obtain reimbursement for sessions or other professionals treating the patient for the purpose of care coordination.

Can the group member be certain that besides the circumscribed instances in which confidentiality cannot be maintained, confidentiality will be guaranteed? In individual therapy, provided the therapist is willing to exercise the necessary care and responsibility, the answer is yes. In group therapy, the therapist can give no such assurance. By definition, other group members are privy to the self-disclosing of each individual member. Whereas the therapist's inappropriate disclosures about a group member can lead to stiff legal and professional sanctions, with some rare exceptions such consequences do not exist for group members. Therapists can and almost always do establish a confidentiality rule by which members agree to protect the identities of the other group members and refrain from exporting the material shared by other members to outside parties. Yet, the therapist can do little to enforce this rule. If the therapist had established that a violation may lead to expulsion from the group, then once a member has broken confidentiality, his or her removal could eliminate future possible incidents. Yet, the violation has already occurred, and the member who is its object may have been hurt by it. The ways in which such damage can occur are innumerable. The following is an example of the harm that can come from a breach of confidentiality:

Kate had revealed in one group session that she was having an affair with her supervisor at work. Lindsey had never revealed in the group that her husband and Kate's husband worked together. Lindsey could not resist discussing Kate's revelation with her husband, particularly because the two men were long-standing adversaries. She swore her husband to secrecy. Nonetheless, he shared this information with a confidante of his at work. Eventually, the rumor passed through the organization until eventually Kate's husband heard it. He was devastated not only about the fracture in his marriage but also about the humiliation at work. He promptly filed papers for divorce despite Kate's expressed willingness to give up her extramarital affair and work on the problems in her marriage.

In some cases, the harm may come not from the sharing of the members' issues but simply from a member being identified as a therapy patient:

Phil was walking down the street with other corporate executives when he encountered a fellow therapy group member, Ralph, after a ball game. Ralph stopped and engaged Phil in conversation about the game. Phil responded amiably but vaguely. One of Phil's companions responded to a humorous comment made by Ralph, and after a bit of a banter between them, the colleague said, "So how do you know Phil? Ralph reddened, obviously disarmed by the question, and anxiously blurted out, "Why, he's in my therapy group!" Weeks later, Phil learned that he would not receive a promotion for which he was a candidate. He always wondered whether his conservative colleagues were troubled by the revelation that he was in therapy.

The two vignettes highlight that violations in member-to-member confidentiality occur in different forms. In the first case, it was far more intentional than in the second case. The range of possibilities for how members might violate confidentiality has implications for how the therapist might create conditions in which such violations are less likely to occur.

In the discussion of risks, it was noted that not all risks the therapist might anticipate are ones that actually materialize in the group. The risk that members might violate confidentiality is one that has been subjected to empirical investigation. For example, Roback, Ochoa, Block, and Purdon (1992) surveyed 100 experienced group therapists about various aspects related to confidentiality, including confidentiality infractions by group members. They found that approximately half reported confidentiality violations at least once during their time of conducting groups. The most common type of violation was the identification of another group member to an outsider (as in the example of Phil and Ralph). The second most common was the discussion outside the group of another group member's sexual activity. In another study, Roback et al. (1996) surveyed group leaders from 33 rehabilitation centers providing services to chemically impaired physicians. The 51 respondents attested to knowledge of 303 incidents of confidentiality violations by members over their careers. Once again, the most common type of violation was inappropriate identification of a comember to an outsider followed by identification of a comember's substance abuse problem to family or friends. Such a violation is especially serious given the irrevocable damage it may cause to the group member.

Davis (1980) also surveyed group therapists and their members. He found that members of groups in which the therapist required member-to-member confidentiality (seven out of eight therapists responding), 42 percent of the group members felt that it was acceptable to disclose confidential information to a friend or family member. Thirty-eight percent admitted to actually having disclosed confidential material to a family member. For 24 percent of the members, this breach entailed revealing the identity of the person who was the subject of the disclosure.

PRACTICAL IMPLICATIONS: The empirical investigations of confidentiality suggest that the risk of the violation of confidentiality is significant. Consequently, it is apparent that informing prospective group members of the risk during the informed consent process is crucial. This risk should be discussed both verbally and in writing. Candidates should also be helped to see that a breach could have negative consequences. Both of these realizations may be difficult for the entering member to achieve. Early on, group members often fantasize that the therapist's control of the group is unlimited and absolute. Consistent with such a fantasy is an assumption that the therapist is capable of preventing violations of confidentiality. Furthermore, if a prospective member contemplates a violation, he or she may see as the most salient aspect of the situation the immediate consequences of the breach. For example, the individual may find most salient the shame that might be evoked by having his or her secrets shared. He or she may not envision the kinds of negative consequences endured by the victims of the violations in our vignettes.

However, merely warning prospective members of the risk is not enough. Because the risk is so significant, therapists must do everything they can to reduce the likelihood of violations in their groups. Five interventions are commonly used to discourage members from committing breaches.

Secure a commitment from the member before entering the group to observe confidentiality. Before obtaining the member's promise, the therapist should explain thoroughly what is entailed by this commitment. For example, the therapist may specify that the member may not talk about the business of the group, even with a close friend or significant other. Yet, the therapist may also permit the member to talk with his or her individual therapist about issues arriving with him or her while not identifying comembers. The therapist should indicate the expectation that confidentiality should be maintained after the group has ended, an important aspect of any confidentiality agreement given that postgroup breaches can be injurious to members. Some therapists turn discussion of confidentiality into process events. For example, they ask prospective group members to identify the person (e.g., friend, family member) they would be most tempted to share information about group members with, the nature of their relationship with the person they would tell, and the most likely topics (e.g., sexual acting out) that would be breached by that individual.

Specify the consequences of violations of confidentiality. Many therapists establish expulsion as a possible consequence of the violation. The therapist may wish to build in some flexibility so that he or she (possibly in concert with group members) can respond with a lesser sanction if it seems appropriate. For example, consider the instance of the group's discovery that a member made an inadvertent violation that resulted in no harm to the member whose confidence was broken except distress. Under these conditions, it may be sufficient for the therapist to encourage a very thoroughgoing discussion of the violation culminating in members' renewed commitment to observing this rule. If a member is asked to leave the group, the therapist's obligation to the patient remains. The therapist must not abandon the group member but must assist the departing member in getting his or her psychological needs met.

The therapist should inform the prospective member of any legal consequences of confidentiality violations. As noted by Roback et al. (1996), in two jurisdictions of the United States, members' breaking of confidentiality is against the law. The Illinois Mental Health and Disabilities Confidentiality Act (740ILCS110) is of a general nature in that it applies to any party who might hear information being given to a therapist by a patient. Hence, it covers group therapy by implication. In contrast, the District of Columbia has a law that explicitly outlaws confidentiality violations by group members (D.C. Law S 6–2002[b]). In the future, other jurisdictions may establish laws to protect group members from violations made by other members. In apprising entering members of the requirement to observe confidentiality, the therapist should discuss and put in writing any legal penalties in the jurisdiction that are associated with shared member disclosures (Kearney, 1984). Another potential consequence is that the member could be sued by another member who is harmed by the violation of confidentiality.

Provide regular reminders to the group members of the confidentiality rule (Slovenko, 1998). Group participants are unlikely to see their observance of confidentiality as a matter of any great importance if the therapist merely raises confidentiality before the member enters the group and never discusses it again. Two especially auspicious occasions for encouraging confidentiality discussions are when new members enter the group and when members happen to encounter one another outside of group. The latter is particularly useful because such occasions are opportunities for confidentiality violation. Members may talk, for instance, about their experience of a conflict between wanting to greet the other member and wanting to steer away from any behavior that might undermine confidentiality:

JOE: I saw you with your friends. I didn't even say "hi" because I was worried you'd have to explain who I am and how you know me.

MIKE: Yeah, it felt kind of weird. For a second I felt kind of rejected, but I realized later that you were just preventing an awkward situation from becoming even more awkward.

Following this exchange, the therapist might point out that a miscommunication about the rejection of one member by another can be cleared up in the group. A violation of confidentiality may not be capable of remedy. A benefit of such a discussion is that members can learn ways to negotiate unexpected encounters. Some populations may require even more frequent reminders. In this case, the therapist could review the group rules at the beginning of every session or have a sign-in sheet with the confidentiality reminder printed at the top (Bernstein & Hartsell, 1998). In all cases, the group should talk about out-of-group encounters before they occur and develop guidelines for handling them.

If confidentiality violations do occur, they should be explored thoroughly by the group regardless of what penalties are administered to the violating member. Roback et al. (1992) surveyed highly experienced group therapists on members' short-term reactions to confidentiality violations by other members. Among the major effects are anger toward the violator, diminished self-disclosure in the group, less cohesion, anger toward the therapist, dropouts, and greater resistance. Such phenomena would suggest that whether or not an infraction produces harm outside the group, it creates a major disruption within. A thorough discussion can underscore the unacceptability of the behavior but at the same time reinstate safety as members see they can approach this event with the same useful exploratory processes as they can any other. Indeed, Roback et al. (1992) found that in some cases, groups led by highly experienced therapists, while showing disturbing short-term effects, eventually moved to a higher level of cohesion.

The therapist should not violate confidentiality (Corey, 1995). Throughout this text, we have discussed the powerful effects of modeling on group behavior. While it may seem perfectly obvious that the therapist's behavior must be exemplary on this score, it should be also acknowledged that occasions will arise to tempt the therapist:

> *Dr. Ramkin's group met weekly on Wednesday evening. On Wednesday morning she came down with the flu. She dreaded the prospect of having to contact all eight members. She considered contacting four members and giving each the phone number of one other member. With the no-socialization rule of the group, members had never exchanged phone numbers. Dr. Ramkin rationalized that this was an emergency.*

In disseminating identifying information that members had not shared themselves, Dr. Ramkin was violating their confidentiality and thereby modeling behaviors at odds with the group rule.

Furthermore, members' calling other members might set the stage for further violations. For example, a member might leave a message such as "tell her that group therapy is canceled tonight" without knowing whether a roommate should be privy to such information.

COMMUNICATION WITH OTHER PROFESSIONALS: Members of therapy groups may receive mental health services from other professionals. For example, a group therapist may be seeing a person who is also being seen in individual therapy by another professional. The term for this arrangement is *concurrent therapy*. This format is discussed in Chapter 14 when it is contrasted with combined therapy, a format involving the same therapist across modalities. When treatment is provided by two or more therapists, the coordination typically requires them to communicate with one another. However, to do so the group therapist must secure in writing the consent (release of information) of the group member beforehand, possibly before the member enters the group. However, it may also occur at some point during the member's tenure of participation. For example, the group therapist may refer a member to a psychiatrist for a medication evaluation. Regardless of when the possibility for communication arises, the therapist should discuss with the member the kind of information that might be shared with the professional concurrently treating the member to avoid violating the member's expectations and thereby preserve trust in the therapeutic relationship. Table 9.2 defines key terms.

In some cases, group therapists operate under the supervision of another practitioner who has legal responsibility for the therapist's work. For example, two psychology interns may conduct a group in an outpatient clinic and report to a licensed psychologist for supervision.

Table 9.2   Key Terms and Definitions

Ethical Dilemma—A circumstance in which the evident courses of action are consistent with one or more ethical principles and inconsistent with another.

Confidentiality—An agreement in a professional situation that the communications of, or information about, the recipient of the service will not be shared outside of the situation.

Privileged Communication—A statutory right given to a group of people to prevent a witness from sharing information in a judicial proceeding.

Because these interns are not yet licensed to practice independently, their on-site psychologist assumes legal responsibility for their work. In this instance, the interns must reveal to each member prior to his or her group participation their trainee status, the fact of their receiving supervision, and the identity of the supervisor. The reason the supervisor must be identified is so that the group member can, if he or she wishes, have access to the supervisor. The prospective group member can also decline membership if he or she has a potentially conflicting relationship with the supervisor, for example, the group member is the supervisor's next-door neighbor.

Privileged Communication: Privilege refers to the statutory right given to a group of people (in our case, the therapy group member) to prevent a witness from sharing information about them in court testimony. In the individual therapy situation, privilege means that the patient has the right to prevent the therapist from disclosing confidential information in a judicial proceeding. Thus, in the therapist-patient relationship, it is the patient who possesses the privilege, not the therapist. While all states recognize some level of therapist-patient privilege (Shuman & Foote, 1999), the scope of the patient's privilege varies from state to state. For example, it may be limited to a certain class of practitioners, such as licensed professionals. It is crucial that the therapist know what privilege the patient has in his or her jurisdiction given the circumstances of the treatment so that the patient can be properly informed about any limits before treatment begins (Haas & Malouf, 2002).

Whether group members possess the privilege is a major question. Generally, the privilege is given to participants in dyadic relationships such as individual therapy. Courts have not tended to uphold privilege when a third party was present. As Slovenko (1998) notes, courts reason that privilege is nullified because communication of information to a third party is in essence communication to the world. If the world can be privy to information, so too should the courts. (For further reading on this topic, the reader might consult Chapter 9, "Group Therapy" in Slovenko's [1998] comprehensive text, *Psychotherapy and Confidentiality.*) Given that group therapy is a multiperson treatment, how privilege would fare when tested in the courts is uncertain, though the privilege of group therapy has been at issue in a few relevant cases.

In the well-known case of *State v. Andring*, the Minnesota Supreme Court upheld privilege in a case in which the session records were sought when a defendant was charged with criminal sexual behavior. Consistent with the thinking of legal commentator Charles McCormick (1972), the court saw the group members as integral to the treatment rather than casual spectators. The court also noted that excluding group therapy from the privilege would significantly limit its effectiveness: Without the guarantee that their communications would remain confidential, patients would be reluctant to make disclosures (Reisner, Slobogin, & Rai, 1999).[4]

While the court's reasoning in *State v. Andring* is likely to be compelling to group therapists, there is no guarantee that it would be so to the court of any particular jurisdiction. Therefore, it would behoove the group therapist to incorporate as part of the informed consent the fact that privilege has not been universally established as existing within the group therapy situation. To do so adequately will require some explanation by the therapist of how such situations might arise, particularly for a member who does not anticipate operating in any legal arena. For entering members who are in legal situations, knowing that their disclosures in a group may enter court proceedings (but only if the information is relevant to the case) could affect their decision on what disclosures they are willing to make. Once again, providing such information about risks helps maintain the member's autonomy.

The therapist can take steps to make it less likely that a member will have disclosures shared in a legal forum without consent. The therapist's records should be written in a way to protect the privacy of each group member. The notes about each group member should not refer to other members in a way that identifies them. Admittedly, this individual-centered approach may not be consistent with how some

---

[4] A similar line of argument led to the upholding of the privilege by an appellate court of California (*Farrell, L. v. Superior Court,* 1988 203 Cal. App. 3d 521). Few recent court decisions have specifically related to privileged communication and group therapy. The few that have been made have been unpublished and hence are likely to have limited impact on future rulings (i.e., Ballard, Personal Communication, May 22, 2001). This discussion should not be construed to suggest that issues concerning privilege never arise in dyadic therapy. Parties in litigation may attempt to bring therapy records of another party into legal proceedings regardless of the therapeutic modality. Whether the therapist-patient privilege holds depends upon a variety of factors including the evidentiary value of the sought-after clinical information (Shuman & Foote, 1999).

practitioners conceptualize a member's activity. The notes should be concise, relevant to treatment goals, and free of extraneous information. A second aspect of the effort to safeguard privilege is the therapist's response to a subpoena of a group member's records. If the member in question opposed the release of his or her records, it would be incumbent upon the therapist to assert the privilege, probably most effectively by obtaining the services of an attorney. Whether the therapist would be successful would depend on a variety of factors such as the nature of the case (e.g., Slovenko, 1998, suggests that privilege is less likely to be upheld in a personal injury case than a case concerning family matters and the jurisdiction in which therapy takes place). A third aspect is to allow the member to have the freedom to share information with the therapist that may not be shared with the group. In a survey of group therapists, Roback et al., (1992) found that when a member threatens harm to someone outside the group, 80 percent of group therapists will manage this situation not only through group sessions but also through individual sessions. Because such a threat may activate mandatory reporting requirements, such a communication has a prominent legal dimension.

Evaluation of Progress and Termination

Throughout, this text has cited outcome research showing that group members can benefit from group in a variety of ways. As discussed in the section on informed consent, a given prospective member cannot legitimately be told that he or she will definitely benefit from group participation. It is the therapist's responsibility to monitor whether group participation is benefiting each member. To aid in such monitoring, every therapist should develop means of assessing the impact of the group experience. Some may rely upon their own observations. Is the member exhibiting new social behaviors over the course of the sessions? Is the array of themes that the member is addressing broadening? Some therapists may incorporate standardized psychological measures of symptoms and other psychological phenomena (such as level of self-esteem) that are administered at regular intervals. Whatever methods are used should be linked to the member's goals for being in the group. For example, if the member entered because of a difficulty in expressing feelings such as anger, the therapist should monitor and document how anger is being addressed inside and also perhaps outside the group.

When a member is no longer profiting from group participation, that member should be encouraged to leave the group and, if necessary, seek assistance from another therapeutic venue whether another group or another modality altogether (Schoener & Luepker, 1996). While for therapists using any modality, terminating a patient can represent a financial hardship, for group therapists the cost may be especially great. In order for the group to possess sufficient interpersonal resources, there must be a critical mass. If the member's leaving pushes the group below that threshold, the therapist may feel exceedingly invested in safeguarding that member's presence. The therapist may also worry that one member's departure may inspire others to leave. The therapist should be aware of such apprehensions to avoid succumbing to them. At times other members may place pressure on a member to remain in the group. They may be motivated by their own fears that the group may disintegrate, their sheer liking of the member, or their perception that the member provides an important resource for the group. Members may exaggerate the risks the member is accepting in departing, the enormity of the work still to be accomplished, or the extent of the progress the member is currently making. Sometimes these efforts amount to coercion. At such times, the therapist has an ethical obligation to support the member in resisting excessive pressure to remain when the group has outlived its usefulness (Corey & Corey, 1997).

At times, members may feel that they are not benefiting from the group. They may believe that they have already accomplished the goals that brought them to the group or may feel that group therapy is not a place where effective work can be done. How should the therapist proceed if he or she disagrees? Where should the therapist's responses fall on the continuum of degree of encouragement to induce the member to remain? The ethical conflict that arises is between beneficence and autonomy. Beneficence is activated by therapist's desire to continue to make available a resource of potential usefulness to the member. Sometimes, a therapist can clearly see that the member has hit a temporary stumbling block that would be removed with continuing work or a narcissistic hurt that would dissipate with time. Beneficence is therefore served when the therapist and other group members share their observations with the member who is intending to depart. Autonomy is served when the therapist and hopefully even the members can see that it is ultimately the member's decision whether or not to remain in the group. Mullan (1987) notes that once the therapist has made a case for the potential merits of remaining in the group, "Contracts that force the patient to stay for a stated time or to give so many weeks notice before leaving or else forfeit a prepayment are all understandable, yet border upon the unethical" (1987, p. 412).

Technology and Group Therapy

Technology has long had a role in the delivery of mental health services. For example, the role of the telephone to deal with the emergency treatment of patients organized at the borderline level has been documented repeatedly (Jerome & Zaylor, 2000; Kaplan, 1977; Lindon, 1988). In recent years, more rapid advances in technology have radically broadened the spectrum of possibilities for using technology in delivering mental health services. Nichelson (1998) calls these new technology-based methods *telehealth*. He writes that telehealth is "the use of telecommunications and information technology to provide access to health assessment, diagnosis, intervention, consultation, supervision, education, and information across distance. *Behavioral telehealth* is simply the application of the same technology to provide behavioral health services" (p. 527).

Behavioral telehealth has begun to influence the practice of group therapy. Therapists may use software packages to administer, score, and interpret instruments used in the initial assessment of a prospective member. They may have members use software packages in completing homework assignments, file insurance claims electronically, or pose a question to a supervisor via e-mail (Janoff & Schoenholtz-Read, 1999).

While most of these applications are reasonably common, some are sufficiently new that as McMinn, Buchanan, Ellens, and Ryans (1999) note, "the dearth of systematic research on the ethics of technology in professional practice make it difficult to anticipate which technologies are creating ethical tensions, controversies, and dilemmas" (p. 165). Without such information, it is also difficult for disciplines and professional organizations to establish standards and guidelines, although some preliminary efforts have been made by such organizations as the American Psychological Association (1997) and the National Board for Certified Counselors (2000).

Even with these guidelines, the therapist entering cyberspace is traveling in largely uncharted territory (Weinberg, 2001).

The ethical principles and decision-making process described earlier in this chapter are of particular use when guidelines and standards are either vague or nonexistent. In considering some new application, the therapist would be well served to systematically and carefully determine whether it creates any ethical dilemmas, identify and weigh the ethical principles involved in the dilemma, identify courses of action that might resolve the conflict, and so on.

In many technology applications, many ethical dilemmas are likely to involve confidentiality. The difficulty of ensuring that member confidentiality is maintained may preclude the use of certain technologies. For example, Humphreys, Winzelberg, and Klaw (2000) consider whether online therapy groups can be ethically conducted. These authors appropriately distinguish online therapy groups from other types of electronic forums such as discussion groups and chat rooms. They outline the different ethical issues that arise for a mental health professional's involvement in each group format. They conclude that at present, the obstacles are major. Two of the problems concern confidentiality: (a) unless videoconferencing is used, there is no guarantee that the person who logs on is the group member and (b) once information is put out over the Internet, it may be accessible to people outside the group. A third problem these authors identify is that because online groups typically involve persons from a broad geographic area, the group therapist would have difficulty executing all of the responsibilities of group leadership. For example, assessing the member's appropriateness and intervening in emergencies might be extremely difficult with the geographically remote individual. Because of these problems, Humphreys et al. (2000) conclude that at present, conducting an online therapy group with the customary ethical safeguards would not be possible except in special circumstances. However, they do acknowledge that technological improvements such as improved encryption and procedural adjustments such as restricting the geographic area of group members may alter the ethical feasibility of online therapy groups. Ultimately, addressing the impediments to ethical online group therapy would be important given the potential of this medium to serve the needs of persons (e.g., the frail elderly) who cannot be transported to a therapy group. In this respect, online groups could ultimately accord well with the principle of beneficence.

The kind of analysis that Humphreys et al. (2000) conducted to determine the feasibility of online therapy groups is what group therapists must do with every new technology advance having potential relevance for this modality. As always, the therapist is likely to do a more effective analysis if he or she operates within a community of group therapists and consults with colleagues regularly to identify any blind spots in his or her understanding of the ethical and legal dimensions of a situation.

Summary

While the major mental health professions have ethical codes that guide decision making in conducting therapy groups, the group therapist is nonetheless likely to confront circumstances in which the correct course of action is not evident. In these circumstances, ethical principles appear to collide: Any given course of action consistent with one principle would seem to violate another. The practitioner is well served both by knowing ethical codes and the law in his or her specific jurisdiction and by having a method by which to resolve ethical dilemmas. This chapter presented one particular method or system, that of Haas and Malouf (2002), in its application to a group therapy situation.

The particular areas of ethical concern were discussed. The first area, competence, was discussed as the sine qua non of all ethical action. The multiple components of competence, such as knowledge of theory, technical skills, self-awareness, and emotional maturity, were outlined. Also described were some of the ways these components can be achieved, such as formal academic training, participation in experimental groups, supervision, and personal therapy.

The second topic was informed consent. The elements of adequate informed consent were described. Among these are the likely benefits and risks of group participation as well as the methods used in the groups. However, it was noted that informed consent should be tailored not only to specific groups but to individual group members. The format of the informed consent, written versus oral, was also considered. Finally, the informed-consent obligation of the group therapist when the group member's participation is not voluntary was discussed.

The third area was that of confidentiality and privilege. In group therapy, it was stressed, the therapist cannot guarantee confidentiality. While there is much the therapist can do to discourage member-to-member violations, there is nothing the therapist can do to prevent absolutely such violations. This description of limitations on confidentiality should be a component of informed consent. Testimonial privilege, or the right to protect one's records from use in a court of law, poses a special problem for group therapy members. Typically, privilege has not extended to circumstances in which a patient has communicated to a professional in the presence of a third party. The fact that the third party is critical to the delivery of treatment may provide a compelling basis for the court to uphold the privilege, but prospective group members must nonetheless be informed about the possible limits of privilege.

The fourth topic, evaluation of progress and termination, covered the therapist's obligation to monitor continually each group member's progress. When group therapy is no longer benefiting a member, an alternate plan should be developed in collaboration with that member.

The final topic, technology and group therapy, brings the group practitioner into territory that is relatively uncharted from a legal and ethical perspective. The group practitioner contemplating the use of technology to enhance his or her group would be well advised to identify any ethical dilemmas involved and to resolve them through a systematic decision-making process. Particular attention should be given to any ways technology may compromise confidentiality.

MODELS OF
GROUP THERAPY

Interpersonal Model

In the next four chapters, the reader is introduced to four different theoretical approaches to conducting groups. Certainly there are many others that I might have chosen. The selection of the particular approaches featured was based on several factors. These approaches contrast considerably with one another in the goals of the models and the interventions that can be used to pursue these goals. Second, they are models that have achieved some level of popularity as reflected by their presence in the literature. Third, they are approaches with fairly wide application in terms of the clinical populations and the venue of the group. At the same time, the models differ in the typical length of the member's participation within the group. For example, whereas the object relations model has tended to be used in longer term group experiences, the cognitive behavioral and problem-solving approaches are often used in relatively brief time frames. The juxtaposition of these models enables a discussion of the important variable of time as it relates to goals and methods.

Through the presentation of the four models, I hope to illustrate a point made in Chapter 2: Therapy groups can be used in the pursuit of a range of goals. The reader also has an opportunity to see how the therapeutic factors unique to this modality can be activated within a variety of group formats. Finally, the reader sees how his or her role as therapist would both change and remain as he or she moved from model to model.

The description of the theoretical approaches follows a recursive outline to enhance the reader's appreciation of similarities and differences between and among the approaches. The first step is a discussion of the goals of the approach. The immediate and ultimate goals may vary for some models. In the second step, the mechanisms identified to instigate change in group members and the therapist interventions used to activate these mechanisms are outlined.

For the reader to see these processes and interventions in action, a vignette is provided. It is important for the reader to understand that in the vignettes, events unfold at a somewhat brisker pace than is characteristic of groups in actual practice. This compactness, typical in textbook and video presentations, enables the student to see the processes with greater clarity than would be the case in a more plodding but realistic depiction. The essential point is that the student should not be discouraged if his or her groups move more slowly than the ones in this chapter.

For approaches that have been developed in a relatively long-term time frame, short-term applications are discussed. The final step is a consideration of the status of the research on the approach. Whether the approach has been demonstrated to be effective and under what conditions is considered. The fifth step, related to the fourth, is the circumstances under which the approach can be used most effectively. At the end of each chapter, references are supplied for the reader who wishes to explore further a given approach. Each of these approaches should be applied to groups only under the supervision of a practitioner who has achieved competence with a particular approach.

Above all, it is hoped that through this survey of four approaches, the reader obtains a glimmering of the richness of this modality. The diversity of approaches enables its application to a wide range of populations, problems, and situations. But amid this diversity, there is unity. There are features that all of these approaches share, features that the reader finds in any effective application of this modality. We talk about these common features upon presentation of the approaches.

Aaron, a 26-year-old man, was referred to a group therapist, Dr. Johnson, by his family physician. This physician told Dr. Johnson that Aaron, whom the physician had seen for six years, had recently presented to him a variety of somatic complaints. He said Aaron had admitted that he had had a number of romantic disappointments and wondered if these developments might not be connected to his physical symptoms.

Dr. Johnson interviewed Aaron and discovered several areas of difficulty. Aaron talked about his puzzlement over a pattern in his romantic relationships with women. Early on, he reported, his experience seemed very positive with the woman in whom he was interested. However, after several months he would sense that she was growing impatient with him and bored in the relationship. Eventually, much to his disappointment and dismay, she would end her involvement with him.

In other areas of his life, Aaron saw himself to be less than successful and fulfilled. He was a dentist in a solo practice. He employed a dental assistant and an office manager. He felt dominated by the office manager, who dictated to him how to run his practice. At times she established office policies with which he silently disagreed. However, he could never even consider terminating her employment, because he needed a highly assertive person like her to negotiate with difficult patients and the insurance companies.

Aaron's attitude toward his parents was one of filial duty. While he strove to fulfill what he saw as his many obligations to them, he derived minimal enjoyment from the relationship. He resented his parents for their intrusiveness. For example, his mother had keys to his condominium and recently had been leaving on his kitchen table the names of physicians other than the one who had referred him to Dr. Johnson because she felt that he was not identifying the malady responsible for Aaron's somatic complaints. Aaron had made some futile efforts to get his parents to respect his privacy but in the face of their noncooperation had never considered changing his locks.

Goals of the Interpersonal Approach

To understand how a group run within the interpersonal approach might help Aaron, it is first necessary to know a bit about the history of the interpersonal approach and how psychological difficulties are understood within it. As the reader will see, the interpersonal approach comprehends a group of models that are adapted to a range of clinical situations. For example, whereas early applications were developed especially for long-term groups, more recent applications have been for the time-limited situation (e.g., Yalom, 1983). Interpersonal models have been created for different clinical venues—for example, inpatient versus outpatient—and different populations—for example, low functioning versus high functioning.

Contributions of Sullivan

All of these applications owe a debt of gratitude to Harry Stack Sullivan, the father of the interpersonal approach. He held that at the most fundamental level a psychological problem is a problem a person has with others in his or her life. Psychopathology is invariably an interpersonal matter. Even those symptoms that do not seem to be inherently social will ultimately be found to have an interpersonal underpinning. For example, in Aaron's case, once any medical explanation was ruled out, the hypothesis could be considered that the basis was psychological, and even more specifically, social.

Sullivan sees development of personality as emerging from the individual's negotiation between the core tendencies to achieve satisfaction and security. These tendencies can and do come in conflict with one another (Maddi, 1972). For example, a person who relentlessly pursues power may achieve a certain level of satisfaction but may also risk the disapproval of others, thereby creating insecurity. Therefore, the lifelong task of the person is to negotiate between these potentially competing impulses to find modes of interaction that maximize satisfaction while minimizing insecurity.

Early in life, the capacity to negotiate between these forces depends, at least in part, on the social environment itself. When the extremely young child receives parental responses that are more disapproving than affirming, a sense of insecurity is evoked. To lessen the insecurity, the child uses a defensive maneuver. One especially important maneuver is the *parataxic distortion.* Parataxic thinking is a characteristic mode of cognition in early childhood when symbols are used in a personal, arbitrary way that does not take into account the perceptions of others. An undue arousal of insecurity leads to the persistence of this immature form of thinking in later life because it enables the individual to defend against aspects of reality that might be disturbing. By ignoring these aspects through what Sullivan termed a parataxic distortion, the individual achieves a sense of security. Yet, the social behaviors attached to his or her parataxic distortions are likely to be ineffective because they are not planned with a sufficient appreciation of others' experiences. Therefore, while the parataxic distortions may bring some measure of security, they do so at the cost of satisfaction or fulfillment in relationships with others.

Aaron, for example, might incorrectly perceive the women in his life as requiring his rather complete accommodation of their needs in order to secure their interest. This perception may be accentuated in longer, more intimate relationships. Aaron's perception is distorted in that it does not take into account any information from his partner suggesting that she would want him to function as an equal partner in the relationship. In Aaron's case, the origin of the parataxic distortion may be a tyrannical parent who insisted on submissive behavior as a condition of affection. By seeing the woman with whom he is romantically involved as being like this parent, Aaron may beget the behavior he expects. That is, in acting in a compliant fashion, he may evoke in his partner an impulse to take charge. However, this oblivion to his partner's needs would likely also evoke considerable hostility (Yalom, 1995).

What might be helpful to Aaron to increase his capacity to have satisfying relationships? It would be beneficial for Aaron to know how he was misperceiving women's needs. His recognition that his passivity induced alienation rather than closeness would be a first step in broadening his behaviors in intimate relationships. This process of comparing his perceptions to those of others is one of *consensual validation*. It involves not so much discarding one's perspective as expanding it by incorporating the views of others. Sullivan noted, however, that typically the identification of a parataxic distortion "is attended by a sharp fall in the patient's feeling of security" (1953, p. 235). However, the benefit of this momentary loss of security is ultimately that the patient "as known to himself is much the same patient behaving with others" (p. 237).

Sullivan laid the theoretical foundation for the interpersonal approach to group therapy because he emphasized the criticalness of the interpersonal dimension of symptoms and psychological problems and the use of the interpersonal context to alleviate them. In short, his position was that at root, psychological problems are problems with other people. It follows quite naturally, then, that to treat them, other people are required.

Other early contributors to the interpersonal approach provided a suggestion of how such interpersonal problems could be addressed. Jacob Moreno, the father of psychodrama, believed that early familial conflicts should be brought into the present through their dramatic enactment. As noted in Chapter 4, Moreno coined the term "here-and-now," which emphasizes the power of group process to produce psychological change. Although psychodrama has developed as an action-oriented approach to groups in its own right, the influence of Moreno's ideas on group therapy in general and the interpersonal approach specifically has been considerable.

If Moreno emphasized the usefulness of group process, Kurt Lewin pointed to a way the group process could be used. Lewin, a social psychologist whose work was discussed in Chapter 4, identified the phenomenon of feedback, in which individuals have the opportunity to discover how they appear to others in the group based upon their behavior during the group itself. As Yalom (1995) noted, "Feedback . . . was found to be most effective when it stemmed from here-and-now observations, when it followed the generating event as closely as possible, and when the recipient checked with the other group members to establish its validity and reduce perceptual distortion" (p. 488). Notice how feedback is precisely what Sullivan saw as necessary to correct parataxic distortions.

While there are a number of other important contributions to the interpersonal approach such as those of Jerome Frank (Frank & Frank, 1991), we now have enough of a conceptual foundation to consider the one person whose contribution to the interpersonal approach specifically and group therapy in general is monumental. This person is Irvin Yalom, whose contributions have been discussed throughout this book. For example, in Chapter 1 we discussed how across different theoretical approaches, group therapy must capitalize upon those processes that are unique to this modality to be maximally effective. Yalom's contribution to identifying those processes is inestimable. At this same time, Yalom developed a specific theoretical approach to conducting therapy that has enormous popularity and, as noted earlier, a wide range of application.

The goal of the interpersonal approach flows directly from Sullivan's position that psychopathology invariably has roots in interpersonal difficulties. Regardless of the nature of the symptomatic presentation, whether it is clearly interpersonal or otherwise, any effective treatment is going to require that the individual's capacity to have fulfilling relationships be enhanced. This objective is the overarching goal of any interpersonal group: to enable the individual to acquire behaviors that will further rather than hinder relationships.

The particular interpersonal goal selected for an individual depends on many factors, including the context of treatment. For example, in the inpatient setting it is not uncommon for individuals to exhibit a high level of withdrawal that can limit the potency of any modality. In this setting, an appropriate interpersonal goal is to foster greater openness to relationships (Yalom, 1983) through the experience of nonthreatening, rewarding interactions in the inpatient group. In a long-term outpatient group, the goals will be likely to have a more specific character based upon whatever have been the individual's long-standing difficulties with others. For example, in a videotape in which Yalom (1990) demonstrates the interpersonal approach, one group member shows a tendency to exhibit condescension and intellectualization when other members express strong emotion. This automatic response was extremely off-putting and interfered with his wish to have closer relationships with others. The goal for him, then, would be to acquire more sensitive, relationship-forwarding responses when feelings arise.

While the primary target of change in an interpersonal approach is by definition relational, the presumption is that positive change in the interpersonal arena can beget positive changes in other realms. Consider once again Aaron's case: In an interpersonal group the goal would be for Aaron to learn about and modify behaviors that are a detriment to his having successful relationships. Yet, one might expect that as Aaron's relationships with women, his parents, and his coworkers improved, the physical complaints that brought him into treatment would lessen. This latter positive change would occur because of the linkage between the interpersonal problems and the other psychologically based difficulties in a person's life.

Change Processes

How might Aaron manage to increase his perceptiveness of himself and others and expand his repertoire of behaviors so that he could enjoy more lasting intimate relationships, greater assertiveness in his work setting, and greater independence in his relationship with his parents? What processes might be deployed to move him toward his goals?

The Importance of Focusing on the Here-and-Now

The reader may recall that Chapter 4 described a variety of therapeutic mechanisms that can be used in the group context. For any interpersonal approach, the therapeutic mechanism par excellence is interpersonal learning. As noted in that chapter, the condition of interpersonal learning is that the group resides within the here-and-now. That is, members must be engaged with their immediate interactions with one another. As Vinogradov and Yalom (1989) noted:

> By directly focusing upon the here-and-now, the leader engages the active participation of members, and in so doing maximizes the power and efficiency of the group. The therapist emphasizes to the group that the most important transactions are the ones occurring in the group room, under the eyes of each and every member. (p. 84)

Yet, on their own members are likely to avoid the here-and-now, occupying themselves with matters external to the group. For example, Aaron might feel a greater willingness to talk about being annoyed with his mother's intrusive entries into his apartment than a member's penetrating invasions into his emotional life.

To understand why such avoidance occurs, we must first appreciate the two potential dimensions of the here-and-now: the activation of affect and the group's doubling back upon itself to process its own activity (Yalom, 1995). Processing involves the group's examination of how members interact with one another and the reasons for their doing so. A process focus is to be distinguished from a content focus, which concerns what is said. For example, if Aaron describes his date with a woman, the content is his description of the event. A process discussion might be an exploration of how Aaron narrated the event to the group.

Yalom (1975), citing an unpublished essay by Miles, notes that for a variety of reasons a process focus in the here-and-now tends to feel far less safe than a content focus on matters external to the group. First, process comments tend to be associated with the criticism of early authority figures. For example, Aaron may associate members' comments about how he relates to them as reminiscent of his parents' expressions of dissatisfaction with his behavior. Such associations are likely to be accompanied by anxiety.

A second factor that Yalom cites is the social taboo against process commentary. Imagine a business meeting in which participants are discussing company sales. Members suggest different solutions for slumping sales. Imagine that one of the participants says to another, "Will you stop jumping down everyone's throat when they give a solution that's different from yours?" With the group's shift from content to process the tension in the group is likely to rise sharply. Members also now realize that their different behavioral styles are being monitored. Members are no longer free to act as they will but now feel a self-consciousness borne out of an awareness of being observed. Process comments belie the rude reality that we are not oblivious to one another.

But in addition to uncomfortable self-awareness, the participants in the committee are also likely to wait with bated breath to see how the confronted member responds. Will this member respond in anger? The fear of retaliation is often a component of people's anxiety about processing their interactions.

Finally, Yalom correctly points out that within a system, the possibility of participants reciprocally commenting on one another's behavior, including that of authority figures, works against the maintenance of the current authority structure. Comments on a leader's behavior, particularly when opinions are shared by a substantial subset of the group, place pressure on the leader to be responsive to group perceptions. Leaders have far greater freedom to behave as they will when they are not accountable to those they lead. Consequently, a member of any group who makes a process comment, especially when such comments are not a well-established part of the group culture, is challenging the leader of the group and thereby takes on any consequences that accrue from such a challenge.

A primary task for the therapist of many types of groups but most intensively and consistently groups run within an interpersonal approach is to help members set aside their understandably self-protective avoidance of the here-and-now. The interpersonal therapist works to support members in immersing themselves as fully as possible in the here-and-now in order to realize the goals of improving their capacities to relate to others.

Techniques for Activating the Here-and-Now

From the moment the therapist first begins to discuss the possibility of group therapy with a group member to the member's last session, the therapist is fully engaged in keeping the here-and-now focus alive in the group.

Pregroup Preparation: For all the reasons described earlier concerning why people in general avoid the here-and-now, a prospective member is likely to harbor the expectation that the group will focus on external topics such as the presenting problems that brought members to the group. For members who are entering a new group together, all with the strong expectation that the group will have an outward focus, the therapist is likely to face an uphill battle in shifting members to an intergroup focus. Members may be stalwart in their unified resistance to this move! On the other hand, an individual entering an ongoing group is likely to be confused by the group's discussion of its own process. For example, I can remember how startled a member was when the group he joined spent four sessions talking about the implications and meanings of members greeting and updating each other in the minutes prior to each session. From this member's perspective the members were absorbed in trivialities. Probably, I failed to prepare my new member sufficiently for the group experience.

Methods of preparation should be tailored to the characteristics of the population from which members are drawn. When members have a high level of psychological mindedness, the preparation may consist primarily in developing a rationale for why the here-and-now is important. For members who may have greater difficulty envisioning a here-and-now process focus, the feedback process should be demonstrated, perhaps through a videotape, and prospective members should be given the opportunity to practice the kinds of feedback statements that would be made in the here-and-now.

Getting the Group off to a Here-and-Now Start: Early group behavior is important because such behavior begins to shape the norms of the group. Because the therapist seeks to have established as normative the group's focus on the here-and-now, he or she should influence members from the very first session to live within the here-and-now of the group.

Yalom (1990) provides an example in his outpatient videotape of how the therapist might move the group in a here-and-now direction. During the first session, the group members were talking about their various concerns that led them to join the group. When the group was almost over, Yalom noted that as the session had been proceeding, members were doubtlessly forming first impressions of one another. He then encourages them to share them with one another. Of course, such an invitation creates potential for the members to share views that are other than favorable.

Morran, Stockton, Cline, and Teed (1998) suggest that members be given opportunities to share their apprehensions about giving and receiving feedback within the here-and-now. Many of the fears that impede members from delving into their experiences with one another can be lessened by recognizing that these fears are shared.

Continuing to Nurture the Here-and-Now: Once members have been oriented to the here-and-now, the therapist must work to keep the group in this domain. Particularly when tensions arise in the group, members are likely to be tempted to flee from them into the relative safety of the there-and-then. Various types of interventions can be used to shift the focus of the group. The following is a sampling of such interventions.

Find in-group analogues to external problems (Vinogradov & Yalom, 1989). As members describe problems arising for them outside the group, the therapist should seek parallels within the group:

> *Aaron enters the group, and in response to another member's observation that he seems despondent, he shares that he had a conversation with a woman immediately prior to the session. He had made a general inquiry about the possibility of their getting together in the next several weeks. She indicated that she would be occupied with various activities in the foreseeable future. Aaron felt that she had dismissed him but hadn't shown him the respect to say directly to him that she wasn't interested in him. The therapist said, "You're describing someone rejecting you but doing so without acknowledging it. I'm wondering if there has ever been a moment in the group when you've had that experience."*

In seeking parallels, the therapist may wish to allow members to develop a theme before bringing the members back into the here-and-now. The reasons for doing so is that the therapist can develop a more articulated hypothesis about what interpersonal issues may be being avoided:

> *Paula, Stewart, and Brittany were in agreement over their displeasure with their coworkers. While their situations varied widely, a commonality was a sense of competition with a person who seemed to have an unfair advantage— the boss's daughter, the good-looking person who offered no substance, the one most able to appear to be doing work while remaining indolent. They saw*

themselves as sharing a sense of being unappreciated and unrewarded by their other coworkers. As they talked, it occurred to the therapist that something similar had been happening in group. A new member had been holding the group's rapt attention by relating a tale of woes. While this member was using the group as an audience, she wasn't doing any work. At the same time, the older members of the group who were entering the sessions with more of a commitment to work were being passed over.

The therapist said, "Possibly in here you haven't received a fair shake either. But at the same time, it may be like work, you haven't felt able to do anything about it."

With an air of relief, the group members talked about resenting the new member for monopolizing the sessions yet feeling that with all of her troubles, interrupting her would intensify her anguish. The member laughed and said she was wondering why everyone let her talk on and on and why no one else had much to say.

Interpersonal therapists vary in the extent to which they allow members to remain outside of the here-and-now. In this case, the therapist permitted the group to focus internally long enough for a theme to emerge. An advantage of doing so is that members can see more clearly connections between interpersonal issues emerging within the group and those outside. In fact, there is empirical evidence (Flowers & Booraem, 1990a, 1990b) that by making bridging comments linking members' behaviors in their everyday environment, positive outcomes can be augmented.

Focus on nonverbal behavior. As members are talking about events and people outside of the group, the therapist might draw attention to their nonverbal behaviors. Such behaviors may convey information about members' reactions to the immediate situation:

Isaiah was a member of a group of homeless persons in an urban clinic. He was a long-standing group member whose gruff candor was endearing to other members. Isaiah, in the present session, had returned after a 3-week hiatus due to his hospitalization. Isaiah had been sleeping in a park when he was attacked by a gang. The beating was very severe but was interrupted after a passerby summoned the police. When group members first learned about the assault, Isaiah was in intensive care and members feared for his life. Upon his return, they quizzed him on the details of the event. They were spellbound as Isaiah related the sequence of events.

The therapist said, "As Isaiah has been talking, we have had our eyes glued upon him. And several members teared up at many points." Members went on to express their past terror that they would lose Isaiah, terror that they relived as he narrated his experiences, but also their joy at his return. The tears apparently contained many unarticulated feelings that became more evident to members following the therapist's comment. Isaiah, listening to these expressions said, "I wouldn't have imagined that anyone would be thinking of me."

Nonverbal behavior is a conduit to the present because it is subject to less conscious self-monitoring than verbal behavior. Members are often unaware of how their immediate reactions play upon their faces and body postures. As such, these behaviors are an artesian well of information for the therapist about what members may be feeling about the proceedings of the group.

Make structural comments. As group members are focusing on topics outside the group, the therapist can comment on the process of the interaction and encourage members to articulate their reactions to it:

Two members were talking with animation about their difficulties with their husbands. Other members sat silently with some looking distracted and the others looking bored. The therapist said, "There seems to be a real divide in the group right now between those who can pursue this topic with zest and others who seem to be elsewhere. How does it feel to have this divide right now?"

In this same interaction, the therapist may not wish to emphasize the varying levels of engagement but rather the two members' degree of connection with one another. The therapist might say, "What do members observe about how Harriet and Tammy are relating to one another?" Perhaps for either Harriet or Tammy this level of engagement is unusual; recognizing the shift might enable an awareness of their own progress in the group.

Understanding the Here-and-Now: As members work within the here-and-now, the therapeutic mechanism being displayed is interpersonal learning. As noted in Chapter 4, two sequentially emerging elements are critical for interpersonal learning to occur. The first is the experiential affective element. Many of the interventions outlined in the preceding section would have the effect of stirring up affect. For example, the therapist's focus on the nonverbal behavior accompanying the assault of Isaiah brought to the surface feelings of joy and relief. However, affect is not sufficient for learning to occur about oneself in relation to others. The other essential element is understanding, and it is achieved by processing the data that emerges from the affective exchanges among members. As Yalom (1993) notes, "The group must examine itself, it must study its own transactions, it must become self-reflective and examine what has just occurred in the group" (p. 180).

Just as activating the here-and-now requires the therapist's possession of a set of interventions, so too does the understanding or illumination of process. The interventions are driven for the therapist's goals for members during this phase. Keep in mind that the overarching goal is to have an individual learn to relate to others in a way that is likely to be more fulfilling than when he or she entered the group. Certainly a member cannot change unless he or she is aware of what needs to be changed. The initial step is for a member to become aware of what his or her social behaviors are. For example, Aaron in the opening vignette of this chapter is unlikely to have a comprehensive and detailed view of how he is seen by others in his life. This is so both because it is inherently difficult for us to see ourselves from other than our own perspective and in areas of interpersonal inefficacy we are particularly likely to have blind spots. So a first order of business is for Aaron to get feedback on how he appears to others. Presumably, this occasion is not Aaron's first opportunity to obtain feedback on his interpersonal style. The research has resoundingly shown that in the initial period of group participation positive feedback is more useful to members (Morran et al., 1998). Therefore, Aaron is far more likely to accept the corrective feedback Susan is ready to give if it has been preceded (in earlier sessions or even better, earlier in that session) by positive feedback.

To be useful, the feedback should have several properties. First, it should be stated in simple, clear terminology rather than jargon (Leszcz, 1992). Second, it should be based upon the person's recent behavior within the group. Third, it should be attached to the emotional reaction of the feedback provider. For Aaron to know he fails to express preferences when the group is faced with a decision is not

Table 10.1 **Characteristics of Useful Feedback**

1. Concrete, or descriptive of specific interpersonal behaviors
2. Immediate, or referencing behaviors within the here-and-now, preferably shortly after these behaviors occur
3. Simple and clear, without jargon
4. Tied to the affective response of the feedback donor
5. Inclusive of behaviors that evoke both positive and negative affective responses

especially enlightening unless he also knows how others react to this behavior. Because the problematic behavior is often rooted in a parataxic distortion, the individual may have some incorrect assumptions about others' responses to his behavior.

Table 10.1 summarizes the characteristics of useful feedback.

Aaron may incorrectly believe that unfailingly acquiescing behaviors make him likable to others. In actual practice, the affect is likely to enter the here-and-now first:

SUSAN: The therapist is giving us the option of whether to bring the new member in in five or six weeks. Just about everyone has said something, but, Aaron, you just sit there. It makes me sick when you're so passive.
THERAPIST: Makes you sick? Could you be more specific?
SUSAN: Makes me really irritated.

At this point, the first stage of interpersonal learning has occurred. Affect has been engaged and Aaron knows what the member's affect toward him is. However, if the exploration were to stop here, it might be more of a negative experience for Aaron than otherwise.

To enable the feedback to be productive, specificity should be encouraged:

THERAPIST: Susan, I'm wondering if you can figure out what precisely Aaron is doing when you notice yourself getting irritated with him. Is it just that he's not saying anything? There are several others here who haven't said much about this issue, but you seem more keyed into what Aaron is doing.

SUSAN: That's true—it's not that he is sitting there. It's the way he nods his head that bothers me. . . . He will—

THERAPIST: [interrupting] Can you speak to Aaron directly?

SUSAN: Right . . . Aaron, you nod your head when people who come down on different sides of the issue speak. I mean, how could both be making so much sense to you when they disagree?

AARON: Well, maybe I agree with both. I mean, couldn't they both have a point?

SUSAN: If I thought that's what was going on, I probably wouldn't get so annoyed with you. If it were, you might say, "Well, I agree with Mike on this score but Todd has a point on this aspect." It seems as though you're trying to please people. It's almost as if when you nod your head, you're saying "I'll support you. Now like me back."

TODD: Hey, let's admit it: we all want to be liked. But the problem is, Aaron, that when I talk and you nod your head, I don't necessarily take it that you really agree with me. In fact, Aaron, I have a hard time knowing what you think on any given topic. You're so agreeable that I find myself believing that underneath, you're having a lot of reactions that are very different from the ones you're showing to us.

Let us return to the therapist's initial effort to encourage Susan to be more specific. Her original expression of vexation had the quality of an affective release. That is, her effort was more to show her annoyance rather than to support Aaron's learning about his interpersonal style. However, the therapist's entreaty to her to give more detail effected a shift in her from an affective to a more reflective mode of work. Susan now had to refine her observations to aid Aaron in increasing his self-awareness. This refinement process is beneficial both for the recipient of the feedback and the deliverer.

The recipient of the feedback benefits in two ways. First, as research has shown, the information is more useful when it is reasonably concrete (Morran, Stockton, & Harris, 1991). From this exchange Aaron can monitor whether his head nodding reflects his actual agreement with the speaker's position, a yearning to curry the speaker's favor, or both. Second, a very clear communication of what behaviors are off-putting or problematic in some other way is an antidote to a pervasive feeling of worthlessness. Rather than feeling a global sense of social inadequacy, the member recognizes specific, troublesome patterns of interaction that can be changed.

The purveyor of the feedback benefits, too, from acquiring the skill of sharpening his or her perceptions. For example, in the preceding exchange Susan realized that her initial account was less than precise. By recognizing the need to refine her observations, Susan strengthens her ability to work out conflicts with others, given that an essential element of effective conflict resolution is each party's possession of reliable information. In this instance Aaron is far less likely to act in a way that is irksome to her once he realizes that the offensive behavior is not his silence but his favor-currying. The provider of the feedback also benefits by learning to state potentially upsetting information in a tactful, sensitive way. This skill can be further cultivated by having the feedback provider reflect upon the success of the communication (Morran et al., 1998). In this case the therapist might say, "Susan, did you feel you were able to share your observations with Aaron in a way that was useful to him?"

One special consideration arises in relation to the feedback Susan provided Aaron. Susan did not merely describe Aaron's head nodding. She also interpreted the motive underlying the behavior, which was to secure others' favor. Which type of statement is likely to be more beneficial to Aaron—the description of behavior or the identification of possible motives? As discussed in Chapter 4, Flowers and Booraem (1990a) looked at these types of interventions and found that group members who frequently received a description of their behavioral patterns and information about others' reactions to them showed improvement over the course of the group, while members who frequently received statements about motives showed an intensification in symptomotology.[1] Similarly, in a preadolescent counseling group, interpretations (defined as statements that explain behavior) led to nonproductive responses (e.g., resistive reactions); feedback ("a direct and honest personal reaction to another person based on observational behavior") led to productive responses such as insight (Shectman & Yanov, 2001).

---

[1] Flowers and Booraem's (1990a) study was a naturalistic one. The interventions were not planned for the purpose of the study but were observed and categorized as they occurred. A question is whether those members who received a given type of intervention more abundantly were distinguished from others in some way. If so, the outcome may be the result of these member characteristics rather than the type of intervention per se.

Do these results mean that motive interpretations have no use? Viewing one of the videotapes in which Yalom functions as the therapist provides opportunities to see a number of effective uses of motive interpretation. In the inpatient videotape, Yalom worked with a male adolescent who exhibited a variety of alienatingly disruptive behaviors. At one point, Yalom makes an interpretation that all of these behaviors may be misguided attempts to connect with others. The interpretation appeared to have a twofold effect that was wholly positive. The member became less disruptive, and the other group members showed more compassion for and sensitivity toward him.

As Flowers and Booraem (1990a) note, interpretations of motives do have great power to stimulate anxiety, and therefore they must be used with some care. In weighing whether or not to make an interpretation about motive or encouraging members to make them, several questions must be asked. First, how is this motive likely to be regarded by the recipient? The interpretations that are likely to have the greatest power to evoke distress are those imputing motives that most people would judge to be negative in some respect. In the example of Yalom's interpretation, a motive was suggested that most would consider healthy and positive: wanting to connect with others. To some extent, how the motive is regarded depends upon how an interpretation is delivered. In the study cited earlier, Shechtman and Yanov (2001) found that interpretations delivered in a supportive way are more likely to lead to productive group behaviors than interpretations expressed in a critical tone. Second, how readily will the person recognize the presence of a motive? Inferences about motives of which a person is unaware often have great potential to be disorganizing because the information cannot readily be integrated into the person's sense of self. Third, to what extent are others likely to identify with the motive? In long-term groups in which members may have come to recognize in themselves and others a whole array of motivational forces, members are more likely to have others resonate with their concerns, known or discovered. What is especially distressing for a member is to have a motive identified that then seems to separate him or her from other members of the group.

The interpretation of and speculation about motives is a natural component of human activity. Members become interested in one another's motives because motives drive behavior. Indeed, for the father of the interpersonal approach, Harry Stack Sullivan, the consideration of motives, conscious and unconscious, is at the center of understanding how personality develops. Rather than discouraging interpretation of motives, the interpersonal therapist should intervene to ensure that such interpretations are maximally useful.

In summary, in the processing phase of here-and-now explorations, the therapist should help members identify patterns in one another and link a member's patterns with the reactions they induce in other members. In some cases the individual can be assisted in recognizing the motives that may be underlying behavioral patterns.

Mass Group Process Commentary

Interpersonal therapists generally accept the notion that all forces that emerge within the group affect the group's work. An example of such a force or phenomenon is group cohesion. The interpersonal therapist will work vigorously to promote cohesion by, for example, providing continuity between sessions, discouraging tardiness and absences, creating a safe environment for self-disclosure and constructive conflict resolution, and so on. Hence, although the interpersonal group therapist may focus on an individual or dyad, he or she will always keep the entire group in mind.

At times, the interpersonal therapist will foster a group's exploration of some phenomenon occurring within the entire group. In most instances, the therapist does so because the phenomenon at issue is impeding the group's work (Leszcz, 1992):

> *Members of the group had been responding in a listless fashion. While this mature group had ordinarily dwelled within the here-and-now, recently the group had had a curious focus upon external events in members' lives. Yet, even this focus, while persistent, was half-hearted.*
>
> *The therapist was puzzled and had no good hypothesis about the concerns that might have prompted the shift in behavior. Nonetheless, he felt that the group was in a flight pattern. He revealed to the group both his impression that they were avoiding something in the group and his uncertainty about what that might be. He saw two members exchange a meaningful look, and he began to suspect that the avoidance was conscious.*
>
> *The therapist said, "This group has addressed many difficult issues in the past and I'm certain we can do so again."*

One of the members who had exchanged glances with another member spoke up. "I think it's hard for us to get into what we're avoiding because we know something that, well, is none of our business."

The therapist looked puzzled. There was a strained silence. A member said, "We heard something about your health . . . not being so . . . good."

Immediately, it hit the therapist like a thunderbolt. The therapist had been recently diagnosed with cancer but was still struggling with his treatment options. Because he didn't know if, when, or how he would need to make special arrangements about the group, he hadn't shared information about his condition with the group yet. Apparently, they had obtained this information from another source. Given that members realized that something was afoot, he felt that giving them some indication of his medical situation and how it might affect them in terms of the continuity of the sessions was in order. The group proceeded to have a rather thorough discussion about not only their reactions to his disclosure but also their anxieties and inhibitions over bringing up the topic.

The group in this vignette was paralyzed by fears over the health of the therapist and, by extension, the health of the group. It is precisely when extreme anxieties prompt flight behavior that mass group commentary is a useful intervention. Notice that in the vignette the therapist did not know what was prompting the flight. Yalom (1995) suggests that the therapist need not necessarily have a highly articulated understanding of the basis of the group's flight. As in this case, it may be useful merely to open up an exploration of what is occurring.

Another circumstance in which the therapist may make a mass group interpretation is when unhealthy norms are developing, behaviors that will not move members toward the goals of the group (Yalom, 1995). For example, suppose the therapist noticed that some members tended to meet 10 minutes or so in advance of the group and rehash the previous session. Such an event could siphon off productive energy and hence could be an untherapeutic norm. Yalom recommends that the therapist clearly label the unhelpful behavior along with the negative consequences and any alternatives to the behavior. The alternative would be to deal with the material in the sessions themselves.

On the score of mass group interpretations, the interpersonal approach contrasts greatly with the next model to be featured: the object-relations model. For the interpersonal approach, mass group interpretations remove obstacles to the group's engagement in its essential work. In the object-relations approach, the group interpretation may be part of the essential work and is relied upon much more heavily than in the interpersonal approach.

Other Therapeutic Factors

While the group is working within the here-and-now, a variety of the therapeutic mechanisms delineated in Chapter 3 are deployed. For example, as Aaron recognized the link between his indiscriminant head nodding and yearning for acceptance, *self-understanding* occurs. Susan's description of her irritation is an act of *self-disclosure*. If Aaron were to explore his inhibitions over directly asserting a position on an issue facing the group, other factors would most likely be deployed. *Universality* might occur as other members related to Aaron's hesitancy about taking a stand. Perhaps another member would talk about having made progress in being able to articulate opinions and beliefs at odds with others. This sharing could *instill hope* in Aaron that he might be able to make headway in this area. That same member may offer some tip or thought about how he handles his apprehensions about others' reactions to his opinions. He might say, for instance, "I realized that people only respect me more for not being wishy-washy." This statement engages the therapeutic factors of *guidance* and *altruism* as the member experiences himself being helpful to Aaron. As members successfully address Aaron's and others' interpersonal issues, the group becomes more cohesive.

Underpinning all of the factors described in the preceding is group cohesion. The interpersonal therapist must be unflagging in his or her efforts to nurture group cohesion. In fact, research shows it is well worth the therapist's effort. For example, Kivlighan and Tarrant (2001) demonstrated in groups of male and female adolescents that therapist interventions directed toward creating a favorable group climate were associated with favorable outcomes. Measures of outcome tapped satisfaction, symptoms, and interpersonal behaviors. Specific features of the climate associated with more positive outcomes were high level of engagement (a dimension combining cohesion and the work orientation) and low levels of conflict and distance among members.

Therapist Disclosure

At various times in the life of a group, the interpersonal therapist engages in a moderate degree of self-disclosure. The therapist may do so to model a behavior for other members. For example, early in the life of a group the therapist may say at the end of a session, "I have a very good feeling about the work we did tonight. I think there was greater openness than before about the fears that are present about sharing reactions that members have toward one another with one another." In this mild self-disclosure, the therapist is modeling the communication of feelings about the group session. This disclosure not only models openness about reactions to the group process but also serves to foster cohesion by suggesting the possibility of members' taking pride and satisfaction in the good work they do together.

Disclosures can also be used to validate members' reality testing. For example, suppose a member walks in late and says later in the session, "I think you were irritated at me." The therapist's denial of such affect or deflection of the observation would undermine the member's sensitivity to others' feelings (if indeed the member were on target).

Finally, the therapist engages in self-disclosure to accept responsibility for any therapeutic errors. Such therapist activity models responsibility taking for members. Let us return to the earlier example of the ill therapist. Perhaps the therapist recognized that he had unduly delayed the announcement in group out of apprehension over members' reactions. The therapist might acknowledge that this worry had caused him to delay the announcement more than was optimal for members.

From the standpoint of the interpersonal approach, the therapist need not be the kind of blank screen that evokes regression. In fact, such a posture is likely to interfere with members' engagement in interpersonal learning because such a leadership style evokes a preoccupation with the therapist. On the other hand, the interpersonal approach recognizes that the therapist has a special role in the group. Certain disclosures (e.g., acknowledging dislike of a group member) may have special potency in damaging members' self-esteem; others (revealing severe psychological problems) may diminish members' confidence in the therapist. Therefore, all therapist disclosures should be made with care.

Interpersonal Vignette

We now consider a more extended segment of the group's life and Aaron's participation within that segment. The featured group is ongoing and has been in existence for 2½ years. Three of the original eight members remain in the group. Aaron, who began group six months ago, continues to be the newest member. The brief segment of a session presented on pages 291 and 292 occurred shortly before the current sessions and, hence, was still in members' minds.

Before we look in upon the group, several other members will be introduced:

- Shayna: A 28-year-old woman who was one of the original members of the group. She originally came into the group because her extreme volatility precluded her having stable relationships. While she had made much progress in achieving a more relaxed and modulated style of relating, she nonetheless had extreme reactions to minor insults and rejections both in the group and outside.

- Susan: This 40-year-old woman, while critical of others and quick to anger, was exceptionally perceptive and focused on keeping the group on task. Her excessively high standards of others created difficulties for her as a manager of a branch office of a bank.

- Derek: This group member, also among the original group, entered the group following the death of his wife. At the time of his entry, he was incapacitated by compulsive checking activities, which had been present to a much lesser extent while she was alive. While the symptoms had abated considerably, he showed a stunning unawareness of others' emotional reactions. Group members found his naïveté charming at times and vexing at others.

- Annette: This member's entrance into the group preceded Aaron's by only several months. She was a member who showed great oblivion to boundaries. Often, she would give highly concrete pieces of advice to members and would place considerable pressure on members to disclose. Members tended to perceive her efforts at closeness as aggressive acts. In relationships inside and outside the group, Annette frequently felt disappointed and shortchanged by others.

- Rasheed: This gay 37-year-old man was in the group because of job-related difficulties. His overt competitiveness with his supervisors at work prevented him from obtaining full recognition of his talents and contributions. At the time he entered the group, he believed that his supervisors' awareness of his sexual preference hindered him in obtaining promotions. Now a year later, he realizes that his interpersonal style played a role in his difficulties.

The Session

SHAYNA: I've decided I'm giving my three weeks' notice. I've been in group for at least two years and I'm tired of coming here every Thursday night. I want my Thursday evenings back.

[There was a brief period of stunned silence.]

DEREK: Man, I didn't see this one coming! Well, let me be the first to wish you the best of luck. So how are you going to use your Thursday evenings?

SUSAN: Whoa! I'm not ready to have a parting ceremony. Shayna, I'm blown away by this announcement. There's nothing that's led up to it. . . . I mean, it has seemed to me that we were in the middle of our work and out of nowhere, you say you're bailing.

SHAYNA: It's my right to leave whenever I want to.

RASHEED: Of course it's your right to leave when you want to . . . that's not the point.

ANNETTE: You're not ready to leave. You're not even close. You still can't hold on to a relationship with a guy for more than six weeks. You still can't go six months without blowing up at work.

SHAYNA: Who are you to tell me what to do? You're hardly in a position to tell anyone . . . Just the fact that I'm here talking about it is something I never would have done two years ago shows that I've come a long way. But you wouldn't know that because you haven't been here that long so before you start shooting off your mouth.

THERAPIST: When members leave the group, it's a big event and arouses some pretty strong feelings. I think Shayna's announcement is having a big emotional impact. Shayna, I'm glad that you have come to realize how important it is to be here so we can look at all of these feelings.

Note: The therapist is seeking to shift group members from an evaluative, critical position to one of openness to their own emotional reactions to a potentially major group event. The decision the therapist must make is whether an escalation between Shayna and Annette might lead to greater available affect or greater defensiveness. The therapist's judgment was that the latter would occur and so the therapist interrupted the interactions. Morran et al. (1998) identify the intervention of *cutting off* as one that must be in the interpersonal therapist's repertoire. Not only should it be used when the feedback is excessively harsh but also when it appears that a protracted period of feedback is overwhelming a recipient.

SUSAN: Okay . . . well, maybe I should say something here because after I left our session least week, I couldn't get the group out of my mind. And Shayna, I was worried and anxious about you in particular because I felt I had said a few harsh things to you just as the session was ending and didn't have time to clarify what I meant. . . . I half expected you not to show up but I didn't expect you to leave the group.

SHAYNA: Has nothing to do with that—

THERAPIST: Maybe it doesn't, but perhaps you did have a reaction to the comments Susan made to you last week.

Note: Given the suddenness of Shayna's interest in leaving the group, the link between her decision and last week's events is likely. However, forcing this point upon her would be unlikely to increase her receptivity to the emotional aftermath of the last session.

SHAYNA: [to the therapist] Would you like being accused of being a fake?

THERAPIST: Not at all: I'd be upset. But I'd also be curious what the person meant by it. And it was unfortunate that because we ran out of time, you were deprived of the opportunity to learn more about what Susan meant.

RASHEED: Shayna, I know you felt hurt and angry. I know it because it has happened in here with me and when it did, I would say to myself, "This is a bad place—get out," and it has especially happened with Susan. Susan, you go on the attack and pulverize one of us but then when we take what you're saying apart and look at it, it turns out that you're saying something helpful and not all that terrible. But it doesn't sound that way at first. And when I left the session, I felt annoyed with you that you began something that you couldn't finish.

THERAPIST: It sounds as though you're saying that Susan has a valuable perspective to offer but you've observed not only from this event with Shayna but your own experience with her is that the timing can interfere with her communication's being helpful.

Note: Rasheed has engaged in an activity that is key to effective group processing: He has made a connection between present and past incidents in the group (Stockton, Morran, & Nitza, 2000). Through this comparative thinking, he has identified one member's behavioral pattern, which the therapist seeks to underscore by paraphrasing his feedback. When the recipient of the feedback may not accurately comprehend it, the therapist would have that group member paraphrase it.

RASHEED: Exactly. Susan, you blurt something out and if there's not enough time to get into it, it ends up being hurtful.

SUSAN: It's hurtful to the target or should I say "victim" and it's hurtful to me. As I said, I spent my whole week worrying about what my little . . . explosion did to Shayna.

SHAYNA: Well, it did upset me because I know I'm more emotional than most people and it makes me feel weaker than everyone else. So when you came down on me for crying . . .

SUSAN: That's the point, though, I don't see you as weak at all. In fact, I think you're quite powerful because you cry so intensively that we cannot do anything but focus on you.

ANNETTE: True! How can we not pay attention to someone whose crying so hard?

THERAPIST: [to Susan] And something about that makes you feel irritated.

SUSAN: I feel irritated because our work in the group comes to a halt once the crying begins. We're not talking about anything; we're not figuring out our feelings. We're just listening to someone cry. And if someone tries to say something consoling, you cry harder.

RASHEED: I don't think that's all of it . . . I mean when did anyone in here ever try to say something soothing to you [referring to Susan]? There must be times when you need it—we all do—but you have this hard edge on you that says, "Stay away!"

THERAPIST: What do you mean by "hard edge"? What does Susan *do* that conveys a "hard edge"?

Note: The therapist is attempting to get members to be a bit more behavioral and specific in their feedback to Susan.

AARON: I don't think I've ever even see you tear up. I think if you did that, I'd be shocked.

ANNETTE: Yea, hard edge means not asking us for nothing! Absolutely nothing!

SUSAN: [turning back to Rasheed] So you're saying that I'm actually envious of Shayna cause she can do something I can't? I did say she is powerful when she cries so perhaps I feel rather powerless that I can't be so . . . commanding.

RASHEED: I don't know about "can't." Maybe "don't" because it's just not easy for you. Just like it's not easy for you, Shayna, to hang in there and keep talking with us once we've gotten into something kind of sensitive with you. Just as Susan says, you cry and then our progress gets interrupted.

THERAPIST: [to the entire group] And what is the consequence of that interruption in terms of how you behave toward Shayna?

Note: Part of the interpersonal learning process is recognizing the interpersonal consequences of one's behaviors (Yalom, 1995). Thus far, Shayna has been given the feedback that her crying evokes anger in Susan. However, she does not yet know either the affective reactions other members have toward the crying or any ways they might treat her differently because of it.

AARON: I keep in some of my thoughts. I don't want to precipitate an outbreak.

DEREK: Yeah, I try to be very gentle in everything I say and if I can't think of a gentle way to say it, I bite my tongue! I really stop and picture how Shayna will react.

THERAPIST: More so than with other members of the group?

DEREK: Definitely.

AARON: Well, yeah, probably.

THERAPIST: And the fact that you must "walk on eggshells," does that make a difference in what feelings you have when you're interacting with Shayna?

AARON: [reddening] I feel a bit apprehensive. . . . I mean I still like you, Shayna, and because I do, I just don't want to cause you distress.

SHAYNA: You mean you baby me?

DEREK: Well, no, of course I do see you as an adult.

RASHEED: See, you're doing it as we speak! Shayna, he's babying you by claiming that he doesn't baby you.

[Everyone laughs, including Shayna.]

THERAPIST: Shayna, I know you've gotten a lot of feedback and I have been wondering what's been going on inside? Does it feel like it did last week?

SHAYNA: Not at all . . . I feel much better than I did last week even though [feigns a glare toward Aaron and Derek] certain people in here have questioned my adulthood.

> *Note:* The therapist is modeling for the group the action of checking out the effects of one's communications on the receiver. The therapist is also monitoring the level of stimulation to ensure that it has not gone beyond what a member can tolerate. The therapist's attentiveness to level of stimulation can also convey to members that they can monitor themselves and make a conscious decision to take a break rather than resorting to an unconscious defensive maneuver such as, in Shayna's case, sobbing.

DEREK: Does that mean you're not going to leave?

SHAYNA: I just don't know. I felt so strong on it when I came in here tonight.

SUSAN: You feel that to change your mind would be to betray your-self?

SHAYNA: Sort of . . . I feel confused. I don't know whether I should leave or not.

THERAPIST: One way of making this determination is to figure out whether you've accomplished the goals you established for yourself in entering the group.

> *Note:* Interpersonal learning is facilitated by encouraging mem-bers to compare their accomplishments in group to their estab-lished goals.

RASHEED: I remember when you came into this group, you said that all of your relationships were very intense and very brief. And boy, were you intense when you came in here. You would be so into your own mood, it seemed as though we didn't matter.

ANNETTE: Yeah, each session I wondered what will set her off this time?

SUSAN: And I have to say, I feel you're much more present and tuned in to what's going on.

DEREK: So you're saying she's ready to leave?

AARON: Can I say something?

ANNETTE: Come on, you don't have to ask permission. Speak when-ever you want. I do!

AARON: I just wanted to say to Shayna . . . Shayna, I don't think you're ready to leave. If you left now, I don't believe that you would have the kinds of relationships that would make you happy. Look at what happened with you just this session and last. Susan may have not been completely tactful . . . but your response was extreme. You were ready to throw the whole thing away. And I just think you'll be ready to leave when someone can get you upset but not send you into a total tail-spin. Because, then, you'll be able to hang in there with other people and your relationships will last.

SUSAN: Wow!

RASHEED: Wow, what?

SUSAN: Wow, Aaron gave a clear and distinct opinion. It happens to be one that I share but the important thing is that you took a stand. Aaron, I feel so much more drawn to you when you're not wishy-washy.

RASHEED: And I liked what you said to Shayna. Did it make sense to you, Shayna?

SHAYNA: It did, but I want to still think about it.

[The session continues.]

In this segment of a session, we see interpersonal work done by Susan, Shayna, and Aaron. The session is not typical of interpersonal groups in that for expositional ease the group's work proceeded more quickly than might often be the case. It was typical, however, in that members worked in a complementary way on the relational difficulties that brought them into group. For example, Shayna addressed her overreactivity to slights and criticism while in concert Susan examined her blunt criticalness of others and difficulty in requesting help from others.

This vignette features a relatively mature group. Members showed a familiarity with interpersonal learning and the importance of focusing on experiences within the here-and-now. Had the group been less mature, we probably would have seen the members presenting there-and-then topics and the therapist intervening to bring the group into the here-and-now. What was incumbent upon the therapist was intervening to ensure that the interpersonal learning process contained not only the first step of interpersonal learning, activation of affect, but also the second step, processing of reactions and interactions. The therapist was active in sculpting the feedback members gave to one another so that it would be maximally helpful. The therapist used modeling, paraphrasing, cutting off, and clarifications to encourage greater specificity in the feedback, and checking out to ensure that the feedback is not overwhelming. The interpersonal therapist needs to call upon a broad repertoire of interventions as members pursue interpersonal learning.

Short-Term Applications

When Yalom (1975) first wrote about his interpersonal approach, he described a long-term therapy situation. An individual would work in treatment for an extended period—in many cases, several years—in order to undergo substantial change in his or her interpersonal functioning. Someone like Aaron with difficulties in various relational realms might spend considerable time in group learning about his interpersonal style and the difficulties associated with it, and practicing new, presumably more effective ways of interacting.

Although the interpersonal approach was viewed by group practitioners as most applicable to a long-term time frame, in fact processes used by this approach such as feedback were originally identified by Lewin and colleagues in groups lasting over a weekend (Sabin, 1981). However, the fact that such processes as interpersonal learning can be activated in a group of brief duration does not mean that the same goals can be accomplished as in a longer-term group. As is generally the case with time-limited group therapy, members are most likely to benefit when the goals of treatment are substantially limited. Yalom (1995) stresses that a brief group experience cannot accomplish the kind of thoroughgoing change that would be expected from long-term group participation.

So what goals can be successfully pursued? The answer to this question depends on how brief the life of the group or an individual member's participation in it is. Yalom (1983, 1995) points out that in some settings the life of a member's participation can be only a single session. Such a brief tenure might occur within an inpatient setting in which patients remain for several days. In a single session or even a handful of sessions, it is folly to hope that a maladaptive relational style can be modified. However, certain goals can be realistically pursued. Yalom notes that a primary goal for such groups is to engage members in a therapeutic process and that this engagement has horizontal and vertical aspects. The horizontal aspect concerns the member's exploration of concerns in a way that will enhance receptivity to, and use of, all other therapeutic opportunities in the setting. For example, a seclusive patient who participates minimally in all of the groups might address her fear of others sufficiently to be somewhat more participatory in all therapeutic situations in the hospital. The vertical aspect involves preparing the member for his or her therapeutic involvement following hospitalization. As Yalom (1983) notes, "an important goal of the inpatient group is to introduce patients to therapy and to provide a therapeutic experience so relevant, comfortable, and effective that they will elect to continue it" (p. 56).

In the inpatient situation, the overarching goal of engaging members in the therapeutic process can be partitioned into subgoals. First, the group member can learn that talking can benefit him or her by providing relief and by revealing that one is not alone with one's experiences. Second, the member can also identify problem areas that can be pursued on an outpatient basis. Patients frequently conceptualize their problems as restricted to their symptoms. A time-limited group experience can help them to recognize the interpersonal problem underlying the symptom. For example, one persona may come to understand that depressive symptoms are undergirded by a fear of expressing negatively toned affects such as anger to others. While the time-limited group experience may not permit substantial progress in acquiring comfort and skill in such expressiveness, it can allow for the realization of the problem. Following brief group work, the individual may pursue the problem elsewhere, most desirably, in a longer-term group experience. Third, the group provides a forum for coping with all of the stressors that can attend hospitalization.

How can this array of goals be pursued in the context of a single session? Imagine a new member coming into an inpatient group. Suppose the therapist were to take a fairly nondirective posture, intervening in the fashion of the therapist in the prior vignette. It would not be at all unexpected for the new member to defer to any more senior member and participate minimally. If the member's group participation were limited to this one session, then the subgoals identified for group involvement would certainly not be realized. On the contrary, the lack of felt progress might actually alienate the member. The member might well be less rather than more likely to pursue group therapy (or perhaps any therapy) in the future.

In order for any appropriate goals to be achieved from a very brief experience, the therapist must assume a more directive stance than he or she might in a longer term frame (Brabender & Fallon, 1993). The direction provided by the therapist entails establishing a structure wherein all members systematically engage in those processes that are likely to move them toward their goals. In determining the particular structure, the therapist should consider the level of functioning of the members. For inpatients who have a modicum of ability to tolerate anxiety, Yalom suggests an *Interactional Agenda* format. Within this format, each session consists of five steps that will be briefly described. A far more extensive discussion is provided in Yalom's text on inpatient group therapy:

Step 1: Orientation and Preparation: The structural features of the group such as frequency and length of sessions are described to members. The goals and processes of the group (for example, the importance of working within the here-and-now) are also presented.

Step 2: Agenda Go-Around: In this step, each member develops a problem area on which he or she can work during that session. This step prevents the kind of circumstance described in the preceding in which a member may remain relatively inactive throughout the session. The agenda ensures that each member will do a significant amount of work in the beginning of the session and thereby set the stage for continued participation. Moreover, the opportunity for the therapist to hear all group members' agendas early on will help the therapist recognize ways members can pursue their agendas in tandem.

To be maximally useful, an agenda must be specific enough that it can be accomplished during the time available. For example, an agenda such as "I want to become more assertive" is unrealistic because it is unlikely to be accomplished during a brief group tenure. Far better would be an agenda such as "I intend to speak up at least once during this session when I have a reaction that is different than someone else's." Accomplishing this more concrete agenda would represent an initial step on the road to becoming more assertive in relationships.

The therapist must also assist the member in constructing an agenda that has an interpersonal focus. For example, a member who says "I want to be less anxious" has created an agenda that does not involve others and, hence, does not use the resources of the group. An agenda with a more here-and-now interpersonal dimension would be, "During this session, I will listen and respond to others rather than being distracted by my worries." This agenda is one that could influence how the person behaves within the group. Moreover, the person could obtain feedback on the extent to which the agenda was fulfilled.

The agenda-setting step has therapeutic value in its own right. By accomplishing this step, members can accomplish what was previously mentioned as one of the foremost goals of brief interpersonal therapy: learning what issues might be addressed on a longer-term basis and to recognize the social dimension of their symptoms.

Step 3: Agenda Fulfillment: In this step, members participate in the here-and-now process of the group while looking for opportunities to pursue their agendas. As noted earlier, the therapist tries to find ways members can weave their agendas together. In some cases the therapist must give members assignments for fulfilling their agendas outside the group.

Step 4: Wrap-up by Therapist: The wrap-up is an extension of the process of interpersonal learning. The therapist engages in a retrospective analysis of the session, focusing on the progress of each group member. In inpatient groups it is not unusual for students or members of the treatment team to observe the group. The group therapist would be obligated to make certain that the appropriate informed-consent procedure is followed in relation to the inclusion of observers and that the observers are fully aware of their confidentiality requirements. By having observers share their impressions of the session, they offer something in exchange for what the members have provided them. Within this format group members are less likely to feel exploited by the presence of observers because they derive something from their presence.

Step 5: Wrap-up by the Entire Group: This second wrap-up step involves all members and the therapists. We can imagine how the conversation of the observers and therapist about the group would capture the members' interest and serve as fodder for discussion during this phase. Members can also use this period to talk about any residual reactions from the meeting. The therapist may check in with some member who may have received a great deal of feedback or who was relatively reticent.

Although this model is designed for radically brief member participation, it retains the defining features of the interpersonal approach, both in terms of goals and methods. The goals are interpersonal, and the method entails use of the here-and-now of the group.

Other Short-Term Applications

The interactional agenda model is for a very specific patient population. Suppose the therapist must create a positive group experience for individuals who are at a lower level of functioning. For these individuals, what would pose a threat to benefiting from sessions is the degree of anxiety evoked by the focus on group process. People at the lowest level of ego functioning are highly prone to a sense of fragmentation in the face of ambiguity and uncertainty (McWilliams, 1994), and an immersion in group process necessarily requires a reckoning with these features. The antidote to any untoward reaction of lower-functioning patients is to provide a higher level of structure. A series of exercises can be conducted in which members have a taste of group process but in a fashion that guarantees that their experiences from moment to moment will be more positively than negatively toned. For example, the therapist might direct group members to engage in some activity together such as throwing a beach ball back and forth and then asking them to reflect upon their feelings about pursuing this activity. To the extent that the therapist perceives that members can handle spontaneity, the therapist might create greater or lesser opportunities for its emergence in planning the exercises. A format for conducting sessions with lower-functioning inpatients can be found in Yalom's 1983 text.

Outpatient groups usually have a longer time frame with which to work relative to the inpatient setting, even if the group is short-term. Whether the group lasts two weeks or six months, the more prolonged opportunity to engage in interpersonal learning enables the therapist to at least contemplate the issue of whether the individual member can make progress in modifying interpersonal behaviors that have not served the individual well, that is, have not led to satisfaction in relationships. As Yalom (1995) notes, the research base has not yet been sufficiently abundant for us to know with any precision what types of changes can be made within different time frames. However, models for doing outpatient short-term work within the interpersonal approach are emerging and being subjected to empirical test. For example, Simon Budman and his colleagues at the Harvard Community Health Plan have developed a model for treating persons with personality disorders over a six-month period. This model is described, and the research on its effectiveness are summarized in the remainder of this section.

Budman, Demby, Soldz, and Merry's (1996) model for individuals with personality disorder was developed with a recognition that persons at this level of ego functioning frequently fail to follow through on long-term treatment. They cite the finding of Waldinger and Gunderson (1984) that only one-third of borderline patients completed individual therapy as judged by a therapist and one-half do not continue beyond six months. Budman, Demby, et al.

reasoned, therefore, that it is more reasonable to conceptualize the treatment of this patient population as intermittent with any one treatment stint constituting an episode within a series of treatment experiences. The interval they established was six months with the option to renew at six-month intervals. They actively use the time limit to motivate members to make positive changes and to lessen dependency and regression.

This model is briefly described by outlining those characteristics that distinguish it from longer term applications. As the following quote suggests, Budman, Demby, et al. remain very true to the interpersonal approach described by Yalom (1995) both in terms of goals and methods:

> *We view the group setting as a place in which maladaptive interpersonal patterns are replayed, recognized, and acknowledged.* At the same time, the group provides a unique opportunity for learning new ways of relating in a relatively safe and contained environment. *Over even a limited period of time, group members can reenact their interpersonal difficulties, receive disconfirming evidence for their negative beliefs, and begin the rehearsal for change. The focus of the groups is primarily in the here and now. Emphasis is placed on within-group behaviors and the members' current lives, with acknowledgment of historical influences as they operate in the here and now.* (p. 336)

There is much in this quote that by now should be familiar to the reader. However, Budman, Demby, et al. realized that the time limit required the following modification of procedures:

- *The therapist takes a more active, directive (but noncoercive) posture than typically is the case in the long-term group.* For example, the therapist will energetically involve members in the interaction, set limits on acting out behaviors, and underscore key issues.

- *Responsibility taking on the part of members is vigorously cultivated.* Members are asked to state their goals for the group and their own criteria to assess their progress. Strengths and competencies are also emphasized both to enable them to recognize that they can take responsibility for their own progress and also to nurture positive expectations about the value of their group participation. The therapist finds examples of how a member has successfully negotiated past difficulties in order to convey that future adversities can be overcome.

- *Pregroup preparation is extremely substantial so that members can derive as much from the group as possible.* Group therapy candidates meet with the group leader to obtain information and to work with the therapist to frame the presenting problem in a way that is consistent with the focus of the group. If the individual is seen as an appropriate candidate and remains interested in joining the group, he or she proceeds onto a pregroup workshop. In this 90-minute structured group experience, the member interacts with other members one to two weeks prior to the group's beginning. Members have the opportunity to learn experientially about some of the processes that will be deployed in the group and to acquire or strengthen the skills that these processes require.

- *An oral summary of each session is provided by the therapist to crystallize learning.* Although the session summaries are only a few sentences, they "are used to tie together the process of the group, to link the content and process of the session to the focus of the group, and to link the sessions to one another over the life of the group" (p. 346). At the end of a member's participation, the therapist writes a detailed letter to him or her summarizing that member's achievements in the group.

- *Homework is sometimes assigned by the therapist or other group members in order to intensify learning.* In addition to the aforementioned features, the model of Budman and colleagues has a strong developmental orientation. Developmental stages emerge with particular clarity when the group has a definite beginning and end. These stages can be used to accentuate and explore a range of interpersonal issues. For example, early in the life of the group members address issues of safety in relationship, an especially poignant concern for personality-disordered individuals who have histories of abuse and neglect. When the group approaches termination, the temporal limit activates issues to loss, abandonment, and death in a powerful way. Members exhibit their characteristic ways of responding to these life changes, and examining these ways can lead to new, growth-producing responses.

A comparison of Yalom's interactional agenda model for inpatients and Budman, Demby, and colleagues' time-limited model for personality-disordered individuals reveals several commonalities. In both approaches, the therapist is more active than in long-term approaches. Both approaches involve an underscoring of the cognitive framework, in Budman, Demby, et al.'s case through the end-of-session summary and in Yalom's through the end-of-session review. Both approaches engage the members in goal setting and thereby promote responsibility. These commonalities are likely to be found in most effective approaches to time-limited group therapy. However, there are important differences. The Budman model places greater stress on developmental stages and the use of the time limit as a resource. The Yalom agenda model entails a more heavily formatted session with perhaps less opportunity for spontaneous interaction. These variations suggest that within every setting there are constraints and opportunities that will affect the ways in which work can be accomplished in a group. We need a plurality of interpersonal models to accommodate the plurality of settings in which such models are applied.

Research Support for the Interpersonal Approach

Much of the research on the interpersonal approach has concerned therapeutic factors. The research has shown unequivocally that across a variety of settings and populations, group members value the mechanisms such as interpersonal learning that are the hallmark of the interpersonal approach (Leszcz, 1992; Yalom, 1995). This research is important because it shows the relevance of the approach to members' self-perception of their needs. Because members see the activities of the group as relevant to their issues, they are likely to invest themselves in the group more fully than if the pertinence of group activities to their problems were less clear.

A good deal of the research on therapeutic factors was considered in Chapter 4. In this section, we consider the empirical support for the basic postulate of interpersonal theory—the connection between interpersonal problems and symptoms. We then move onto three lines of research that address the effectiveness of the interpersonal approach in modifying interpersonal style and secondarily, altering symptoms.

Theoretical Postulate of the Interpersonal Approach

As noted earlier, Harry Stack Sullivan's premise was that all psychopathology is relational. Gotleib and Shraedley (2000) reviewed the evidence for interpersonal hypothesis and found that across a variety of disorders, it is substantial. These reviewers cite evidence that depressed individuals, for example, have more impoverished social networks relative to controls. Ingram, Scott, and Seigle (1999) document specific interpersonal difficulties in persons with unipolar depression such as engagement in excessive reassurance seeking from others (Segrin & Abramson, 1994), self-disclosure at a level inappropriate to the situation (Jacobson & Anderson, 1982), and on a more general level, a lower level of involvement with, and responsiveness to, others (Segrin & Abramson, 1994). Depressed individuals are also more likely to be rejected by others (Joiner & Metalsky, 1995; Sacco & Dunn, 1990).

Other types of psychological disorders have also been linked to interpersonal problems. These include schizophrenia (see Hooley & Candela, 1999, for a comprehensive review of the various interpersonal impairments associated with schizophrenia), eating disorders (Tiller et al., 1997), agoraphobia (Carter, Turovsky, & Barlow, 1994), panic disorder (Marcowitz, Weissman, Ovellette, Lish, & Klerman, 1989), and substance abuse (e.g., Frieze & Schafer, 1984). The diagnostic criteria of the personality disorders generally include interpersonal deficits.

In summary, the association between psychopathology and interpersonal problems is extremely well established. What is less clear is whether interpersonal difficulties (a) set the stage for the emergence of a disorder, (b) are a consequence of the disorder, or (c) are related in a more complex way to the disorder. While research continues to address the relationship between the two, currently, there seems to be ample empirical justification for establishing as a major thrust of group treatment across a great range of diagnoses the goal of improving the individual's capacity to relate to others.

Effectiveness of the Interpersonal Approach

What evidence is there that participation in an interpersonal group leads primarily to an enhanced ability to relate to others and secondarily to other kinds of change such as symptom relief? The studies that address this question are sparse probably because of a variety of factors. First, measuring interpersonal change is challenging. A full picture of interpersonal functioning entails not only self-report but the observations of others, presumably important others. Such information should be garnered well after the group has ended to determine the sturdiness of change. Such an empirical pursuit requires access to resources that clinician investigators in many settings may not have. Second, the popularity of the interpersonal approach has led it to be integrated with other group methods in order to accommodate the special needs of different clinical populations. For example, Lubin and Johnson (1997) tested a model they developed for trauma victims that has interpersonal and educational components. Although these investigators obtained positive outcomes, they cannot be attributed uniquely to the interpersonal components of the model. Similarly, many psychodynamic/psychoanalytic approaches such as the loss model researched by Piper and colleagues have many elements of the interpersonal approach. Third, much of the research energy in contemporary group therapy is directed to the cognitive approach, which is described in Chapter 12.

Nonetheless, support for the interpersonal approach can be obtained from three types of research. The first is from a comparison of the meta-analytic studies covered in Chapter 1. As Fuhriman and Burlingame (1994) point out, those studies featuring meta-analytic analysis of groups whose focus was on process tended to have favorable outcomes relative to individual therapy. These studies capitalize on the hallmark of the interpersonal approach: interpersonal learning within the here-and-now. The outcome measures in these studies were highly varied and included interpersonal and symptom measures. In contrast, meta-analysis on groups that did not use the unique features of a group fared more poorly relative to individual therapy.

The second type are those outcome studies on groups explicitly run according to the interpersonal approach. An example of a study pertinent to the material on time-limited formats presented in the last section is one by Budman, Demby, et al. (1996), who attempted to determine the usefulness of the model developed for personality-disordered individuals participating in the Harvard Plan. Members of four different groups were tracked over an 18-month period of group participation. (The study began with five groups, but one group dissolved prematurely and was excluded from the study.) Although the sample initially consisted of 49 members, the dropout rate was substantial: The final sample consisted of only 21 members. This experience, which was consistent with the attrition rates obtained by others, motivated Budman and his group to create the six-month renewable interval format in their succeeding application of this approach. An extensive outcome battery was used with a number of measures reflecting various aspects of interpersonal functioning. These measures were administered at the beginning and end of treatment and at regular intervals in between. A major limitation of the study is that there was no control group of any sort. Fortunately, this particular population has characteristics well-known to mental health professionals: Spontaneous and sustained improvement in the area investigated would defy all expectations.

The researchers found enhanced psychological functioning in many realms over the 18 months. The number of diagnostic criteria that the members met for personality disorder lessened substantially. Positive self-esteem increased steadily over group participation. Most importantly for our purposes, interpersonal functioning was markedly improved as reflected in an inventory of interpersonal problems and another inventory on social adjustment and improvements continued over the entire 18-month period. Curiously, on scales of perception of social support and satisfaction in relationships with friends and intimates, no change was observed. This pattern of positive and negative outcomes suggests that some types of interpersonal changes may be more responsive to this treatment than others. This finding points to the importance of incorporating in future research measures that systematically tap the person's capacity to negotiate different kinds of relationships (e.g., ranging from the more casual to the more intimate, from the more professional to the more personal).

A handful of other studies is consistent with Budman, Demby, et al.'s (1996) investigation in supporting the effectiveness of the interpersonal approach in instigating interpersonal change. Using another quasi-experimental design, Albrecht and Brabender (1983) tracked change on a composite measure of a number of specific variables, some of which reflected interpersonal change. The purpose of the study was to determine if dual diagnosed inpatient members with substance abuse derived as much benefit from participation in an interpersonal group as other members. In fact, members overall

showed considerable change from pretreatment to posttreatment regardless of the presence or absence of a substance abuse diagnosis. As
noted in Chapter 2, after participation in an interpersonal group,
chronic patients exhibited more flexible behaviors in relation to a
goal and greater accuracy in perception (Beard & Scott, 1975). Sullivan would have seen both of these developments as moving the individual in the direction of psychological health. Beutler et al. (1984)
showed the value of an inpatient interpersonally-oriented group in
reducing symptoms.

Not all findings have been positive. Jones and McCall (1991)
found no difference in adult male offenders' willingness to join other
groups following their participation in an interactional agenda versus
psycho-educational life skills group. However, the authors' description of the group process suggests a laissez-faire style of leadership at
odds with Yalom's recommendation of an active therapist posture.
They write, "attention would frequently focus on an individual for
unspecified and often long periods of time" (p. 89). Cloitre and Koenen (2001) found that participants with both posttraumatic stress
disorder and borderline personality showed a worsening on measures
of anger after participation in a 12-week interpersonal group, and a
lack of improvement on other interpersonal and symptom measures.
In contrast, members with PTSD without a borderline personality
disorder showed a significant reduction in anger, depression, and
symptoms of PTSD but little change on interpersonal measures related to symptoms of PTSD and on interpersonal measures related to
assertion and control.

The third type of support is derived from studies that pit components of the interpersonal approach against components of other
approaches. In this chapter, we have already had examples of this
type of study. For example, Flowers and Booraem (1990a) found that
members' receiving descriptions of their behavioral patterns and the
impact on others of those behaviors obtained more from the group
experience than members receiving motive and historical interpretations. This finding is exactly what would be predicted by the interpersonal approach. This type of elemental research is especially helpful
because it not only provides validation for the approach at large but
also assists the group therapist in fine-tuning its application.

From these three types of research, there is sufficient evidence
to conclude that the interpersonal approach can result in positive
change in the person's capacity to relate to others. However, how

member and situational characteristics as well as the time frame available affect the type of change achieved and the durability of change is a matter for future research.

Summary

This chapter summarized what is perhaps the most influential theoretical approach to group therapy. Not only have many group therapists paid primary allegiance to this orientation, but many others have integrated the concepts and methods of interpersonal theory into an alternate approach.

The goal of the interpersonal approach is to positively affect all aspects of psychological functioning by enhancing the person's capacity to have fulfilling, effective relationships with others. The means to this end is members' use of the here-and-now of the group to achieve interpersonal learning. Much of the training of the interpersonal therapist is in mastering the techniques associated with the two stages of interpersonal learning, the activation and the understanding of the here-and-now. The interpersonal approach has been used in both time-limited and time-unlimited formats, although the goals and methods must vary somewhat for successful application of each. Much of the research on the interpersonal approach has focused on therapeutic factors rather than outcomes. Nonetheless, there is support for the connection between symptoms and interpersonal problems and for the success of the interpersonal approach in fostering healthy change in the person's capacity to relate to others. Future research will be needed to elucidate what types of relational changes are possible within different time frames.

Psychodynamic Group Therapy: An Object-Relations Approach

11

Chapter

Arabella, a 32-year-old woman, had recently begun individual therapy with a new therapist. In taking the history, this therapist learned that Arabella had had a string of therapists since she was 15. By speaking with her last therapist, reading treatment summaries, and considering the patient's own account, the therapist detected a pattern in the preceding treatments. In an initial rosy period Arabella would rejoice in finally having found the right person to treat her. While in some cases fairly protracted, these periods would be punctuated by brief episodes of fury at the therapist for some disappointment or felt rejection. Her last therapist recounted that on one occasion after she saw another patient leave his office, she railed against him for allowing the encounter to occur. Over time, such episodes would increase in frequency until eventually the relationship would sour because of her experience of a major loss inside or outside the therapy such as an extended absence by the therapist or a boyfriend's disaffection.

Arabella had had a history of unstable attachments. When she was only a year old, her father, a wealthy Argentinean, emigrated to the United States with her British mother. After only a brief time in the new country, he left both of them. Following his departure, her mother had bouts of severe depression for which she required periods of psychiatric hospitalization over 2 years. While her mother was in the hospital, Arabella would be in the custody of her father, who entrusted her to nannies. During her childhood, her mother attempted to create stability by sending her to boarding schools, but by high school Arabella refused such arrangements.

In her high school years, drinking, drugs, and promiscuity became staples of her lifestyle. However, she developed an interest in theater, which continued into her early 30s. Since she was frequently unemployed as an actress, her father covered her living expenses. She lost roles by throwing tantrums during rehearsals. Her manner was extremely flirtatious, and she could attract suitors easily. Yet, she drifted in and out of relationships much like a limited gig in a production. She complained of loneliness and emptiness.

Arabella's new therapist felt that group therapy might be invaluable in her treatment. He believed that the group setting might be ideal given her tendency to end therapy when she felt any significant disappointment with the therapist. He reasoned that Arabella might be able to hold on to some positive tie with a group. Arabella eventually did enter a group with a different therapist while continuing in individual treatment.

We now consider the object-relations approach, which is a set of models within the psychoanalytic/psychodynamic school of thought on personality, psychopathology, and treatment. It is similar to interpersonal theory in that its influence has been broad: Concepts emerging from the object-relations theory on groups have permeated the group therapy field as a whole and have influenced approaches to group treatment that are not formally object relational. Although some of the concepts of this approach are complex, and at least rudimentary grasp of them helps the reader understand other approaches within the psychodynamic school. The reader will recognize that some of the concepts we have already covered—particularly those in Chapter 3 on group development—have their roots in the object-relations school.

Stated briefly, the object-relations approach holds that Arabella's difficulties—her loneliness, depression, and angry episodes—are connected to a lack of maturity in her internal images or representations of herself and other people. The sometimes confusing term "object-relations" pertain to these representations. Object-relations are the interrelationships between the self or internal pictures (representations) of the self and others, or internal images of others. The "object" is an entity perceived as other than the self. While the object often is a person (or image of a person), it need not be. For example, this text that I am writing certainly is an object. Moreover, representations may be constructed of only certain aspects or components of a person or thing. Suppose Arabella recognized only those aspects of others that met her needs. If so, her representations of others would be *part objects*.

A basic tenet of object-relations theory is that through a process of *internalization* human beings form paradigms or templates of social experiences. Early experiences with caretakers especially shape these schemes. Object-relations theory holds further that these internalizations then shape future social experiences, serving as a framework for organizing social data. For example, the schemes or representations of other people that Arabella formed in her earliest relationships are likely to shape her social experiences into adulthood. If she experienced her earliest figures as depriving or inconsistently caring, she will carry these expectations with her and behave toward others accordingly.

Yet, just as representations affect how current interactions are cognitively registered, so too does the tenor of interactions affect representations. Suppose Arabella manages to have a significant long-term relationship with a person who responds with a consistency that had little precedent in her experience. Her paradigm itself might undergo revision to accommodate this new input. Hence, the relationship between representations and experience is reciprocal and dynamic.

Goals of the Object-Relations Approach

As the reader has probably gathered, from the preceding example, representations of self and other people are a critical target of change for the object relations. However, to understand in more specific terms the types of goals a member would pursue in an object-relations group, a consideration of the somewhat complicated history of object-relations theory is necessary.

Conceptual Foundations

Although different theoreticians have taken contrasting positions on critical issues, each has contributed to the richness of this approach as it is practiced today. Many of these contributions have also had an influence on other psychodynamic approaches such as self-psychology and systems-centered approaches. In describing the ideas of these contributors, greatest emphasis is given to those ideas that have had greatest influence on how group therapy is practiced today.

Melanie Klein: While having significant roots in Freud (1917/1957) and other early psychoanalytic writers, object-relations theory truly began with the work of Melanie Klein, an English psychiatrist. While Freud speculated on the intrapsychic life of a child based on his work with adults, Melanie Klein worked with children directly in the context of play. Her direct observation of children's play led to a conclusion that was dramatically at odds with Freud's: Children's primary interest is not drive gratification or the control of sexual impulses. Rather, their fundamental concern is in their relationships with significant persons in their lives and modulating the feelings arising in these relationships (Cashdan, 1988). This relationship focus revealed to Klein that the infantile internal world is composed not merely of a bundle of drive states but of human relationships. Klein's departure from Freud—the primacy of human relationships over drive states—established the theme or red thread that runs throughout the often-differing views of object relationists. It also built a bridge between psychoanalytic theory and a group perspective (Ashbach & Schermer, 1987). For what Klein was suggesting was that treatment must concern itself primarily with human relationships, a view completely compatible with those group treatments emphasizing the here-and-now exploration of relationships within the group and their changes over time (Alonso & Rutan, 1984).

Klein took a special interest in the infant–mother relationship because of its critical and all-consuming character for the infant. It is here that we come to a revolutionary idea of Klein's. For Freud (1905/1953), the infant comes to construct an idea of mother through her connection with drive gratification. Klein held that some primitive unconscious scheme of mother is present at birth. This primitive maternal representation, she believed, organizes the child's interactions with the real-world mother. Klein saw the infant as having other innate ideas (breasts, penises, wombs) or fantasies that concern the somatic universe in which the infant dwells. While Klein's views on innate notions have been subject to much criticism (Ashbach & Schermer, 1987), her emphasis on the role of phantasy in human development is an inestimable contribution (Spillius, 2001).[1] Her notion that the infant's relationship with the

---

[1] Klein sees phantasy in different terms than Freud. For Freud, phantasies are the result of blocked unconscious wishes. Phantasies originate in consciousness and partially fulfill the wish in disguised fashion. For Klein, phantasy is an unconscious activity present at birth and continually taking place alongside all of the person's activities (Spillius, 2001). Klein used the *ph* spelling of phantasies to distinguish them from conscious fantasies. Yet Spillius (2001) notes that because it is sometimes difficult to distinguish the conscious from unconscious contents, the *ph* spelling currently prevails.

mother serves as the foundation for all later relationships has been in various ways embraced by object relationists.

The mother–infant relationship and the infant's own intrapsychic development are shaped by the interplay of two forces: libido, or the creative self-preservation impulse, and the death instinct, or self-destructive urge. How the infant negotiates between the two forces changes, Klein held, as the infant matures. She described two successive positions that the infant assumes, each moving the infant to greater relational maturity. The initial position was termed *paranoid-schizoid*. During the first few months of life, the infant feels beset by danger precipitated by the loss of the security of the uterus and the pain of childbirth (Cashdan, 1988). The infant also feels under siege by her own death instinct, by the conflict between the death and life instinct, and by the discomforts of being abjectly helpless. Klein's infant at birth possesses the wherewithal to defend itself against the anxiety generated by all of these sources. The infant in part projects part of her own death instinct outward and sees herself as being attacked by fantasized internal and external objects. (The previously introduced term "part object" is perhaps more accurate here in that the infant is conceiving of an entity that will ultimately in the course of healthy development be recognized as only part of a whole object.) With projection, it is no longer the self attacking the self but external agents attacking the self. The material the child uses for the creation of these persecutory agents is the inborn unconscious fantasies of bodily parts as well as experiences with real external objects such as the mother's breast. While the idea of the infant's being attacked by all of these fantasized internal and external agents may not seem much of an improvement upon the infant's original psychological situation, it actually is so because through these acts of projection, the danger is made more peripheral and less encroaching. The infant also turns part of her death instinct into aggression and experiences herself as attacking these persecuting agents (Segal, 1974).

What a menacing, dreadful world it would be for the infant if her world were populated only by these ferocious internal and external objects! However, the infant also projects outward her libido, or life-sustaining instinct, and in doing so ensures the presence of good internal and external objects. For example, the infant can recognize a good, sustenance-providing breast. But immediately a problem arises: Were the infant to see that the mother's breast, the one that is experienced as devouring, is the same breast that sustains life, the infant would be beset by the overwhelming anxiety that the aggressive, devouring qualities will destroy the good. To alleviate this anxiety, the infant performs a defensive separation of the good and bad aspects of internal and external objects called *splitting*. The good breast is experienced by the infant as an altogether different breast than the one attacking her. Because it is bereft of all that would tarnish its perfection, it is an idealized breast.

We have seen how projection and splitting are important to the infant's psychological survival during this period. However, another operation plays a crucial role in spurring the development of the child's internal life. When the child projects her negative and positive feelings onto external objects, she retains an identification with these objects. As real experience with these objects accumulate, they influence their corresponding internal, fantasy representations. In other words, based upon how the real objects behave, the internal schema of the objects is altered accordingly. If good experiences with external objects prevail over bad, the self's tie to the good and bad internal objects strengthens and weakens reciprocally (Segal, 1974). It is precisely this imbalance of power that sets the stage for the child's progression into the next position.

As the infant moves into months 5 and 6, increased perceptual-cognitive abilities make the splitting of positive and negative aspects more difficult. Moreover, the child's increased buildup of positive ties with the mother renders less immediate the threat that the negative elements of the infant's response to the mother could overwhelm the positive. In this more mature depressive position, the infant comes to recognize the whole object. She is no longer merely a breast or another body part but an entire person. This shift is actually visible to those in the infant's social environment because they see that the infant can now recognize her mother. Increasingly, the infant is cognizant that the mother who is associated with frustration is none other than the mother who brings pleasure. With this unification of the various aspects and parts of the mother, a new psychological experience, ambivalence, is born; the infant can have simultaneously positive and negative feelings toward her mother and other figures. The integration of the positive and negative means that no longer does all-good mother exist. Because this all-good mother has been banished from existence through the infant's own integrating activity, the infant's sense of loss is laced with guilt

(Segal, 1974). Also emerging is the infant's awareness of her dependence on the mother and the mother's relative independence from the infant. This awareness creates anxiety, as does the infant's concern that the aggression toward the all-good mother will be repeated toward the whole-object mother. Hence, the infant in the depressive position, while having faced loss, fears further loss.

The depressive position remains throughout life and appears most clearly and pronouncedly in circumstances of loss. The position is stronger in those people for whom the positive side of ambivalent feelings of the object is sufficiently weak to bring into constant question the individual's tie with the object. These individuals typically have an insecurity in their relations with others, a vulnerability to regression into a more primitive mode of object-relations, and a difficulty handling everyday stressors.

While the depressive position is always to some extent resident in the person, even partial progress through it confers extraordinary benefits on the growing child. The capacity to integrate the diverse characteristics of objects promotes the growth of the ego, the part of the personality responsible for adaptation to the environment, because it enables the infant to see the world more realistically. This greater attunement to reality and ability to distinguish reality from fantasy provide a firmer basis for the formation of adaptive responses to the environment. The child's experience of loss in relation to the ideal mother is a formative experience for the development of empathy for others. It also leads the infant to an awareness of her own impulses, their effects on others, and their need for modulation. The wish to restore the ideal object gives rise to creative strivings.

What ramifications does Klein's theory have for the goals that would be pursued by a member in a group run according to the object-relations approach? Within this approach, psychological health is a consequence of development; psychopathology is stunted development resulting from the child's inability to negotiate conflict successfully. Through treatment of any sort, group or individual, the individual is helped to continue to pursue the developmental process. Essentially, the goal of any object-relations treatment is to help the person to grow up intrapsychically and interpersonally. The Kleinian perspective also qualifies the group as an especially good medium for spurring development because the Kleinian infant is radically interpersonal, influencing her social environment and building up her internal world by obtaining information from the social environment. The group provides a milieu in which these activities can be carried out maximally. Klein's thinking also suggested processes and resources by which these goals could be pursued; these will be considered in the next section.

Donald Fairbairn and D. W. Winnicott: While Klein effected the decisive shift in personality theory from infant drive gratification to the pursuit of relationships, a number of theorists developed the implications of this shift for understanding both personality development and psychopathology. Two of them were Donald Fairbairn and D. W. Winnicott, who removed the gauze of fantasy between the mother and infant. The way in which Fairbairn and others such as Mahler (1972) and Winnicott (1958) departed from Klein only increased the applicability of object-relations theory to the group modality. If Klein gave primacy to objects, Fairbairn, like Sullivan, gave primacy to real human relationships (Greenberg & Mitchell, 1983). Both believed that the human being could not be reasonably described apart from his or her relational context. For Fairbairn, innate ideas do not shape relationships with objects; rather, direct experiences with others become introjected and form the inner objects of the infant.

While Fairbairn saw as central to the everyday well-being of the infant the very mechanisms such as splitting that Klein described, a crucial difference is the motive for their operation. Recall that Klein believed that mechanisms such as projection and splitting were used to protect internal and external object-relations from the virulence of the infant's instinctual life. In contrast, Fairbairn saw the activation of these mechanisms as necessary to compensate for deprivations in the infant's relationship with the mother. The child goes inward to protect its relationship with the mother in the midst of the mother's inevitable failure to perfectly gratify the infant. Specifically, in response to frustrations with the mother, the infant introjects a representation of an object that she splits into an ideal object and a depriving object. The depriving object is further split into a depriving or rejecting object and an exciting object. Whereas the depriving object represents the frustrating aspect of the mother, the exciting object symbolizes the tantalizing aspect of the mother, the part of her that withholds the nurturance for which the infant craves.

How do these rather complicated splits serve the adaptation of the infant? By internalizing the negative aspects of the relationship, the infant can safeguard the positive tie with the mother. Internalizing an ideal object provides double insurance. It enables the infant to defend against the anguish associated with the depriving object and provides a compensatory realm of gratification when the contacts with mother are too little fulfilling. Yet to the extent that the infant must create an internal world to defend against and compensate for what is or is not occurring in the relationship with the mother, the infant is that much less available to connect with the mother and other real-life figures. As Greenberg and Mitchell (1983) note, for Fairbairn, the internalization of the negative aspects of the relationship with the parent sets the stage for later relational pathology:

> *It is the experience of these internal object relations and the projection of them onto the outside world that produces pathological suffering within human experience. Love objects are selected for or made into withholders or deprivers so as to personify the exciting object, promising but never fulfilling. Defeat is orchestrated again and again to perpetuate the longing and need of the libidinal ego for the fulfillment of the promise of the existing object.* (pp. 173–174)

A further consequence of this internalization of negative elements is that the individual fails to mature in a relational way. The frustration of longing for adequate nurturing keeps the individual locked in a dependent posture as he or she pursues relationships, unable to establish with others the give and take of healthy adult relationships (Cashdan, 1988). Like Klein, Fairbairn believed that psychological problems bespeak the need for further development, a need that any adequate treatment must address.

Donald Winnicott integrated the contributions of Klein and Fairbairn (Rice, 1992). Winnicott, like Fairbairn, emphasized the real interaction between mother and child as critical in the child's psychological development. Like Klein, he gave the child a very active role in shaping the interactions. Like both Klein and Fairbairn, he believed in the centrality of the human relationship to not only the development but the existence of the infant and expressed this emphatically in the notion that there is no such thing as an infant apart from the mother.

While Winnicott's (1965) contributions to object-relations theory are many, two have particular impact for group therapy: the holding environment and the transitional object. The *holding environment* describes the emotional atmosphere created by the mother so that the infant is able to maintain a state of well-being and to develop to his or her fullest extent. This concept of holding is broader than Bion's construct of containing (Shields, 2000) and refers to a variety of maternal functions. For example, the mother monitors the infant's environment to ensure that the infant is not over- or under-stimulated. The mother may use a word to describe the infant's experience, thereby uniting or integrating the fragments of the infant's world. The mother achieves synchrony with the infant in presenting an object to satisfy the infant at the moment the infant experiences this need, referred to by Winnicott (1971) as the moment of illusion. These illusory experiences contribute to a sense of omnipotence that ultimately leads to the sense of agency necessary for vitality in work and play (LaMothe, 2000). All of these are ways of holding the infant. Holding involves being present and available but nonintrusive when the infant does not have an active need.

The term *transitional objects* refers to symbols of an object's presence, specifically an object such as a caretaker on whom the child depends. Transitional objects are particularly important when a child has not yet achieved object constancy, the recognition of the continued existence of an object even in its absence, but is en route to doing so. While absence of the mother evokes anxiety in the infant, the presence of the transitional object—an object associated with the mother—subdues the anxiety. Transitional objects are important in development because they make separation less traumatic and thereby support the child's use of progressive rather than regressive processes.

Wilfred Bion: The theorist who played the seminal role in applying object-relations theory to the life of a group was Wilfred Bion, who paved the way for the development of an object-relations approach to group therapy. Bion described the propensity of members to not only interact with one another but move toward one another in the development of common behavioral patterns. It is precisely these common patterns that are the basic assumption groups described in Chapter 3. While Bion described three basic assumption states, each corresponding to a different behavioral pattern, they are all a consequence of regression; underlying each basic assumption state is a primitive mode of cognition and affect. In the basic assumption states, members behave as if a specific unconscious fantasy were true, a fantasy that in their lives outside the group they recognize cannot be realized. These fantasies are generated to enable members to defend against certain psychotic-like anxieties the group stimulates. That is, members become intensely fearful of some impending catastrophe, and the fantasy is an imagined way to avert it. Members' anxieties concern the very threats that Klein outlined when she described the schizoid-paranoid and depressive positions that infants assume in the course of normal development—threats such as the annihilation of the self or the destruction of the loved object. These basic assumption groups exist in contrast to the work group, in which members' activity is goal directed and based upon mature cognition.

Why should the experience of being in a group stimulate these kinds of primitive anxieties? Why is regression such a regular feature of group life? Bion's (1962) explanation for these phenomena was that the act of joining a group is highly stressful and thereby induces a massive regression, that is, a regression to an infantile mode of functioning. As a consequence of this regression, the individual member perceives the world as part objects with different part objects being activated at any point in time. The group, too, is seen as a part object by its members. Bion held that the notion of the group as an entity is a construction in the minds of the members to cope with the reality of being among an aggregate of individuals (Brigham, 1992). The specific part object that is activated is a maternal entity. The group has the all-encompassing swaddling quality evocative of the mother of one's infancy. Yet because the group is experienced as an infant experiences her mother, it is not the whole mother with good and bad qualities, the mother who is recognized with the resolution of the depressive position. Rather, it is the shifting mother of infancy who at one time is idealized for her pervasive goodness and at another reviled and feared for her aggressiveness.

The power of the group to evoke maternal imagery creates the potential not only for regression but also for growth. Remember that for Klein the infant, rather than tolerating the full weight of his or her self-destructiveness, splits off this part of self and projects it onto the mother. Yet rather than merely placing this psychological part on the mother, she attempts to influence the mother actively, seeking to evoke in the mother the experience corresponding to the projection. The infant maintains her engagement and identification with the mother such that she recognizes how the mother seems to receive the projection. For example, if a mother spending the afternoon with a cranky infant becomes a tad cranky herself, that fact will not be lost upon the infant. Essentially what the mother is doing is holding on to or containing these threatening psychological elements until they can be safely reowned by the infant. Moreover, when the infant reintrojects these elements, they are now neutralized by the presumably healthy mother's more mature, integrated experience of them.

According to Bion (1959), a similar process occurs within the group. Through projective identification, members place upon the group as a whole or a subset of the group (such as an individual member or subgroup of members) some psychological element of a basic assumption state that has been activated as a consequence of the regressive process. The group is then used to contain these elements in the way the mother contains them for the infant. As Kibel (1992) notes, "Containment is important in treatment, since it permits the projective fantasy to be processed, toned-down, and ultimately corrected" (p. 146). When members reintroject the split and projected elements that have been contained by the group, they are able to integrate them with other psychological elements within themselves. It is precisely the member's newfound integrative nondefensive response to his or her internal life that constitutes psychological growth. Essentially, through the group experience the member can be transformed by the opportunity to redress early developmental issues.

Let's consider an example. Remember how in the basic assumption of fight/flight group members frequently engage in an act of projective identification in which they project hostility onto a member of the group, the therapist, or the group as a whole and then experience this party as an aggressor. Why would members want to create an enemy? Isn't life more tranquil without one? The dynamics of this basic assumption state are essentially those of the paranoid-schizoid position described by Klein. Members feel a pressure to rid themselves of their hostile impulses because they fear these impulses will be destructive to themselves or someone else. While it may be more disturbing to have an enemy out there, it is more threatening to have a destructive force within. In the group, creating a repository for hostility enables members to feel safer until such time as they can reclaim the hostility, acknowledging it as part of themselves rather than defending against it.

According to Bion, groups do not always reside within the basic assumption. The group also has a work group mode in which more rational, logical processes prevail. During such a period, members are more productively reflective and more attuned to reality as most would define it. Progress occurs when the resources of the work group are brought to bear in understanding the phenomena of a particular basic assumption state that has been activated.

Contemporary Theorists: Bion wrote far more on group dynamics than on group therapy. As Yalom (1995) has pointed out, efforts to translate his work straightaway into an approach to group therapy have been largely unsuccessful. A primarily limitation of Bion's thinking when used to inform interventions in a therapy group is its failure to take into account the individual group member (Scheidlinger, 1960). It was for a rather large group of later object relationists to translate object-relations and group dynamic concepts into terms that can be implemented within group therapy.

A seminal concept was the relationship between individual development from an object-relations standpoint and group development. Many observers of group life, from as early as Bennis and Shepard (1956) and as recently as Rice (1992), have noted that the basic assumption states emerge in an orderly rather than random fashion. The regression of members leads the group to follow a developmental path that resembles infantile development. Moreover, the various phases and subphases correspond roughly to the basic assumption states outlined by Bion.

Emerging early in group life is the dependency basic assumption group, corresponding to Klein's schizoid position in which the infant experiences a sense of fusion with an all-good, all-nurturing, all-protective mother (Alonso & Rutan, 1984; Rice, 1992). As noted in Chapter 3, members at this time reveal their wish to fuse with a larger entity through a variety of behaviors such as their unquestioning attitude toward the therapist's authority and their exaggeration of similarities among members and minimization of differences. As Kernberg (1976) noted, "Members feel united by a common sense of need, helplessness, and fear of an outside world they dimly experience as empty or frustrating" (p. 251). From an object-relations perspective what is occurring is that the members build up a sufficiently strong network of positive representations—

representations of the group's goodness and safety—to be able to permit them to continue their work into the next subphase.

Group members then move on to Klein's paranoid position (Alonso & Rutan, 1984), where they attempt to hold on to themselves and the group as a whole as good and the therapist as the repository of all that is evil and deficient. This emotional reaction is Bion's fight/flight group, in which splitting, projection, and projective identification predominate. During this period of group life, members export those internal contents—impulses, affects, and cognitions—that are experienced as threatening or otherwise unacceptable. The therapist becomes a container for these unwanted elements. In serving as a repository, the therapist allows members to consolidate their network of positive representations of themselves, one another, and the group as a whole. The strengthening of these positive representations is a critical step in enabling members to progress to the next developmental challenge in which they will reown their negative projections (Kernberg, 1976; Kibel, 1993).

The group next performs the work of the depressive position as described by Klein (1935). The hallmark of this phase is the integration of members' positively and negatively toned representations of themselves and others. This period, more than any prior one, possesses the characteristics of Bion's work group in which members' interactions are guided to a lesser extent than previously by unconscious fantasy and wishes and to a greater extent by realistic perceptions of the social landscape. Members can now show greater specific attunement to one another and thereby be able to offer to one another positive and negative feedback based upon their here-and-now experiences. They can also now feel genuine caring for one another, such that when they give feedback, it is with the intent to help one another, at least in part. As Safan-Gerard (1996) noted, "The pace is slower as people are now truly learning from experience and need time to assimilate what they are learning" (p. 182). Also, because of this genuine caring, members learn how to make reparation to one another for present and past injuries, a capacity contributing to their achievement of stable attachments.

Work in the depressive phase allows for an expansion of the range of relationships explored. Members need no longer to be exclusively absorbed in the dynamics of the parent–child dyad but can move into an immersion in triadic relationships, which enables an exploration of Oedipal dynamics. As Alonso and Rutan (1984) note,

"Jealousy takes over from envy and triangles abound. Sexual attraction, competition for the leader's or another member's favors, and castration anxiety related to new levels of growth and creativity are all relived in the new group transferences" (p. 1378). Members' work on peer-based transferences in this mature phase contributes to their ability to form intimate, lasting relationships.

Group development, when understood in object-relations terms, enables members to readdress the succession of conflicts faced by the infant in the normal course of intrapsychic/interpersonal development. The group affords a member an opportunity to resolve conflict better than had occurred during infantile development by using the resources of the group. Bion recognized that individuals enter the group with different developmental vulnerabilities. His term "valency" refers to the propensity of an individual to take on certain roles in the group based on the period in which the individual encountered impediments to reckoning successfully with the challenges of that period.

For example, a group member who remained locked within the paranoid position of individual infantile development would have a proficiency in the use of splitting, projection, and projective identification. His or her readiness to use these defenses would likely make him or her a prime candidate to act as a leader of the protest phase of the group's development. However, this member would also have the opportunity to do critical work as the group transitioned out of the paranoid phase into the depressive period. Specifically, this member could participate in the reowning of projections as members move toward integrating their perceptions of others they perceive as good versus bad. Such work would enable this individual to relate to others in a less suspicious and hostile fashion; others would be seen as more benevolent and less threatening. Moreover, this person's self-experience would be more stable because the person's conscious view of himself or herself would comprehend a greater array of personality elements than prior to his or her work in the depressive period. As such, the individual would be less likely to need to revise radically the view of the self based upon the sudden emergence of some unsuspected new element (Kernberg, 1976).

The goal of the object-relations approach to group therapy is to enable the individual to undergo development in relationships with the self and others by reliving the successive intrapsychic interpersonal conflicts of infancy and early childhood, and resolving them in a more adaptive way than the member did then. We have spoken in general terms about how members use the resources of the group to manage the anxiety of reowning their projections and projective identification and to undo splits in the perceptions of self and others. The next section will address in more specific terms the therapist's activity that enables members to fulfill the goals of the object-relations model.

Change Processes

The three elements used by the object-relations therapist to forward the goals of the group are (a) the creation of a holding environment, (b) transference, and (c) countertransference.

Holding Environment

Like the mother creating a growth-promoting environment, the group therapist cultivates an atmosphere where both group development and individual development can take place. To develop a holding environment (Winnicott, 1945), the therapist establishes regular features in the group such as consistent temporal boundaries and a constant location. The therapist encourages members to observe the boundaries by, for example, arriving on time and announcing anticipated absences. The therapist also creates safety by an emphasis upon confidentiality (Tuttman, 1992).

The therapist holds the group through his or her empathetic attunement to members' negatively toned emotional reactions but most especially those painful experiences associated with shame and guilt. The therapist also holds the group by providing words to describe members' affects and impulses. In Chapter 5 we discussed how providing labels for member' experiences is an activity within the therapist's cognitive function, and an example was provided of how the therapist's labeling of the affect state of jealousy dissipated the tension among members and enabled the member to feel more centered. The group therapist engages in this activity in the same way that the Winnicottian mother names the infant's reactions, thereby helping the infant to have a more cohesive identity-fostering experience of himself or herself.

Transference

A hallmark of any form of psychodynamic/psychoanalytic group therapy, with the possible exception of self-psychology, is the use of transference to forward the goals of treatment (Alonso & Rutan, 1993; Freud, 1910/1977). Transference occurs when members' experiences and behaviors within the group are determined by the unconscious mobilization of the conflicts of infancy and childhood. For example, members' perceptions early in group life that the therapist is an omnipotent, all-gratifying caretaker expresses an unconscious wish rooted in the earliest phase of object relatedness when the infant experiences a sense of merger with the mother. Within the classical definition of transference (Freud, 1912/1958), a transference reaction was seen almost entirely as a distortion. A more contemporary perspective, highly congruent with object-relations theory, is that transference is a highly relational phenomenon in which both the individual experiencing the transference reaction and the person or entity evoking it make a substantial contribution to it. For example, because at the beginning of the group's life group members face actual dangers such as loss of self-esteem, the fear that members typically experience is realistic.

From an object-relations perspective, there are multiple types of transference, any one of which may be the most fertile line of investigation at the moment. Members may have transferences to the group as a whole. Such transferences involve a construction of the group in primitive, part object terms, such as when the members see the group as having the soothing qualities of the pre-Oedipal mother (Scheidlinger, 1974). There are also transferences to the leader or to the other group members (peer transferences). Peer transferences can be to either an individual member or a subgroup of members. Different object-relations theorists vary in the extent to which they emphasize each type of transference, but most agree that all have a role to play in an object-relations group and each adds to the richness of the group experience (Alonso & Rutan, 1993). As Winnicott would say about the mother with respect to the infant, the synchronous group therapist recognizes the level of intervention most needed by the group at different points in its life (Rice, 1992).

How might these three types of transference be used to foster members' development? The object relationist is likely to use a range of interventions to help members move to more mature means of responding to the challenges that each phase poses. As we discussed in the theory section, the object-relations approach explores the existence of group dynamics in which each individual participates. At times these dynamics are played out through members' organization into subgroups, each of which may represent a different side of a conflict. To foster the group's and the individual's development, the object-relations therapist uses interventions at various levels, depending upon what is likely to be most helpful to the group at the moment (Horwitz, 1994).

While group-level interventions have often been regarded as the hallmark of object-relations therapy, in fact such interventions are used alongside individual and subgroup interpretations. Yet the groupwide statement is especially warranted in some circumstances. At the most general level, a groupwide statement is typically indicated in the presence of a group-level resistance, much as in the interpersonal approach. However, within the object-relations approach, resistance is defined in more specific terms than in the interpersonal approach. Resistance is the protracted use of primitive defenses in the absence of the reflective activities that allow members to own discarded parts of their internal life. That is, resistance is the group's becoming locked in a defensive pattern. The defensiveness is related to transference in that the use of primitive defenses leads members to organize their contemporary group experiences with the schema of an early developmental era. That is, members transfer early self and object representations onto the present. Because members' engagement in group-level resistance is a regular feature of group life, so, too, is the necessity of group-level interventions. In the following vignette a group-level resistance took hold of the group:

> For several weeks the members had become intently focused upon certain perceived shortcomings of the therapist. Prominent among these was the assumption that the therapist pushed the group to approach painful issues. The tone of members complaints was a kind of passive whining rather than a full-fledged attack. More recently members had been edging toward acknowledging a sense of anger toward and disappointment in the therapist that a few associated with resentment over deprivations from early caretakers.
>
> A new member entered the group. The member was a reasonably confident person who asked various members rather astute, penetrating questions about their reasons for being in group. The group members reverted to

their earlier mode of criticizing the therapist, but now their focus was on the new member, who was portrayed as a kind of vulture purging upon their vulnerabilities. The new member's discomfort unsurprisingly escalated. Members seemed intent by their incessant lamenting to rid themselves of this perceived persecutor.

Perhaps because of the anxiety of having a new member or simply the fear of going forward, these group members retreated to an earlier mode of handling affect. This mode entailed the use of projective identification in which they disowned anger by creating a persecutor. The strength of this group-level reaction not only jeopardized members' making the important step of acknowledging anger and integrating it into the rest of their conscious selves. It also threatened the successful installation of the new group member. Hence, this circumstance would invite a group-level comment by the therapist.

What form should such a group-level intervention take? Possible interventions vary according to the extent to which the content of the therapist's group-level communication involves material that is fairly accessible (as in a therapist's intervention that labels or clarifies members' experiences) or material that is not within consciousness (in the form of an interpretation). The therapist in our example might point out the nature of the group's defensive activity (projective identification), the psychological element against which the group is defending (anger), and the anxiety that requires the use of the defense (guilt over the destructive effects of anger). Each of these elements can be explored over time and with much greater specificity. For example, what is the root of members' anger? Is it envy of the new member? Apprehension over the felt demand to move to a new developmental stage? In fact, for individuals, there may be a somewhat different motivation. All of these concerns can be explored once the therapist has instigated the reemergence of a work group by successfully challenging group-level resistance.

A groupwide intervention is also useful when the organization or structure of the group is shaped by members' internal conflicts (Kibel, 1993). When members subgroup around different sides of a conflict, typically they are dramatizing the conflict that a few (if not all) members are experiencing internally. For example, early in group life members typically subgroup into dependent and counterdependent factions. The conflict between whether to lean on others or fend for oneself is an inescapable human dilemma that can be a sticking point for many (if not all) group members. When members divide into dependent and counterdependent subgroups, they act as if only the members of the alternate subgroup have a particular psychological element (e.g., "Those other members are so dependent; we're not like that at all"). The mechanism at play is projective identification. Each group is projecting onto the other a discarded part of the self. So, completely disavowing that part, the members of the subgroup receiving the projection are maneuvered into experiencing it that much more acutely.

When presented with the situation, the therapist might deliver a group-as-a-whole interpretation,[2] helping members to see that the subgroups represent different sides of an internal conflict. Further, the therapist can point out the defense (projective identification) that leads to externalization of the conflict.

The goal of group-as-a-whole intervention is to restore the work climate in the group. Because the group-level intervention by definition is at a general level, it does not necessarily produce significant change in the individual group member. However, by altering the group dynamics, it creates an atmosphere in which individual interpretations can be made that do capture the specificities of that person's internal life. These more custom-fit interpretations of an individual's specific ways of using a given defense or the particular fantasy that is the impetus for the defense are the means by which change in individual members is effected (Kibel, 1993). In our example of the group whose members scapegoated the new member, for one or more members the threat of the new member may be fear of regression instigated by identification with the member's baby position in the group. For another member it may be sustained by envy over imagined good things that the new member possesses. The group-level intervention can move the group to a plane where these individual dynamics can be addressed.

---

[2] Other models of group therapy would deal with this same subgrouping structure with other types of interventions. Systems-centered therapists (Agazarian, 1997) encourage the consolidation of subgroups and differentiation, according to the model, which increases members' proclivities to identify with the position of the members of the other subgroup. With this identification comes the greater recognition of the previously disavowed content within themselves.

Group-level interventions, however, make two other contributions to the goals of the group. First, they develop the group's cohesion by encouraging members to recognize their connection to one another, their movement together. A cohesive group is one that can serve as the needed holding environment for development to take place. Cohesion also enables the group to realize its potential as a transitional object. When members feel a secure attachment and commitment to one another, they can call up the image in order to apply the understandings derived from group experience, particularly in times of difficulty in their lives outside the group. Second, groupwide comments cultivate members' awareness of the universality of various human affects and urges. As members see that certain psychological experiences are simply part of what is in every person, they find them more acceptable and thereby less in need of being split off from the conscious self (Kibel, 1981).

Once the group-level intervention has successfully effected a shift where members can be reflective about what transpires in the group, then work at the individual or interpersonal level is likely to be fruitful. The aim of such work would be to examine the very specific defenses, wishes, fantasies, and interpersonal behaviors that characterize members' experiences with each other. Let us return to out group with the new, scapegoated member:

> *The therapist had delivered an interpretation to the effect that the introduction of the new member had aroused anger in a member. Members' discomfort with the anger led them to deny it and place it upon the new member, whom they saw as excessively aggressive toward them. Members were silent for several minutes. Bertha then noted that she had been trying to restrain herself with this new member because she felt she had made certain withering comments to the last new member that had caused her to leave precipitously. Other members were mystified by this revelation: They themselves had not seen her role as especially crucial in regard to that member's career in the group. Bertha, surprised and strengthened by members' supportive feedback, went on to describe how she felt that her comments to certain other members had irrevocably alienated her from them. These members were surprised by her inference, which apparently she had harbored for some time. One member said to her, "It's as though you think you have a death finger. When you point at someone, the relationship dies." Bertha's eyes widened and she said, "Exactly right." She went on to talk about her belief that her*

older sister, who died of meningitis at two years of age shortly after she, Bertha, was born had received an infection from her.

In this vignette, it is not the therapist but the members who are doing the individual interpretations. While certainly the individual therapist makes interpretations at various junctures, the members themselves participate in this process. As in this case taken from an actual group, members can be extremely astute and penetrating in their observations of one another, in part, at least, because they identify with the therapist's empathic stance.

In this vignette, Bertha's phantasy of having something akin to a death finger was identified. The theoretical section discussed the notion that unconscious phantasies are all-important because people live them out in their contemporary relationships. Phantasies identified in group frequently concern the feared consequence of expressing some impulse or affect. Bertha's unconscious fear was that the direct emergence of anger is associated with the destruction of other people. When phantasies are identified, both Bertha and the other group members can subject them to reality testing. For example, members could remind Bertha of instances in which her direct expression of anger did not have the feared consequence and may have even forwarded both the relationship and the well-being of the person who was the target of the anger.

In this reality-testing process, the individual member engages in a great deal of interpersonal learning, as would a member in an interpersonal group as described in Chapter 10. Bertha, for example, will learn about how others react to her direct versus indirect expressions of anger. The difference is that the object-relations approach places a greater emphasis upon the unconscious phantasies that underpin members' interpersonal behaviors. Both models focus on members' contemporary experiences in the group. Key to the object-relations perspective is the notion that schemas based on past relationships operate within the present and are modified by present interactions. Nonetheless, the object-relations therapist may be less ready than the interpersonal therapist to refocus members when they delve, as they will, into relationships outside the group and historical relationships. As Tuttman (1992) noted, "Most object-relations leaders encourage their groups to proceed by means of spontaneous exploration, free-as-possible communication without prearranged agendas

Table 11.1   **Functions of Group-Level Interventions**

1. Foster group cohesion

2. Increase members' tolerance for their impulses and affects

3. Alter group dynamics by diminishing the strength of group-level defenses

or restrictions regarding subject matter" (p. 256). Whatever the manifest subject matter is, the object-relations therapist attempts to understand it in terms of members' present relations with one another.

Table 11.1 summarizes the characteristics of group-level interventions.

Countertransference

Countertransference is a key tool of the object-relations group therapist. In Chapter 6 we discussed the distinction between objective and subjective countertransference (Ormont, 1991). To review, subjective transference corresponds to the classical definition of countertransference. It occurs when the therapist's own conflicts influence his or her experience of and behavior toward a group member, a subgroup, or the group. Objective countertransference, on the other hand, is that part of the therapist's reaction that is more universal. It is how many others (not necessarily everyone) might react to this individual.

Objective countertransference is useful simply because it helps the therapist recognize how other people experience this group member. This notion is essentially that of the microcosm. Beyond this aspect, the object relationist would hold that objective countertransference is a conduit to the member's inner world. As we have discussed previously, because of the regression that group participation induces, projective identification is a major mechanism shaping the interactions among members. The countertransference reactions of the therapist may be the result of members' use of projective identification in which one or more members attempt to rid themselves of a particular psychological content by placing it upon the therapist (or another member) and maneuvering the therapist into having the experience corresponding to the element.

Therefore, by understanding these internal elements, the therapist comes to realize what elements within themselves members find most threatening at the moment.

Yet to make sense of these projective identifications, the therapist must be able to analyze his or her own feelings and determine what within the member they are reflecting. Heinrich Racker (1972) assisted group therapists with this task by drawing a distinction between concordant and complementary identifications. A *concordant identification* occurs when the therapist experiences a psychological element that the patient regards as part of himself or herself. A concordant identification is the therapist's empathic grasp of how the patient feels to be himself or herself. These types of identifications flow naturally from the alliance between therapist and patient and are often more noticeable by their absence than by their presence. In the group setting the therapist may establish a concordant identification with the group as a whole or any subgroup. Not all concordant identifications are projective identifications. Those that are reveal to the therapist the warded-off aspects of self-representations.

A *complementary identification* occurs when the therapist identifies with an object in the patient's internal world. For example, the therapist may be seen as an all-good, omnipotent parent. The member may treat the therapist with such reverence that the therapist begins to take on these qualities. An important point here is that the projecting member has induced the therapist (or any other person in the group) to become a worldly reflection of the internal object. This member is likely to engage in similar activity outside the group. Therefore, complementary identifications teach the group not only about each member's internal life but also about how he or she structures the social world and pulls responses from others.

An important function of the therapist from an object-relations perspective is to contain those projections that are currently intolerable to the group member. If the therapist does so, members will eventually be able to reown the rejected contents but now will be able to experience them admixed with the therapist's tolerance of them. However, these projections that the therapist is invited to contain are often associated with discomfort. Moreover, as the projective identification is under way, the therapist typically may not recognize it as such. Like all human beings, the therapist is motivated to reduce or avoid discomfort. Therefore, the therapist risks engaging in defensive activity to avoid the identification. One way the therapist can accomplish this defense is by using one type of identification to fend off another:

> *A relatively new group therapist had been conducting a group for 3 months. The first few weeks had a strained quality as the members struggled to relate to one another and the therapist labored to facilitate them in doing so. Eventually, the group members were able to identify the common concern of extreme loneliness and sense of alienation. As members recognized this shared concern, their comfort in the group increased.*
>
> *Dr. Bin announced that in three weeks she would be taking a vacation and had to cancel two group sessions. The group members expressed surprise and disappointment over the upcoming hiatus. Members talked about their expectation that they would be back to "square one" when it resumed. One member rather archly asked Dr. Bin whether the group needs are taken into account when she decides when to schedule a vacation. Another member said she wondered whether she would feel like returning after the break.*
>
> *Dr. Bin spoke to her supervisor about her distress over members' reactions. She revealed that she felt very guilty about interrupting the group and saw it as a selfish act. She was so beleaguered by her feelings of recrimination and fears that members would label her as "selfish" that she was unable to follow carefully the group process. She said that increasingly she had been questioning whether she had the necessary personal qualities to be an effective group therapist.*

The object-relations theorist might examine this situation as follows: Dr. Bin formed a complementary identification with the group's images of an abandoning caretaker. Although she had provided a reality component for some sense of loss on the part of members, the members had elaborated on this material, making it a catastrophe. The extremity of the response is telltale: It bespeaks members' responsiveness to internal templates that have been not created but activated by present experiences. Dr. Bin's response was also noteworthy in that it, too, was disproportionate to the reality of the present. Therapists do take vacations, and most typically their vacations are planned based on personal considerations. The therapist's degree of guilt was simply out of proportion to her actions. While she committed no offense, she felt that she had. Possibly the therapist's response derived from her own conflicts (subjective countertransference). Yet the group played a substantial role in maneuvering the

therapist into having an experience that complemented their own reactions. That is, in response to members' projection of the image of
an abandoning caretaker onto her, the therapist felt neglectful. Moreover, in her distractibility and self-questioning, she did remove herself from the group. Through projective identification the group
induced her to behave like an abandoning caretaker.

The awareness of a given complementary identification clears
the way for the therapist to have other types of identification that
may be useful to the group. Recognizing the identifications being
formed frees the therapist from being locked in an identification. Realizing an identification creates some measure of distance that enables the therapist to respond constructively to it. Moreover, the
awareness of a complementary identification enables the therapist
to clear the way for concordant identifications. When, as in our example, the therapist is so fettered by harsh self-accusations created
by the complementary identification, she would have great difficulty forming a concordant identification with members' sense of
sadness. In fact, when operating on an unconscious complementary
identification of this nature, the therapist's desire to diminish her
guilt would lead her to discourage the expression of either sadness or
the sense of deprivation to which it is attached.

In this example, several types of therapist reaction were manifested, such as guilt and self-doubt. However, object relationists hold
that the range of potential therapist reactions is no narrower than
the range of human experiences: Group therapists may at different
moments feel joy, hatred, lust, confusion, exhilaration, triumph, exasperation, and so on. To object relationists and psychodynamic
therapists in general, all of these feelings in isolation or combination
can be valuable signposts to the nature of the group members' experiences, conscious and unconscious. Greene, Rosenkrantz, and Muth
(1985) demonstrated in a cotherapy situation, the differences in reactions of the two therapists may also have diagnostic value. For example, radically different emotional responses may belie the group
members' use of the defense of splitting. The object-relations theorist would see as a key possession for the therapist a tolerant, noncondemnatory attitude toward any and all of the contents so that
they are the objects of exploration rather than defense. To achieve
this posture, object-relational thinkers see protracted periods of self-
exploration both in therapy and in supervision as critical for the
group therapist.

Psychodynamic/Object-Relations Vignette

This group had been meeting for a year with some turnover in membership. In the last session the therapist had wondered aloud whether members had been offended by an offhand quip she made in the beginning of the session. She speculated that members' disjointed, emotionally flat communications had perhaps been an effort to block the reaction to this moment of insensitivity. The members responded in a jocular way, making sport with the therapist for thinking they were so fragile. At one point Arabella did a rather good humorous imitation of the therapist's earnest style. However, right before she left the group, she said, "Sorry, I didn't mean to offend you."

The Members

The reader has already met Arabella, who has been in the group a year. Four additional members in this eight-member group were:

- Gill: An artist in his mid-30s who was in the middle of a custody dispute. He was court-ordered into therapy in order to have visitation rights with his latency-age children. His former wife alleged that he was verbally abusive. While Gill acknowledged difficulties with anger control, he asserted that his former wife exaggerated the problem.

- Lisa: A woman with paraplegia in her late 20s who suffered injuries from a car accident a year earlier. She had been in the group only two months. In her first month of group sessions, she was very withdrawn and indicated that she did not want to discuss the accident until she was ready.

- Kate: A Roman Catholic nun in her early 70s who had been having recurrent bouts of depression since her retirement from being clinical director of a hospital several years earlier. In her community, she had trouble with relationships with other sisters because she presented herself as having authority over them.

- Ellen: This administrative secretary in a law firm experienced loneliness because of her inability to sustain a long-term intimate relationship with a man. Ellen is in her mid-30s and is worried that if she does not establish a relationship soon, she will not be able to have children.

The Session

KATE: Did you call that new specialist? It just bothered me so when you mentioned there was this new research protocol—some hope for you—and you didn't do anything. So did you call?

LISA: I went to call but that was the beginning of the week and I was told the principal investigator wasn't in and he was the one I had to speak to . . . and then at the end of the week I got busy so . . .

KATE: Sometimes we have these chances given to us but we have to do the rest. . . .

GILL: You mean "given to us by God," don't you? But you didn't want to say that.

KATE: Why does that matter?

GILL: Because I'm onto your bringing subliminal God into the room.

ARABELLA: [laughing] I like that . . . subliminal God.

KATE: She's a young woman—she can't walk. She has some hope—and you're worried about hidden messages?

ELLEN: [to Gill] I think she's right. But *you'd* rather just give her grief than earnestly address a member's problem.

GILL: I am earnestly addressing a member's problem—I'm addressing her problem—Kate's, I mean.

KATE: My problem—are you trying to say *God's* my problem?

GILL: Maybe but if she's being fed this stuff about a cure, she's never going to do it fully.

THERAPIST: It's almost as if you're afraid to have her hope . . . as if disappointment would be the worse thing.

GILL: Yeah, my image is these poor people who traipse around to different statues around the world hoping to get a cure for cancer—having the disease is bad enough . . . but then all of those letdowns.

Note: The therapist's intervention with Gill was a simple clarification. Yet it brought out a dimension of his reaction that was not obvious in his sarcastic demeanor toward Kate: his effort to protect Lisa. Rather than having his response construed as mere hostile indifference by Kate, Ellen, and others, members are able to see the caring that underpins his pugnacious response. From an object-relations standpoint, it is important for members to experience the altruistic aspect of themselves, an opportunity uniquely afforded by group therapy. By doing so they build up and strengthen their positive representations of self so that at a later point each member will be able to integrate those positive representations with those that are negatively toned without undue fear that the former will be destroyed.

LISA: Honestly, sometimes I'm not sure myself. You're right: it can be a letdown.

Note: Lisa's acknowledgment of this aspect of her suffering was unprecedented and in part was facilitated by her recognition of Gill's empathy with her.

KATE: Now I'm getting irritated. I don't think there's one person here—well, except the doctor, of course—who knows the medical field better than I do. If Lisa doesn't go along with her physician's recommendations, he may lose interest in doing anything beyond the most basic medical management.

ARABELLA: [to Gill] She has a point. You can't afford to insult these people.

THERAPIST: Am *I* one of those people? Perhaps you and maybe others were feeling that way after our last group?

Note: The therapist listened to the material in terms of its symbolic value. The discussion of figures of authority can often have implications for members' thoughts and feelings about the therapist. In this case, the connection is especially compelling because of the therapist's offensive comment.

ARABELLA: I regretted doing the imitation. In the moment, I knew I could get a laugh. But, really, I made fun of you. Actually, it bothered me all night . . . but then I got over it [giggles].

Note: Arabella's description of her regret is an emotional characteristic of the depressive position in which there exists a concern that the direction of anger toward the loved object will destroy the object. Arabella's laughter at such a moment is a hypomanic defense against the regret.

ELLEN: [to Arabella] Well, I hope, you noticed that *I* didn't laugh—I found it completely irritating that you did that.

GILL: So you were the good little girl who should get all the teacher's love?

> *Note:* Through his derisive, devaluing tone, Gill is both expressing and hiding his envy over Ellen's capacity to more directly express her dependency needs and thereby have them satisfied. A question in the therapist's mind might be what feared consequences Gill associates with the direct expression of dependency such that he feels he cannot risk such behavior. While the exploration of envy is important in the group, it must be approached with some delicacy because of its intimate connection to shame.

KATE: Maybe you should get off her case.

THERAPIST: Ellen, I think that you have in some way a similar worry to Arabella's. Just as she wants me to know that she didn't really mean to offend me, you want me to realize that you wouldn't join in on something that could be offensive. And maybe there's a worry for both of you—and perhaps for others—about how I might change if I were to be offended. . . .

GILL: I don't think you would change per se . . . you might leave the session in a bad mood and take it out on your husband, if you have one. Of course, if I really got on your nerves, you could report back to the judge and I'd either have to stay here longer or not see my kids.

> *Note:* Gill is talking about one fear connected to his expression of anger: The object may retaliate.

KATE: If she took that action, it would not be because you got on her nerves. It would be because it is her professional duty.

ARABELLA: Guys, I'm becoming sorry I made any big deal of this at all.

THERAPIST: Well, you did say it bothered you after the group—that's a big enough deal and it was helpful that you mentioned it so we could see what significance last week's events had not only for you but also for other members. What went through your mind about it?

Note: The therapist is reinforcing the work climate of the group and providing encouragement to elaborate upon the feared consequences of expressing a feeling.

ARABELLA: Well, I just replayed the end of the group in my head and I tried to picture your expression to see if you looked hurt. I actually thought you did just a little bit. But I got distracted from that because I decided I'd call my mother. I had this fight with her Sunday evening. It was about my taking money from my dad. She says she wants me to be more independent, but I think it's because she feels inadequate because she can't help me financially. After the conversation, I didn't hear from her for four nights and that's unusual.

GILL: What did you think?

ARABELLA: Well . . . where my mother is concerned, I can never be sure . . . she won't . . . she can get pretty low—

GILL: You mean she'll kill herself?

ARABELLA: No—she's never tried that, but she can get so depressed. . . . I mean she hasn't for many years—but I can't feel secure that she won't again . . . that I won't receive a call from some hospital administrator to tell me she's just been admitted.

[Arabella went on to talk about how, in her childhood, a constant preoccupation was whether her mother would need to be hospitalized. She described herself as acquiring a special skill in monitoring her mother's mood state.]

THERAPIST: And perhaps some worry like that is creeping in here—that if the group crosses me that something bad will happen—that I'll take some action against you or will become hurt and defeated. Perhaps it is because of these concerns that the group had a difficult time even considering whether the group had a reaction to my would-be humor last week. Because talking about any irritation with me seems so dangerous, the best strategy may appear to deny it altogether.

LISA: I feel that way about the woman who takes care of me. She's extremely kind, but there are certain things that she does that bother me. I never want to tell her because she does so much for me, and tries hard.

KATE: It's just a matter of diplomacy—if you say it the right way, I'm sure she'll take it the right way.

GILL: And what is the right way for her to take it?

KATE: For her not to become upset, for her not to abandon her commitment to Lisa out of a feeling of not being appreciated.

GILL: You people worry entirely too much about how other people think or what they're likely to do. Look at Lisa. She's in a wheelchair—her life is total discomfort—and yet she can't say one thing to her nurse to just have a little bit of relief.

KATE: I didn't say she should keep quiet—merely said she should take care in expressing what might be construed as a criticism.

ARABELLA: Gill, you have such a chip on your shoulder. Every time you speak, it's with this edge. Why are you getting so irked?

GILL: I don't know—it's just the whole conversation . . . [drifts off]

THERAPIST: Well, I think you gave yourself and the rest of us a clue when you said that it was all of this worry about others' reactions—and maybe we could make it more specific—that it has to do with the people who are in charge—people in authority—like me.

GILL: I hate having to fawn over someone like I hear everyone in this room wanting to do. Just picturing myself doing it disgusts me. I might just as well walk around in despair with a pacifier stuck in my mouth.

ARABELLA: What a great image!

THERAPIST: So sometimes when you think of yourself being concerned with what these people-in-charge think of you, you feel like a baby.

ARABELLA: And that's how you've been seeing us—as whining babies. And so you can't join us . . . because you're trying to cling to the adult Gill—but in case you haven't noticed, you're beginning to annoy us with your haughty I'm-so-mature attitude . . . well, you're annoying me anyway.

GILL: Good, I like to be annoying—especially to you. [Arabella laughs.]

THERAPIST: But what Gill's telling us that he keeps himself apart in a way that might annoy other members when to join in involves doing things that will put him in that baby position. I wonder if others can relate to not wanting to feel like a baby again.

Note: Within the psychodynamic approaches to group work, including the object-relations approach, it is important that the member can connect his or her interpersonal behaviors with indulging impulses and affects. Here the therapist is making explicit the connection between Gill's distancing in the group and his fear of regression.

LISA: I completely understand what he's saying about the baby thing. I am totally dependent on a host of people, all of whom I must mollify and placate just so that I can . . . survive. Yet . . . [becomes tearful], I haven't survived. It's almost as if I don't exist anymore because . . . I don't recognize who this person is.

GILL: [almost to himself] You said it . . . that's it . . . I'm afraid I won't exist anymore.

ELLEN: [to Lisa] I can see how you could have that feeling, but on the other hand, what I see is that despite everything you've been through, you come here every week, and subject yourself to even more discomfort . . . just so you can go forward with your life . . . that's hardly being a baby.

GILL: Yeah, it's pretty cool.

[The session continues.]

In this session, segment members are doing work in the depressive position. The predominant concern of the members is how to reconcile their negative feelings for the therapist with a sense of having damaged the therapist through this reconciliation. A first hint was when the group could not have even a superficial discussion about the therapist's off-the-cuff comment while at the same time not being able to pursue anything else in earnest. Also supporting this hypothesis was Arabella's anxious inquiry at the end of the session. In the next session, the one featured in this vignette, the members begin discussing the risks Lisa incurs in failing to comply completely with her physician's directives. The group could have pursued this topic in many ways, but they did so along the lines of depressive position conflicts. Specifically, the group focused on whether Lisa, by not being a perfect patient, by exercising some autonomy, would in effect damage his professionalism by making him less committed to her.

Members' work in the depressive position has the potential for reaping many benefits. For example, Arabella's lack of a stable connection with a caretaker in her early life because of her mother's depression prevented her from achieving relational maturity. As the reader sees from the vignette, she strove mightily to relate only to that part of the therapist that was acceptable to her. This investment ensured that her relationships would be transient because once she could no longer deny the negative aspects of the other person, she would be forced to abandon the relationship. This dynamic accounted for her inability to sustain a long-term relationship with an individual therapist. However, the group has experiential opportunities for Arabella that the individual therapy situation lacks. We can see that Arabella can hold on to her positive tie with other members while she and other members are exploring their negative reactions to the therapist (and other authority figures). She also can come to realize that her feelings, impulses, and fantasies are really quite ordinary and therefore far less dangerous than she had imagined. As Arabella uses these special resources of the group, she is able over time to tolerate seeing the therapist and others in their wholeness, that is, in both positive and negative terms, an achievement of supreme importance for lasting relationships.

Object-relations therapists do not necessarily presume that all members are doing the same work during any given period of the group's life. We can see that different members have varying catastrophic fantasies about the consequences of integrating positive and negative representations. Each member brings uniqueness to the negotiation of this developmental hurdle based upon his or her particular background. For instance, Arabella is more focused than others on the parental figure becoming depressed based upon her experiences with her mother. Gill's thinking is much more characteristic of the paranoid position—the fear of the therapist attacking him. Nonetheless, he was able to do meaningful work despite possibly having somewhat different dynamic concerns than other members. The role of the therapist is to be attentive not only to group-level themes but to individual variation to encourage the latter to emerge.

For example, the therapist listens for subtle differences in how members elaborate upon a group-level theme and invites them to clarify and further describe their own perspective.

In this session, we see how the therapist used that key tool of psychodynamic work—countertransference. However, because we were privy only to verbalizations rather than the therapist's internal reactions, we don't know how the therapist's use of countertransference played a role in the group's movement. We might wonder whether the therapist's recognition of the effect of her joke was delayed because of a complementary identification with members' image of the all-good therapist who simply would not make an inappropriate comment. A complementary identification would lead the therapist to collude with members' silence in relation to the error. However, having insight into her enactment of this identification may have liberated her sufficiently to be able to form a concordant identification with members' disappointment in discovering that she departs from the ideal. Whatever contemplation occurred for the object-relations therapist over the session, analyzing countertransference patterns would be a crucial activity in understanding the group dynamics.

Short-Term Applications

Like the interpersonal approach, most psychodynamic approaches to group therapy (including an object-relations orientation) were developed for a long-term frame. The goal of most psychodynamic approaches—to effect healthy intrapsychic change and help the individual mature internally—would seem to demand a long duration of participation. Yet awareness is growing that psychodynamic approaches can make a contribution in short-term time frames (Rutan & Stone, 2001). This point is also true for models informed by object-relations theory.

A major factor determining what goals can be established and what methods might be used is how much time is available. When members' typical duration of participation is extremely brief, for example, several sessions, it is unrealistic to expect that emotional maturation is possible through group participation. However, brief therapy often occurs when the individual has experienced a crisis or a set of stressors that have led the individual to regress. Accompanying whatever symptoms the person may have is a decrement in everyday level of functioning. The individual, because of regression, uses more primitive modes of cognition and defenses. These more immature modes of thinking and coping with affects and impulses are typically less serviceable and spawn further adaptive difficulties. A worthwhile goal for brief object-relations group therapy is to assist the individual in recovering his or her premorbid level of functioning.

Kibel (1981) has proposed such a model for the treatment of inpatients organized at the borderline level (see Chapter 2) who are being treated over a brief stay. The goal of Kibel's model is to help members to reconstitute, that is, to return to their premorbid level of functioning. What this means for borderline individuals is the reacquisition of the defense of splitting. While ordinarily we may not think of splitting as an effective defensive maneuver, it does provide the individual who uses it habitually with a certain measure of well-being. That is, it assures the person of some positive experiences of self and others, even though these experiences may be confined to limited periods. An individual who loses access to splitting is overrun by negative feelings about the self and others. Projection and projective identification become much more pronounced. As the individual uses others as repositories for his or her negative feelings, relationships deteriorate.

Kibel's model is applicable to the circumstance in that group therapy takes place within a larger treatment program, typically the unit of a hospital in which patients reside and participate in their therapeutic activities. In this model, the therapist listens to the material that members discuss in the session as a symbolic reflection of concerns that they have in their lives in the unit.

For example, if members complain about bosses at work or other authority figures outside the treatment setting, the therapist might think about and share how these expressions of discontent might be reasonable reactions to difficulties with the authority figures in the unit. Such an intervention helps members to bind and channel their hostility to immediate figures. Such an intervention is an antidote to the pervasive hostility they experience toward self and others, a hostility that leaves no room for pleasurable experiences. At the same time, members are given abundant opportunity to interact positively with one another, thereby helping them consolidate their positive representations of self and others.

Both types of interventions are aimed at the reinstatement of splitting and with it the capacity to function at the level members did prior to the regressive episode. The goal of moving members to a new developmental level is left to group therapy occurring in a longer time frame. Like Yalom's Interactional Agenda Model, Kibel's object-relations model can be useful even if a member's participation is for only a single session.

In short-term group therapy, treatments last from a period of several weeks to approximately a half a year. Such a temporal circumstance may allow for some developmental progress to be made in highly circumscribed areas. Piper et al. (1992) provide an example of a short-term group format directed toward specific goals. This group, described in Chapters 2 and 7, is designed for individuals who have undergone pathological loss reactions (reactions that substantially compromise the person's ability to function adequately and to enjoy life; the grief may be absent, inordinately intense, or prolonged). Piper et al. contend that a significant subgroup of individuals who have pathological loss reactions are those who have developmental vulnerabilities in relation to loss. That is, their early experiences in negotiating the separations that are part of normal development were less than successfully and therefore did not prepare them adequately for later losses.

Piper et al. describe their model as a psychoanalytic rather than an object-relations model per se. However, these writers make such extensive use of object-relations theory in the design of the model that it shows us the potential of this orientation for short-term work. For example, Klein's (1948) notion of pathological loss reactions being rooted in the person's failure to achieve ambivalence (the integration of positive and negative qualities in the representation of the object) is one of the guiding notions of the treatment. Piper and colleagues establish as the goal the group members' overcoming of their pathological reactions to loss by resolving in a more satisfactory way the conflicts associated with loss.

In this 12-session outpatient group, the stages that naturally emerge over the life of a group are tapped for different exploratory opportunities. Piper and colleagues conceptualize the group as consisting of these stages (beginning, middle, and end) with each stage potentially activating a set of loss-related conflicts unique to that stage. For instance, the beginning stage activates the conflict between the yearning to establish intimacy and fear that by doing so the member would incur some significant risk. Such a risk might be the pain associated with the recent loss. It might also be the risk, identified by Bowlby (1963), that new intimacies challenge the mourner's denial of the permanence of the loss. Members might resolve this conflict by establishing connections among themselves but on such a superficial level that they retain a sense of safety.

In helping members to resolve their conflicts in an adaptive way, the therapist adopts a particular role. The therapist assumes a passive or nondirective role at the beginning of each session in order to allow a regressive process to unfold. As explained earlier, regression is key to surfacing those conflicts that psychodynamic group treatment is designed to address. The therapist maintains neutrality in refraining from offering judgment or personal disclosures. One consequence of this neutrality is that the therapist keeps conflicts active by failing to ally with a particular side of a conflict. The therapist engages in interpretive activity, drawing attention to one or more sides of a conflict, sides that may be conscious but are often unconscious. Particular emphasis is given to those shared conflicts related to loss. While the therapist's interpretations may concern transference phenomena, they are by no means limited to these.

All of these therapist activities are fairly typical in long-term psychodynamic groups. What distinguishes the therapist in this short-term group from the former are two behaviors. The therapist in the short-term group frequently calls attention to the limited time available for the group's work. As the ending of the group draws near, the therapist reminds the group of this fact. A second behavior is that the therapist, when appropriate, highlights the limitations inherent in short-term group work such as the fact that members must constantly share the group's and therapist's attention with the other group members. Both of these types of interventions are designed to underscore the features within the group that can engender loss reactions, thereby making these reactions that much more available for the group's study.

Not only does the therapist perform functions for the group but so do the group members by taking on roles. A role is a set of behaviors that represent a conflict or an aspect of a conflict. In displaying these behaviors, the member does so not only for himself or herself but for the other members of the group. Piper and colleagues distinguish this use of the term "role" from its use by Yalom (1995), who emphasizes the defensive function the role performs for the individual rather than the group. For example, one common group role Piper and colleagues identified was "the apparition," wherein the presence of the member occupying this role is unpredictable. This role allows the member to give symbolic expression to the previously described conflict in the group between becoming intimately connected to one another and maintaining a safe distance. When the therapist interprets this role, he or she does so in terms of the significance of the behavior for the group—not merely for the individual.

While only a thumbnail sketch of this model can be offered here, the reader is referred to Piper et al.'s text (1992) for further description of the model and many rich clinical examples of its applications. We consider the outcomes associated with this model in the next section.

Research Support

The goal of the psychodynamic orientation in general and the object-relations models specifically is intrapsychic change. As discussed in Chapter 2, intrapsychic change is measured indirectly and with some difficulty. Moreover, until recently psychodynamic approaches were used only in short-term situations, situations that are more conducive to investigators. For these reasons and possible others, research evaluating the effectiveness of psychodynamic approaches is extremely limited. Yet there appears to be a burgeoning awareness among psychodynamic group therapists of the need for such research both to learn whether a given psychodynamic approach is effective and what elements are critical to its success (Piper et al., 1992). Recently, measures of object-relations constructs have been developed. For example, measures of splitting by Greene (1990) and colleagues (Greene, Rosencrantz, & Muth, 1985) are available for research on therapy groups.

A number of studies have demonstrated the effectiveness of psychodynamic groups in general. Greene and Cole (1991) demonstrated the utility of a psychodynamic group format relative to a structured, task group with borderline inpatients. Lothstein (2001) in a naturalistic study described the success of psychodynamic group in lowering the recidivism and relapse rate of a group of sex offenders over a 10-year period. However, many studies in the literature, while claiming to use a group approach informed by psychodynamic theory, do not make clear which constructs most inform the group structure and therapist interventions. The findings, whether positive or otherwise, are ambiguous because the various psychodynamic approaches differ from one another in important ways.

In this section, two studies are discussed in some detail because they extend the discussion from the former section on the short-term dynamic loss group and provides an example of a study with methodological rigor and clinical utility. Piper et al. (1992) compared research participants, all of whom were suffering from complicated grief reactions, who were assigned to one of two conditions: a short-term therapy group (as described in the prior section) or a wait-list control group. The research participants were initially evaluated for their levels of psychological mindedness, which is "the ability to identify dynamic components and relate them to a person's difficulties" (p. 148). Research participants were paired according to their levels of psychological mindedness, gender, and age and then randomly assigned to the experimental and control groups.

Members of the experimental group participated in the 6-week experience. During the course of this group the investigators applied a measure of psychodynamic work to members' activity. The authors defined psychodynamic work as "the attempt to understand the problems of one or more members of the group, or the group as a whole, in terms of conflict among dynamic components" (p. 149). In including both the psychological mindedness and psychodynamic work variables, the investigators were assessing not only the effectiveness of the approach but identifying factors that might be critically linked to effectiveness.

The investigators assessed participants on a battery of measures before and immediately after treatment and again 6 months after treatment. Eighteen different variables from a variety of areas were assessed using pretest–posttest analysis. These included interpersonal functioning (on which 10 variables focused), symptomatology, personal targets, life satisfaction, and self-esteem. The investigators found that patients who participated in the short-term loss group showed greater improvement across a variety of areas than those in the control condition. Areas of improvement included self-esteem, life satisfaction, personal targets, and symptomatology. Changes in interpersonal functioning were contingent upon the nature of the relationship. While improvement in sexual functioning was noted, positive change in work relationships, friendships, and close associates was not observed.[3]

The investigators examined whether the two variables, psychological mindedness and psychodynamic work, were related to outcome. Psychological mindedness did not predict outcome for any measure. However, psychological mindedness was related to remaining in the group: Those members who left tended to be low in psychological mindedness. While psychodynamic work was associated with positive change in several interpersonal areas such as relationships with family of origin, most correlations between psychodynamic work and interpersonal variable were disappointingly nonsignificant. Piper et al. (1992) note that a limitation of their way of measuring psychodynamic work was that it was restricted to members' verbalizations. The investigators acknowledged that much work can occur internally.

Piper et al.'s (1992) study provides support for the usefulness of a short-term psychodynamic model with loss patients, one which is informed by object-relations notions. The positive change observed across a spectrum of key areas such as self-esteem, life satisfaction, and symptamotology is especially impressive. While the two variables, psychological mindedness and psychodynamic work, did not have the strength of association with outcome that were predicted, the authors obtained information that could enable them to refine their efforts to study the essential mechanisms of the group treatment in future investigations.

In a second related study, Piper et al. (2001) compared time-limited, short-term interpretive and support group therapy in the treatment of individuals with complicated grief reactions. In the interpretive therapy members were assisted in achieving greater insight into repetitive conflicts associated with loss and to acquire greater tolerance for ambivalence toward lost figures. The investigators found that members of both groups showed a lessening of grief symptoms and general symptoms. However, members in the interpretive group showed a greater decrease in general symptoms. In contrast to the prior study, members who were higher in psychological mindedness

---

[3] The reader may recall that in Chapter 10, the Budman, Demby, Soldz, and Merry (1996) study failed to reveal positive changes in similar measures. Again, it appears that a consideration of what types of interpersonal change can most readily be reflected through group treatment is a topic of paramount importance.

had more favorable outcomes in both groups. Another variable, quality of object relations, also proved important. Members with higher scores on this scale obtained more favorable outcomes in the interpretive group, while members with lower scores did better in the supportive group. This finding is understandable given the developmental theory presented early in the chapter. The interpretive group seems to require that members do work in Klein's depressive position. Members who show a lower quality of object relations may not be ready for this work.

For all forms of psychodynamic group treatment, including the object-relations approach, efforts must be undertaken such as that of Piper et al. (1992) to demonstrate the efficacy of the approach. Furthermore, we must learn what intervals of treatment are necessary for different types of changes and what are the mutative or change-producing features of the treatment when it is successful.

Summary

This chapter examined one particular application of the psychodynamic theory to group therapy—the object-relations approach. The goal of treatment according to psychodynamic theory is to effect a positive shift in the person's intrapsychic functioning, which in turn enhances the person's well-being potentially in all important areas. Object-relations theory focuses on the internal templates of self and others that are formed from the individual's early relationships. These templates shape an individual's present experiences but can also be altered by present experiences. The goal of the object-relations approach is to provide the person with experiences within the group setting that will lead to more mature representations of self and objects.

According to object-relations theory, the group provides an ideal setting for modifying representations because it activates a process of regression. Accompanying this regression is the emergence of infantile conflicts—wishes, anxieties, and defenses. Members are able to readdress these conflicts within the process of the group and potentially resolve them more satisfactorily than they did during infancy and early childhood. In assisting group members in this work, the therapist creates a holding environment in which support and safety are provided as members revisit these early issues. The object-relations therapist uses the resources generally tapped by the psychodynamic therapist—transference, interpretation, and countertransference. In using transference, the object-relations therapist recognizes that dynamics exist on the level of the group, the subgroup, and, the individual. Moreover, transferences can occur to the group as a whole, the therapist, a subgroup, or an individual member. At any moment in the group's life, the exploration of one type of transference may be of greatest therapeutic advantage. The challenge for the object-relations therapist is to recognize when interventions on the group, subgroup, or individual level are likely to be most fruitful. Countertransference is a major tool of the therapist. Because therapist's reactions are determined not only by the therapist's own conflictual concerns but by the group's projective identifying activities in which the group's unwanted contents are deposited within the therapist, the therapist's impulses, affects, and phantasies are signposts to the members' unconscious lives.

Although object-relations applications have primarily been long term, brief and short-term models have recently been designed for particular clinical situations. Kibel's brief inpatient model and Piper, McCallum, and Azim's short-term model for loss patients were described. The body of research on psychodynamic approaches and to an even greater extent object-relations applications is limited. Yet, a small group of studies offering support for psychodynamic approaches does exist. Two studies with promising results on the Piper et al. model were presented.

The Cognitive-Behavioral Approach

Buddy is a freshman in college. He is an African American student in a predominantly White university. Two weeks after arriving at school, he received a letter from his long-standing girlfriend indicating her wish to sever the relationship. She acknowledged that she wanted to have the freedom to pursue new social opportunities in her college setting. Two months later, Buddy was unable to focus on his academic work, so preoccupied was he by this rejection. He made two friends among the other majors in engineering but confided in neither about the dissolution of the relationship because he feared that they would see him as weak.

Buddy was distressed to be receiving Bs and Cs. He attributed his low grades to a lack of ability in his chosen area of engineering. He had a meeting with his academic advisor, who encouraged Buddy remain an engineering major, pointing out to him that his high school grades and standardized test scores provided substantial evidence for such intellectual work. Buddy was reminded by this experience of the self-doubt he had before college when he imagined he was not "college material." Only the encouragement of his high school counselor enabled him to pursue higher education.

In the interview, it was learned that Buddy had some mild vegetative symptoms, including hypersomnia and lack of appetite. When the interviewer inquired about Buddy's family life, Buddy said that he remembered his childhood relationship with both his mother and father as extremely positive and it remained so through the present. However, he said that his parents' relationship was flawed by his mother's dissatisfaction with his father's lack of ambition and his father's resentment over his mother's demands.

12

Chapter

In 1976 Aaron T. Beck proposed an approach to treatment that is based upon a cognitive model of personality. This model asserts that how an individual feels and behaves is a consequence of how the individual cognitively structures the world (A. T. Beck, 1976) and the ways he or she makes meaning of events. Buddy, for example, is experiencing psychological discomfort because of how he understands events in his life. To lessen Buddy's discomfort, it is necessary to alter his cognitions about events and how he develops his cognitions.

Cognitive therapy is the product of the weaving of several intellectual strands. A critical influence on cognitive therapy is behavior therapy. As Freeman (1983) notes, from behavior therapy was derived the use of the scientific method. Both the efficacy and effectiveness paradigms (Howard et al., 1996) have been used, with each contributing to the advancement of this treatment approach. Controlled experiments have been done within the efficacy paradigm to show the favorableness of outcomes of cognitive interventions when compared to a control group or other treatments (Persons, Davidson, & Tompkins, 2001). In fact, the accumulation of controlled studies on cognitive-behavioral therapy not only in individual but group treatment is considerable. Within the effectiveness paradigm have been investigations on individual patients to track their progress in treatment. Results from such monitoring provides feedback to the individual practitioner to see if any needed corrections may be made in the patient's treatment. Freeman (1983) also identifies the focus on behavioral change as well as a set of techniques for effecting change. A number of these techniques, such as behavioral-rehearsal, homework assignments, self-monitoring activity, and role-playing are discussed later in this chapter.

Another major influence on cognitive-behavioral theory is psychoanalysis. A well-known historical fact about Aaron Beck, one of the seminal contributors to the cognitive approaches, is that he was a traditionally trained psychoanalyst, graduating from the Philadelphia Psychoanalytic Institute in 1956. Although Beck found many aspects of psychoanalytic treatment lacking, he selectively incorporated certain aspects of it. From psychoanalysis, most especially the writings of neo-Freudians such as Horney and Sullivan, he obtained a very close focus upon the texture of experience and the effect of ideas, all of which may not be fully in awareness, on feelings and behavior. From Kelly's personal construct theory (1955) he derived the notion that a person can function within his or her own mind as a local scientist. Piaget's work on the cognitive development of children and adolescents helped him to consolidate the notion of schemas, a construct key to model for intervention (Wright, Thase, Beck, & Ludgate, 1993).

The initial application of cognitive-behavioral therapy was on an individual level, with particular focus on the depressed outpatient. However, the possibility of cognitive-behavioral group therapy suggested itself as group therapists representing other theoretical orientations described in their writings the difficulty of treating depressed patients in groups of persons with heterogeneous diagnoses. Hollon and Evans (1983) among others hypothesized that it might not be the modality but rather the approach within the modality that was lacking. They reasoned that for this population, more of a problem focus than a focus on process (typical of more psychodynamically and interpersonally oriented groups) may be needed. They pointed out that early attempts to use cognitive therapy with a depressed sample (e.g., Gioe, 1975) had yielded very promising results. While these early efforts were primarily focused on persons with depression, they gradually expanded to other patient populations with positive results, as are discussed in the section on research.

Initially, cognitive behavioral therapists were struck with the potential efficiency of group treatment. They also realized that members might make some contribution to one another in the reality testing of each member's beliefs. Nonetheless, cognitive behaviorists would characteristically ignore the process aspects of the group (Rose, Tolmen, & Tallant, 1985). As was noted in Chapter 1, meta-analyses featuring studies in which individual therapy was compared to cognitive therapy performed in a group in which group process was used minimally tended to favor the former (Fuhriman & Burlingame, 1994). Satterfield (1994) pointed out that generally group formats emphasizing the development of cohesion in the group showed superior outcomes to those that did not. In recent years there has been a burgeoning awareness that the process aspects of the group constitute a set of resources to the cognitive-behavioral group therapist. Consequently, the therapist is far more likely to incorporate the group aspect in conducting cognitive-behavioral groups than was once the case. Nonetheless, a perusal of current articles on group cognitive-behavioral therapy quickly reveals that many applications continue to be primarily individual cognitive-behavioral therapy in a group.

Before we begin to consider some of the key theoretical constructs and postulates, a clarification is in order about the use of the term *cognitive behavioral therapy*. Many approaches fall in the classes of cognitive therapies and behavioral therapies. This chapter primarily features the approach of Aaron Beck and those who sought to develop his approach of treating cognitions in order to modify feelings. However, integrated into this presentation will be the contributions of other cognitive-behavioral thinkers who developed their own approaches within this broad orientation. Among these contributors are Albert Ellis (1962, 1992), Donald Meichenbaum (1977), and Arnold Lazarus (1976).

Conceptual Foundations

The cognitive model on which cognitive behavioral therapy is based offers a conceptualization of the process by which people develop psychological problems. This model holds that how a person feels and acts depends upon the idiosyncratic meaning a person assigns to a situation. It is not the situation itself that directly elicits feelings. Taking the example of Buddy once again, within the cognitive model, the girlfriend's breaking up with Buddy would not be seen as the cause of his sadness and despondency. Rather, this model would see his cognitions (that is, thoughts and images) as critical antecedents of his feelings about the dissolution of the relationship.

How might these cognitions be characterized? Imagine Buddy receiving a test back in class with a C grade. At the moment he looks at the grade, a thought will quickly pass through his mind about the significance or meaning of the grade. While someone else might think, "Next time I'll study harder and do better," given what we know of Buddy, we might expect his conclusion to be, "I'm just not smart enough for this!" Buddy's cognition at that moment is referred to as an *automatic thought*. Although such thoughts are not unconscious, they can occur with such rapidity as to be barely noticeable to the person. The fleeting character of this mentation is important because part of the therapeutic process will be to capture them. By capturing them, it is possible to critically evaluate them. For example, Buddy could address whether obtaining a low grade on a test, particularly under the condition of his preparing for it while distracted, is adequate evidence for its validity.

Suppose Buddy were not the only student in the class to receive a C on that test. Would we expect that all students receiving Cs would have identical automatic thoughts? By no means! One student may say, "I must be smart to get a C given how difficult this test was" or "I'll do better next time." What accounts for the differences in the automatic thoughts people generate? The cognitive model holds that individuals, early on in life, form beliefs that function as a kind of lens through which life events are seen and understood. The beliefs formed by the person are rooted in childhood events, especially with parents but also other significant figures in the child's life such as friends and teachers (Ingram, 2001). These assumptions, or *core beliefs*, are a conceptual substrate that, while not unconscious per se, are so engrained as to be undetectable to the person. The reader may notice how the core belief in cognitive theory functions in a similar way as the parataxic distortion of the interpersonal approach and the representational schemes of the object-relations approach. An example of such a core belief might be, "I'm hopelessly inadequate."

Patterns of core beliefs coalesce into schemas, which are "the deepest patterns in a person's life, integrating one's history, family of origin, beliefs about oneself, and one's most powerful emotions (both expressed and unexpressed)" (White, 2000b, p. 56). If we compare the automatic thought with the core belief, we find the latter more general than the former, and the schema is more general still. The greater specificity of automatic thoughts arises out of their responsiveness to the situation at hand. If Buddy were in some alternate situation, he would develop automatic thoughts that would have some different content but would have consistency with the more situation-independent core beliefs. The automatic thoughts and core beliefs are connected to each other through conditional beliefs that are statements capturing the individual's understanding of what cause-and-effect relationships exist in their worlds. They arise from core beliefs but have an if-then character (White, 2000a). For example, Buddy may have the unremarkable conditional belief, "If I don't study at all, I won't succeed in school." More probably, Buddy's thought content would be in the order of "No matter how hard I try, I won't be successful." Whereas the former response might predispose him to exert himself so as to be academically successful, the latter might prompt him to become despondent upon encountering the first small difficulty in a course and give up.

As the preceding example suggests, conditional beliefs have the power to affect feelings and behavior. The sequence is as follows. Core beliefs set the stage for the generation of conditional beliefs. These beliefs are applied to situations and expressed in the form of automatic thoughts. The automatic thoughts precipitate emotions, which then give rise to behaviors. The behaviors may also be accompanied by physiological responses (J. S. Beck, 1995). For example, Buddy's sleep and appetite disturbance may be a consequence of his cognitive appraisal of his academic and romantic situations.

Because they are rooted in core beliefs, conditional beliefs can be relatively stable. Yet, like the representational schemes of the object-relations approach, they can be updated by the individual's contemporary experience. Cognitive behavioral therapy (CBT) and group CBT is a means by which such updating occurs. Through group CBT, members can examine conditional beliefs and modify those that are no longer serviceable in their current form. In this process of *cognitive restructuring* (Meichenbaum, 1975, 1977), some conditional beliefs may be narrowed. For example, instead of saying, "No matter how much I try, I won't be successful," the person might say, "When I am preoccupied with other matters, my studying isn't that effective." The individual may have certain conditional beliefs connected to more positive core beliefs that simply are not holding sufficient sway in the person's thinking. For example, Buddy may have a conditional belief such as "I can count on my perseverance to get me through" that is tied to positive core beliefs concerning his competence. Through his work in treatment, this belief could be given greater focus than others and thereby greater power to influence his feelings and behaviors.

CBT treatment, a problem-oriented approach, is not designed merely to alter the individual's current automatic thoughts and conditional beliefs in the present. If so, the positive effects of CBT would be only short term. While distress would diminish (an important goal of the approach), the person would be at risk of facing a situation that would activate negative core beliefs giving rise to negative conditional beliefs and automatic thoughts. What CBT seeks to do is to teach individuals skills enabling them to track and modify their cognitions ongoingly. Part of this process entails learning about certain cognitive distortions that may characterize the person's thinking. An example of a distortion is a *mental filter*, in which a negative detail of a circumstance is emphasized in awareness at the expense of an appraisal of the big picture (J. S. Beck, 1995). Table 12.1 lists these cognitive distortions.

In the short run, then, the goals of group CBT are to provide symptom relief and alleviate distress by modifying automatic thoughts and conditioned beliefs. In the long run CBT assists the

Table 12.1   **Thinking Errors**

Although some automatic thoughts are true, many are either untrue or have just a grain of truth. Typical mistakes in thinking include:

1. *All-or-nothing thinking* (also called black-and-white, polarized, or dichotomous thinking): You view a situation in only two categories instead of on a continuum.
   Example: "If I'm not a total success, I'm a failure."

2. *Catastrophizing* (also called fortune telling): You predict the future negatively without considering other, more likely outcomes.
   Example: "I'll be so upset, I won't be able to function at all."

3. *Disqualifying or discounting the positive:* You unreasonably tell yourself that positive experiences, deeds, or qualities do not count.
   Example: "I did that project well, but that doesn't mean I'm competent; I just got lucky."

4. *Emotional reasoning:* You think something must be true because you "feel" (actually believe) it so strongly, ignoring or discounting evidence to the contrary.
   Example: "I know I do a lot of things okay at work, but I still feel like I'm a failure."

5. *Labeling:* You put a fixed, global label on yourself or others without considering that the evidence might more reasonably lead to a less disastrous conclusion.
   Example: "I'm a loser. He's no good."

6. *Magnification/minimization:* When you evaluate yourself, another person, or a situation, you unreasonably magnify the negative and/or minimize the positive.
   Example: "Getting a mediocre evaluation proves how inadequate I am. Getting high marks doesn't mean I'm smart."

7. *Mental filter* (also called selective abstraction): You pay undue attention to one negative detail instead of seeing the whole picture.
   Example: "Because I got one low rating on my evaluation [which also contained several high ratings] it means I'm doing a lousy job."

8. *Mind reading:* You believe you know what others are thinking, failing to consider other, more likely possibilities.
   Example: "He's thinking that I don't know the first thing about this project."

9. *Overgeneralization:* You make a sweeping negative conclusion that goes far beyond the current situation.
   Example: "[Because I felt uncomfortable at the meeting] I don't have what it takes to make friends."

10. *Personalization:* You believe others are behaving negatively because of you, without considering more plausible explanations for their behavior.
    Example: "The repairman was curt to me because I did something wrong."

11. *"Should" and "must" statements* (also called imperatives): You have a precise, fixed idea of how you or others should behave and you overestimate how bad it is that these expectations are not met.
    Example: "It's terrible that I made a mistake. I should always do my best."

12. *Tunnel vision:* You only see the negative aspects of a situation.
    Example: "My son's teacher can't do anything right. He's critical and insensitive and lousy at teaching."

Reprinted with permission of The Guilford Press. From Judith Beck's (1995) *Cognitive Therapy: Basics and Beyond* (p. 119). Originally adapted with permission of Aaron T. Beck.

individual in acquiring those skills necessary to assess cognitions to ensure that they are accurate and of a nature to further the individual's well-being.

Interventions and Techniques

Group CBT is a typically short-term intervention that entails the use of a highly formatted or structured session in pursuit of the goals described previously. This section on intervention covers three topics: (a) the nature of the relationship between the therapist and group members, (b) the format of the sessions across the course of the group, and (c) the use of group factors in CBT.

The Patient–Therapist Relationship

Patients often enter treatment expecting that progress will be made by passively accepting whatever the therapist provides. In fact, the reader may recall from Chapter 3 that behavior consistent with such an assumption is the hallmark of the initial phase of group development. Critical to movement toward the goals of any approach is for the members to assume responsibility for their work in the group. Yalom (1995) refers to responsibility taking as one of the existential factors that he includes in his list of therapeutic factors.

In group CBT, the treatment relationship is defined in a way that encourages responsibility taking by the group members as early as possible. The treatment relationship is characterized by a *collaborative empiricism* between therapist and group members, with the hierarchical dimension of the relationship de-emphasized (Thase & Beck, 1993). To forge a successful collaboration, the therapist must manifest warmth, accurate empathy, and genuineness. The therapist must also clearly convey the rationale for the various procedures used because the member can be a more active, equal participant if the therapeutic process is demystified. Such explanations are given in the preparation and the early phase of group participation. However, throughout the group treatment the therapist should remain receptive to providing direct answers to the members' questions. Through a continuous exchange of information the therapist and group members can function as an investigative team addressing the array of problems they identify. Hence, the collaboration has an empirical character.

In pursuit of a collaborative relationship, the CBT group therapist is likely to take a different stand than the object-relations therapist on the issue of self-disclosure. When the CBT group therapist can identify examples from his or her own life of a point being made, such examples may be offered judiciously (White, 2000b). For example, Stern (2000) notes that in a parent-training CBT group, the therapist's disclosure of his or her difficulties in parenting is an antidote to the shame members often feel in describing their struggles.

The collaboration is also nurtured in the ways in which the group therapist involves the members in the treatment. For example, White (2000a) discusses the importance of member input in establishing the agenda. Providing input on the elements of the agenda gives members an opportunity to collaborate not only with the therapist but also with one another. In this vein White (2000a) writes, "members often have not had the experience of cooperating with others to plan the use of shared time. To do so in a group setting requires skills of being assertive, listening, waiting one's turn, and seeking what is best for everyone" (p. 20). In many other ways collaboration is encouraged, and these shall be outlined as we the various technical components of group CBT.

Both the requirement of collaboration and other demands of group CBT create a need for a particular leadership style on the part of the therapist. When leading a CBT group, the therapist must be active in moving members toward the goals of the group. Group CBT does not allow for a passive or laissez-faire leadership style. Nor does it permit a style in which the leader makes many reflective comments about the group, because such interventions could unwittingly strengthen the maladaptive thoughts expressed by members (Thase & Beck, 1993).

The concepts of transference and countertransference described in relation to the object-relations theory are not irrelevant to group CBT. Cognitive-behavioral therapists recognize that group members may exhibit responses to the therapist or other group members that have their origins in early experiences. As Freeman, Schrodt, Gilson, and Ludgate (1993) note, such reactions can provide information helpful in identifying schemas. These writers also encourage the CBT therapist to limit those transference responses that could undermine the treatment by using the same techniques that would apply to any dysfunctional schemas.

Reciprocally, countertransference occurs when the therapist has intense cognitive and affective reactions to the patient. With certain populations, certain types of reactions may be especially common. For example, in applying group CBT with individuals dually diagnosed with substance abuse and personality disorders, the therapist may hear about behaviors that are illegal, abusive, or manipulative and may have a critical response (Greanias & Siegel, 2000). In response to such strong reactions, reactions that could interfere with the therapist's effectiveness, the therapist should through self-exploration and supervision strive to modify the thoughts that adversely affect his or her capacity to be fully collaborative. Relatively absent in the Group CBT literature is the diagnostic use of countertransference (as described in Chapters 6 and 11). The future investigation of how CBT group therapists might tap their own reactions to understand better members' affects and systems of meaning may lead to the incorporation of a new tool in the therapist's list.

Temporal Factors

The CBT group can either be close-ended, in which case the group meets for a fixed number of sessions, or open-ended entailing members' coming and going at different times. In the former case, the number of sessions is an important element of the group design; in the latter, the number of sessions can be tailored to the individual. Generally, in CBT groups, number of sessions ranges between 10 and 20. Contextual factors play a role in determining the length of the group. For example, in a hospital setting, average length of hospital stay is a crucial factor (unfortunately, in some settings, the brevity of hospitalization precludes the conduct of CBT groups altogether). The goals of the group also affect the length. The greater the range of skills fostered, the longer the group needs to exist to provide members adequate opportunity for their acquisition. The size of the group is also a factor: more populous groups require more time to be productive.

One option is the close-ended format is for the member to enter a new group if there is still work to do after one group experience has been completed. Thompson et al. (2000) describe a group format developed for older adults. Thompson and colleagues' approach seeks to help members acquire various skills (such as problem-solving and self-assertion) that will lead to the long-term lessening of depression. The group is designed to run 10 to 12 sessions. At the group's end, a given member may show a reduction in depressive symptoms but a continuing difficulty with the use of a skill, perhaps in a certain type of social situation. The therapist then recommends that the member join another group, possibly one that focuses more intensively on cultivating the relevant skill.

Structure of the Sessions

The clearest picture of group CBT can be obtained by tracking a group through an individual session. Distinguishing the CBT approach from the object-relations approach and most applications of the interpersonal approach is the use of an agenda to organize the session. Agendas are used because they aid the patient's understanding of the workings of cognitive-behavioral therapy. They increase the efficiency of treatment in the group setting and guarantee that all members will get sufficient air time. The therapist enters the session with a broad agenda or game plan and through collaboration with group members, it is made more specific.

As the session proceeds, there may be many opportunities to digress from the therapist's and members' agenda. Clinical judgment is required by the clinician as to how to respond to such opportunities—whether to adhere to or deviate from the plan (Persons, Davidson, & Tompkins, 2001). Given the interplay of personalities in a group, spontaneous emotional events will inevitably occur. These here-and-now events and their analysis can be powerful vehicles for change for all of the reasons outlined in Chapter 4. In such instances, the temporary abandonment of the agenda in favor of the hot emotional concern may well be in order (B. Zahn, personal communication, February 1, 2002). At the same time, the therapist must be vigilant that a possible digression from a segment of an agenda is not itself an avoidance of an issue that may be anxiety arousing for members or the therapist. In either case, the therapist's judgment takes into account the potential of each direction to foster not only intellectual but also affective engagement. Unsurprisingly, practical factors enter into the extent to which the therapist can treat the agenda flexibly. The longer the life of the group and each session itself, the smaller the number of group members, the greater can be the therapist's latitude to give spontaneously emerging events in the group their due.

The typical format of the session varies according to whether it falls in the beginning, middle, or end of the group's life. Each format will be described in turn. The reader should note that the session structures described are offered only as examples. The patient population, problem area, time frame, or other variables related to the content of treatment will bear upon the optimal format. This sequence is modeled after that of Hollon and Evans (1983) with some modifications.

Preparation and First Session: Before the beginning of the group session, the member may be given some reading material to become acquainted with the cognitive approach. For example, in groups in which members are being treated for depression, the pamphlet *Coping with Depression* (A. P. Beck & Greenberg, 1974) can be very helpful. (The author used this pamphlet with depressed inpatients. While many found reading this material useful, others could not take the initiative to complete the reading until treatment was well under way.) The therapist may introduce other types of bibliotherapy related to members' presenting problems. While the sessions themselves can provide much training in the cognitive-behavioral model, it is often useful in the preparatory interview to address any apprehensions the member may have about beginning the group (J. S. Beck, 1995). Some CBT therapists provide extensive preparation for group members. For example, Greanias and Siegel (2000) developed a model of group CBT treatment for individuals with dual substance abuse and personality disorder diagnoses. Members in the orientation learn to give and receive feedback and are presented with expectations about attendance and homework assignments. The notion of collaboration is cultivated. Finally, policies about expected behaviors such as those pertaining to the use of drugs or alcohol and group attendance are described.

In the first session, members are typically given an instrument that provides baseline data on whatever symptom areas the group is addressing. For example, members may be given the Beck Depression Inventory (BDI-II), the Beck Anxiety Inventory (BAI), or the Hopelessness Scale. For adolescents or children the Beck Youth Inventories may be used. Information from such inventories is helpful in monitoring the member's progress and attending to problem areas that might not emerge otherwise. For example, a member may be having sleep difficulties and not think to report them in the group. Suicidal issues, a concern with a depressed population, can be carefully but unobtrusively monitored through such an instrument as the BDI-II, which specifically queries the individual on suicidal intent (White, 2000b).

A group member may oppose the therapist's request to complete such instruments. The therapist handles the opposition using an approach that may be useful whenever the member shows an unwillingness or hesitancy to comply with some aspect of the treatment. The therapist should always be ready to restate the rationale for the various components of the agenda. If the member is still unwilling to complete the forms or some other aspect of the treatment, then the therapist should employ the very techniques in which the member is being trained. That is, the members' cognitions can be identified and subjected to a process of testing. For example, perhaps through exploration, the member will reveal a fear that the monitoring will show a lack of progress. If so, this fear of failure could be entered as an agenda item for systematic investigation.

Members are told that *mood monitoring*, achieved by completing such instruments or by rating their mood state on a scale from 0 to 100, will be a regular part of the group. Moreover, they will be given a chart so they themselves are able to see their progress (White, 2000a).

The concept of the agenda is then introduced to members with the explanation that agendas ensure that the sessions will address the concerns most critical to members and most essential to their progress. It might also be noted that by setting agendas, members gain experience in defining their problems in a way that they can be addressed in the group (Freeman et al., 1993). They are told that it will be a regular feature of the sessions so that in future sessions they can give some thought to what they would like their agenda items to be. The therapist may then list his or her own agenda items for the session, which should include the statement of individual problems and what expectations members may have for treatment (J. S. Beck, 1995; Hollon & Evans, 1983). Then, members are given an opportunity to add their own elements to the agenda as the therapist records the items.

Members then review the ground rules of the group. Many of these ground rules, such as responsibility to maintain confidentiality, will pertain to all types of groups. Other rules may pertain to the operating procedures of the cognitive-behavioral group, for example, the rule that each member honor the go-around format so that each has an opportunity to receive the group's assistance. Some ground rules may be highly specific to the population being treated such as McCutchen's (2000) ground rules for members in a group she designed for individuals with dissociative disorders. Members are urged not to dissociate in the sessions, to ask another person whom a member is suspecting of dissociation whether he or she is doing so, and to report whether another member is triggering dissociation in him or her.

The discussion of rules may be followed by the discussion of members' expectations and goals for the group. Individuals being treated for depression often will have negative forebodings about their treatment and can profit at this early point from the factor of universality: Members recognize that they share in their negative prognostications, seeing that they represent more of a cognitive bias than a truly objective appraisal of their likelihood to benefit from the group experience. They are also likely to find heartening the overlap in problem areas, which can be an antidote to beliefs that they are alone with such difficulties. As members are talking about their presenting issues, it may be helpful for them to have the opportunity to describe their own explanations for their difficulties because such an opportunity may enhance their receptivity to new ideas.

The group then moves onto a more didactic segment of the session in which members are educated on the principles of CBT. The therapist introduces the most fundamental axiom of CBT—that the meaning assigned to external events rather than external events themselves cause feelings that in turn affect behavior. The therapist can then use the material members had presented in the earlier go-arounds to illustrate this point. Suppose for example, Buddy was in the group and had earlier in the session explained to members that since his girlfriend had ended the relationship, he was overwhelmed with a sense of dejection. The therapist might return to Buddy's case at this time:

THERAPIST: Buddy, perhaps we can use what you shared as a case in point. You said that you felt utterly despondent because your girlfriend left you. The possibility I would like you to consider is that in between losing your girlfriend and your depressed feelings was a particular perspective you had on this event. There were some thoughts you had about the breakup, and I would like you to consider the possibility that it was these thoughts that made you depressed.

BUDDY: I just don't recall having any thoughts . . . now, it's a haze.

THERAPIST: When you told us about the event of opening her letter, you used the phrase "like some kind of loser"? What was your thought about that?

BUDDY: I was thinking that she must see me as a loser . . . in comparison to guys she's meeting there . . . at her university.

THERAPIST: And perhaps you were saying to yourself something like, "I must be a loser if she wants to end our relationship."

BUDDY: I suppose I did say that to myself.

Here the therapist can help the member realize that automatic thoughts occur so rapidly that they are elusive. Members should be encouraged to recognize CBT concepts by having them generate their own examples of the connections between thoughts and cognitions. As members present situations and analyze their cognitions they complete Thought Records that assist them in identifying and modifying automatic thoughts. Although there are different types of Thought Records, a typical format is one in which there are four columns. In the first column of the Thought Record, the *situation* associated with the troublesome reactions, is described. In the second column, the *feelings* of the member in the situation are listed. In the third column, the *thoughts giving rise* to the feelings are listed and in the final column, the *coping responses* that might be made in the situation. Persons, Davidson, and Tompkins (2001) also suggest including a column (after the situation column) in which *behaviors related* to the situation are listed. They see this inclusion as consistent with Beck's view that a symptom such as depression is made up of behaviors, emotions, and thoughts.

While some members may pick up this conceptual system quickly, for others it will be more difficult. To not only assist the latter but also to demonstrate a skill that members must acquire to obtain lasting benefit from the group experience, the therapist engages in Socratic questioning (White, 2000a), which is a series of questions designed to help the member come to important realizations about cognition, affects, and behaviors, and their interrelationships.

Through Socratic questioning the therapist can maintain more of a collaborative relationship than could be achieved were the therapist to lecture to the member. Socratic questioning takes different forms depending on the phase of the group and the activity the group is pursuing. At this time the effort of the therapist is to show the link between cognitions and feelings. One point of departure in the group's life is to mindfully ask members to recount some situation in which they experience distress. Members' memories are likely to be activated by having heard other members describe upsetting situations. Once the member has provided a situation to explore, the therapist can conduct a line of questioning to help the member recognize his or her automatic thoughts:

DANYA: I don't know—I just felt overwhelmed with sadness when I dropped her off for her first day of kindergarten and I haven't been able to snap back since . . . it's just bizarre!

THERAPIST: It only seems bizarre because we haven't figured out what your thoughts were. When we do figure out your thoughts, I bet your feelings will make more sense to you. Picture yourself back in that schoolyard. Imagine that moment—tell us again how did you say that it occurred, that your daughter got into the line and walked away.

DANYA: It was like a final parting. I wanted her to turn around and ask me to come in, but she looked so self-sufficient and . . . actually . . . happy.

THERAPIST: So right at that moment, you said to yourself . . .

DANYA: She doesn't need me anymore.

[The therapist writes Danya's automatic thought on a blackboard.]

LaVERNE: Of course she still needs you!

THERAPIST: [to LaVerne] You're bringing up a very important point: Some of the thoughts that we have don't jibe with how things actually are. We'll be getting to that very topic next. [to Danya] Can you see, Danya, how that thought that your daughter no longer has a need for you would lead you to feel extremely sad?

[The therapist draws an arrow next to Danya's automatic thought and writes the words "very sad."]

The therapist here is using the very useful technique of having the member imagine the situation to gain greater access to automatic thoughts. The therapist would continue with this process of getting Danya to expand because as Hollon and Evans (1983) note, as members elaborate they are likely to get closer to their dysfunctional beliefs.

Once members identify their distorted thoughts, they can be assisted in replacing them with more adaptive cognitions (Rose, 1999). For example, Danya would develop statements that could evoke positive feelings, for example, "My daughter's independence shows that I've done a pretty good job" or "It will be fun to share with her this new era of her life and help her with new challenges." The latter statement would address her anxiety that entrance into school signified the loss of Danya's parental role. Dysfunctional beliefs can also be identified by looking for themes among automatic beliefs (J. S. Beck, 1995).

As forecasted by our therapist in the last vignette, the next step is for members to obtain their first experience in testing out automatic thoughts and dysfunctional beliefs. Note that at no time does the therapist directly challenge a cognition of the group member because to do so would violate the collaborative empiricism that should characterize therapist–member interactions (J. S. Beck, 1995). Rather, the therapist directs the member with the help of the group to consider what evidence exists to confirm or disconfirm the thought. This step becomes more of a focus in later sessions, when members have mastered certain fundamentals of CBT.

As the group session nears its end, three important steps remain. The therapist summarizes the session to underscore the most important points. Then homework assignments are set through another collaboration of therapists and group members. Homework is a regular feature of the group CBT for a variety of reasons. Many of the benefits of homework were described in Chapter 5, such as intensifying the treatment and of encouraging members to take responsibility for their progress in the group. Moreover, homework has been found to improve outcomes (Neimeyer & Feixas, 1990; Burns & Spangler, 2000). Members are most likely to be compliant with homework assignments when therapists follow up on homework in the next session (Bryant, Simons, & Thase, 1999). For this reason, the therapist should factor in the time needed to review assignments in determining the amount of homework members will receive. The therapist should also exercise care in tying homework closely to the work the member is doing in the group (Persons et al., 2001).

At this early phase of the group treatment, homework often consists of having members complete a thought record (A. T. Beck, Rush, Shaw, & Emery, 1979). As described previously, this record requires members to analyze situations using the cognitive model of thoughts, feelings, and behavior as they unfold in a given situation. As White (2000a) points out, not only do these assignments give members practice in the cognitive model, but the sharing of them with the other group members can invigorate the group.

The final task is for the session to be summarized initially by the therapist and in subsequent sessions by the members. At this time members offer feedback on any aspects of the session. In providing the therapist with feedback, the members gain practice for a later time when they will provide feedback to one another. Moreover, the therapist's opportunity to respond nondefensively to feedback is likely to strengthen the member's trust in, and willingness to collaborate with, the sessions.

Subsequent Sessions: The structure of the sessions following the first is essentially the same as the steps outlined above with a few changes. In our relationships outside of treatment, we typically begin our interactions with a check on the well-being of the other person ("How are you?"). At the beginning of each session, we do the same but in a way more systematic and less perfunctory so that it serves as an adequate springboard for work later in the session. In addition to having the member complete one or more questionnaires relating to the target problem, the therapist has the member report on his or her mood over the past week. As J. S. Beck (1995) explains, through this mood check the therapist can show concern, monitor progress, and obtain examples to strengthen members' grasp of the cognitive model. However, if the material a member introduces at this time requires more in-depth discussion, it is placed on the agenda as an item requiring the group's attention later in the session.

A review is conducted of the prior session. Members can offer any reactions to the group process, cognitive theory, or any other aspect of the group. The therapist, too, can offer reactions and observations that highlight the immediate experiences and behaviors of members and thereby signal that this domain is available for the group's exploration within the framework of the cognitive approach:

THERAPIST: Harriet, last week after we had spoken with Danya, you mentioned having had a similar experience when your son left for college. We spent very little time talking about it, and later in the session you were less active and appeared downcast.

HARRIET: Yes, sometime in the session I began to question whether anything could help me.

THERAPIST: And I wonder if you began to have that questioning after you mentioned the circumstance of your son leaving for college.

HARRIET: Well, I often feel that what I put out is just not that interesting! I basically am a boring person and I don't really expect anyone to pay attention to me.

In this interaction, the therapist's probing leads Harriet to reveal not only an automatic thought but also a belief about herself that would be likely to beget negative feelings. The therapist can then put Harriet's belief on the agenda for further pursuit. The natural process of the group and the requirement on members to share the group's focus invites feelings of hurt, rebuff, disappointment, and so on. These difficult feelings become resources when they are used in real time in the group for the application of the cognitive model. Like other theoretical approaches, the model is strengthened through the group's use of the here-and-now.

After each member has given some indication of his or her status, the group proceeds to build its agenda. This activity occurs on a group level, with members deciding together what their priorities are. For example, agendas that members have in common might be given a high place on the agenda. At the same time, the therapist must have input so that the individual needs of members are not neglected. For instance, the therapist should ensure that Harriet's problem, which had been scantily addressed in the last session, would be placed on the agenda of the current session.

Homework from the last session is then reviewed. Difficulties with the homework can signal the need for additional agenda items. For example, an agenda item might be the member's role-playing a particular behavior that proved too challenging to do outside the group. As Persons et al. (2001) note, some therapists may want to have the homework review prior to agenda setting. Reversing the order may prevent the homework from being given short shrift, a particular concern when members enter the group with crises they wish to discuss.

The next element of the session is often its centerpiece: Members work on their agenda items. Certain agenda items require further clarification and translation into a problem format so that a solution is possible. While helping members to fulfill their agenda items, the therapist can also present additional concepts of cognitive theory and cognitive techniques. Particularly important among these techniques are those methods by which members may test their beliefs.

Members learn to test their automatic thoughts, core beliefs, and the schema in which the former cognitions are embedded through a process of gathering evidence. For example, Harriet believes that she has nothing to say that will be of interest to others. Notice that the underlying core belief "I am boring" is an extreme statement. It is likely a consequence of a thinking error—a tendency to overgeneralize. By gaining familiarity with the different types of thinking errors or cognitive distortions, members can identify such problems in their own thinking. After the various thinking errors are learned, they can be applied to newly emerging automatic thoughts.

The next step is for Harriet to assess the evidence for her belief. It is here that the interpersonal data within the group can be tapped. The therapist might begin by offering evidence at his or her disposal and offering members the opportunity to do the same:

THERAPIST: Harriet, you drew the conclusion that what you said was not that interesting because after talking about your point briefly, I moved the group to another activity. You took my behavior as evidence for your belief that you are boring. But I'd like you to know that I was aware that the time for the session is running out.

The therapist might invite others to give Harriet their impressions. The reader may wonder about the possibility that members may give Hannah confirming evidence for her belief. It is indeed possible that members would not altogether contradict her self-perception. Nonetheless, what characterizes members' negative beliefs is their extremity. Even if members were to say that Harriet at times did not compel their interest or that she showed certain behaviors that may lead to their disengagement, they would be making a statement less extreme than Harriet's own. In fact, by not completely negating Harriet's statements, members' feedback may be more credible and thereby more influential. Keep in mind that the goal is not to have members develop wholly positive thoughts about themselves, the world, or the future but rather thoughts that are more in keeping with reality. Once these more adaptive, realistic responses are identified, they can be used to counter the dysfunctional thoughts.

The evidence for a dysfunctional cognition need not be drawn exclusively from the group. The individual generally will be asked to examine his or her life outside of the group for relevant data.

Throughout the session, the therapist may create experiential opportunities for members. For example, the therapist may divide the group into pairs and instruct them to practice a coping response in relation to their partners. Harriet, for instance, might be instructed to have a conversation with another member and to work on summoning interpretations of her companion's reaction other than the usual conclusion that he or she is bored. An advantage of such exercises is their power to stimulate affect within the here-and-now (B. Zahn, personal communication, February 1, 2002). Upon returning to the larger group, members can explore the thoughts that intervened between the situation and the feelings generated. Of course, this is the process, now familiar to the reader, of interpersonal learning.

After the group has completed working on its agenda, it moves on to the assignment of homework. Members will continue to monitor thoughts and feelings. They will also be asked to perform experiments on their automatic thoughts and dysfunctional beliefs. For example, Harriet might be given the homework assignment to have three conversations, each with a different person, and to monitor on a scale from 1 (no attention) to 100 (total absorption) the extent to which they attended to her. The group would also help Harriet anticipate the obstacles to performing the task. Her anticipation could be facilitated by the technique of *cognitive rehearsal,* in which the individual cognitively walks through the successive steps of a given task (A. T. Beck, 1976). For example, perhaps it would be discovered that Harriet did not routinely have three conversations a week because of an isolated lifestyle. Therefore, the group would need to work with Harriet on the task of having interactions. A behavioral rehearsal might also occur in which Harriet might practice a conversation in the group. Harriet might be taught (along with the rest of the group) and encouraged to use relaxation techniques.

The final steps involve summarizing the major points of the session and soliciting feedback.

Termination Sessions: Termination is a focus from the first session of the group (Brabender & Fallon, 1993). The therapists encourage members to see that the skills they are developing are designed not only to reduce symptoms in the present but to assist them through times of stress after they leave the group. Nonetheless, as the group nears its end, focus on concerns related to termination intensifies. Members take stock of what work has been done and what remains to do. If residual symptoms remain, or if new problems have been identified,[1] members design their own programs to carry on the work. In the last sessions members identify what situations or stimuli lead to the emergence of dysfunctional beliefs. This identification enables them to know when to be on high alert and when to deploy their cognitive skills, a process referred to as *relapse prevention* (J. S. Beck, 1995).

To augment relapse prevention, a given group format may entail *booster sessions.* Especially in a close-ended group, the opportunity to meet again at some later time enables members to keep their skills sharp and derive the social support that the group provides (White, 2000a). In the last sessions, the logistics of the booster session may be worked out.

As the group approaches termination, members increasingly move closer toward their schemas, the cognitive substrate of all more immediate and situation-dependent cognitions. This work involves the use of the cognitive techniques described earlier in relation to automatic thoughts and dysfunctional beliefs. However, treating schemas leads to the creation of an internal cognitive environment in which these latter cognitive contents are less likely to emerge.

The Use of the Group in Group CBT

The CBT group therapist can use the resources of the group to enhance members' capacities to derive benefit from the group in many ways. An especially critical set of interventions are those designed to increase the cohesion of the group (White, 2000b). The points at which the therapist can foster cohesion are various. The therapist can encourage the development of cohesion by using a closed group

---

[1] White (2000b) writes about the phenomenon in which the abatement of depression in individuals for whom this is the chief presenting problem leads to the stronger appearance of other psychological problems at termination time. In some instances, such new manifestations might necessitate a referral for an additional course of therapy.

form in which all members begin and end at the same time (Satterfield, 1994). Providing opportunities for members to identify with one another's experiences fosters cohesion. The reader sees examples of such strong identifications in Buddy's interactions with a female member in the vignette that follows this section. Also fostering cohesion is the group problem solving that occurs when, for example, the entire group participates in the design of a behavioral experiment for a member.

Another resource is interpersonal learning. In this regard, group CBT holds a great advantage over individual CBT. Training members to be local scientists who actively, ongoingly test their hypotheses about themselves, their futures, and the world is best done if the individual can use the here-and-now of the group as the hypothesis-testing venue. The inevitable diversity of personalities in a group enables the individual to receive different types of feedback. Harriet, for instance, may find that some find her interesting while others do not. Moreover, the hypothesis-testing process can be directly observed as Harriet assesses whether others are interested or at least attending to her.

A third set of resources are the developmental stages. We know that structured groups are in no way immune to developmental phenomena (Stockton, Rohde, & Haughey, 1992). Each stage invites the emergence of certain types of cognitive schemes. For example, in Phase II members' issues related to dependency, anger, and authority emerge with wonderful prominence. Automatic thoughts such as "If I criticize the therapist, she won't help me" become available for scrutiny. The therapist's attentiveness to developmental-stage issues will help the therapist be sensitive to schema-based themes as they emerge in the group.

Group CBT provides members with abundant opportunities to deploy the therapeutic factor of altruism. Members throughout the course of the group can be helpful to one another in identifying automatic thoughts and dysfunctional beliefs. They can participate in the design of appropriate homework assignments for one another. They can serve as participants in role plays for members engaging in behavioral rehearsal. These activities are an experiential antidote to the sense of helplessness that members, particularly those who are depressed, have upon entrance into the group. Bowers (2000), writing about a group for members with eating disorders, notes that opportunities for altruism help members to move beyond an unhealthy level of self-focus.

Clinical Illustration

The group featured in this example was an outpatient group that was currently in its fourth out of 12 sessions. This co-led group was set in small university town. While many who attended were students, the group also drew people from the community. The reader has already met one of the group members, Buddy. Others include the following:

- Amber: A 20-year-old college student who is depressed at school because she had been forced to give up her major in dance because of tendonitis. She feels that now that she can no longer be a professional dancer, life is not worth living.
- Abdul: A 22-year-old Muslim man who works as a cook in the university food service and attends classes part-time. He complains of test-taking anxiety despite a high level of academic performance.
- Ira: This 45-year-old bank manager complained of feeling exhausted at work and "burnt out." He spoke about the conflict among his supervisees as leading him to experience doubt about his managerial role.
- Harriet: The reader has met this 54-year-old woman. Harriet has had episodic depressions since her child left for college three years ago. However, a recent episode was sparked by family financial pressures that would require her to obtain employment after being at home for over 30 years.

This session segment will feature the group in its agenda-working period. The therapist reads the next item on the agenda while standing at a blackboard. On the board are four columns: Situation, Automatic Thought, Feeling, and Alternative Thought:

THERAPIST: Our next agenda item is to help Amber get a handle on the distress she felt this afternoon when she went to the majors fair. Amber, can you tell me a little more about what you were feeling?

AMBER: I went in there and freaked! I just . . . I don't know . . . I just went wild . . . I don't mean in a public kind of way . . . just in my head.

[Notice that Amber has described both the stimulus and the response in vague terms. The therapist's strategy will be to get her to articulate both more specifically.]

THERAPIST: Let's go back and replay this event in slow motion. Tell us moment by moment what happened when you entered the fair?

IRA: What kind of fair was it?

[The group has developed a norm of members' speaking out spontaneously.]

AMBER: It was a majors fair—they have representatives there of all of the majors at different tables. It's something they have every year for the people who haven't declared a major yet . . . or for the ones who want to . . . or have to change.

THERAPIST: So you walked in and . . .?

AMBER: I saw about 50 different tables and the table right in front of me were the psychology people. And I got this sick feeling.

THERAPIST: Sick?

AMBER: I don't know . . . like scared. You see, my roommate is a psychology major and we talk about her psychology courses and I really find it interesting . . . but . . .

BUDDY: But you're afraid you can't do it, right? That's exactly how I feel about engineering, but unfortunately for me, I've already chosen it.

[Members' freedom to speak out enables the therapeutic factor of universality to operate. Moreover, members can be quite skilled at identifying one another's automatic thoughts.]

THERAPIST: So maybe you had a very quick thought on seeing the psychology table . . . perhaps a thought along the lines that Buddy was saying?

AMBER: It's a little vague to me now, but it was something like, "Just something else I won't be able to do."

[The therapist writes her statement on the board under the column labeled "Automatic Thought."]

THERAPIST: The "something else" being ballet.

AMBER: [tears up] It just seems impossible starting something else when I screwed up so badly on this.

THERAPIST: So it sounds like you're saying, "Because I did not succeed at ballet, I will not succeed at anything else." I think how we can all see how I thought like that could result in some pretty painful feelings.

COTHERAPIST: Does anyone recognize what kind of cognitive distortion this is? Harriet, you're nodding your head? Do you have an idea about it?

HARRIET: Well, I was just looking at that list you gave us. Isn't that overgeneralization. I mean, Amber thinks because ballet didn't work out, nothing will work out. And that's just not true!

THERAPIST: Exactly right, Harriet. Amber is making a prediction about the future based upon this one experience. What are the consequences of this distortion?

ABDUL: She can't move forward with her life. Dance isn't a possibility anymore but she can't get involved with anything else. It keeps her stuck! And it makes her miserable.

COTHERAPIST: What might be a more helpful thought?

HARRIET: Can I say something?

AMBER: [laughs lightly] Of course, Harriet!

HARRIET: [tentatively] Well, my daughter was in ballet too—I mean she didn't go into it in college but . . . I know it takes a great deal of discipline. And the fact that you got tendonitis—it's just an unlucky thing. But your discipline—practicing day in, day out, ignoring distractions—that's something that you can take to anything you do . . . psychology included!

IRA: I think Harriet has a great thought there.

THERAPIST: So the more adaptive thought is that Amber showed important skills in her pursuit of ballet that she can take with her whatever she does.

[The therapist is pursuing the second step of cognitive restructuring: helping the individual to develop adaptive thoughts.]

AMBER: Yeah, but I keep thinking . . .

BUDDY: What if I fail again?

AMBER: [laughs] What, are you my personal mind reader?

BUDDY: I just know what you're going through because of my having been dumped by my girlfriend.

ABDUL: [incredulously] That has something to do with selecting a major?

BUDDY: Actually, it does. You see, it's not three strikes you're out—it's two strikes you're out.

AMBER: If he dates someone else and she jilts him, he's a failure, a loser . . . just like me if the next major doesn't pan out.

THERAPIST: Buddy, you're bringing up a problem that is actually one of our agenda items. You said that you wanted to explore why you aren't beginning to date again. Maybe we could work on that item and at the same time continue to deal with Amber's issue.

BUDDY: Like we are saying: two strikes and you're out. If I get rejected again . . . [his voice trails off]

THERAPIST: Yes, let's think about that. What are the consequences of being rejected by another woman?

BUDDY: Well, then I'd know I'm a loser.

THERAPIST: That would be your thought about it. And what we've learned is that we can examine and change our thoughts when they don't jibe with how things actually are. But besides the possibility that you would have that about yourself, what else would be a consequence? What if you do have another breakup initiated by *her?*

[Here the therapist is decatastrophizing, or using the what-if technique.]

BUDDY: I don't really know . . .

THERAPIST: Can others help?

ABDUL: Well, it would mean he would have to keep trying to meet new people. Now that can be a little rough, at least it is for me.

HARRIET: It would mean he would have had a relationship and that wasn't right because if it's not right for her . . . well, it's not right for him, either.

AMBER: So he would be available to find someone who was.

[Amber and Harriet are using the technique of reframing: They are helping Buddy to recognize the positive side of a negative experience.]

THERAPIST: Certainly we all recognize that having a relationship end can be sad. However, I was hearing something in both how Amber and Buddy were thinking with this two-strikes-you're-out idea.

IRA: They're both catastrophizing. The truth is nothing awful is going to happen if Amber picks psychology as a major and it doesn't work out or if Buddy dates a girl and it doesn't work out.

[The members themselves identify more functional cognitions that Amber and Buddy can adapt. The therapist writes them on the board.]

BUDDY: Shouldn't we be turning to your agenda item next?

[The therapist agrees that it is time to move onto the next agenda item but notes that the homework Buddy and Amber will do take into account the work each did on their fears about taking the next step on overcoming loss.]

THERAPIST: Ira, our next agenda item is working on the inhibitions you felt in giving Abdul feedback on his homework.

ABDUL: I could tell he had more to say but he wouldn't say that.

THERAPIST: How could you tell?

ABDUL: He was puckering his lips in a funny sort of way—not as though he was going to kiss someone but like he couldn't hold his words back . . . but couldn't say them, either.

AMBER: I noticed that, too! It looked like you were afraid the words would escape from your mouth.

THERAPIST: [to Ira] What about that?

IRA: I've just gotten to know Abdul, so why should I go out of my way to offend him?

ABDUL: Man, I'm here to get input!

THERAPIST: Abdul, how did you feel when you saw Ira puckering his lips.

ABDUL: It irritated me because it was obvious he was holding back. And when I asked him and he shrugged his shoulders as if nothing was going on, it was even more irritating.

IRA: I think people get irritated with me quite a bit, especially at work.

THERAPIST: And that's why it's very important that we understand better what went on in here. When Abdul discussed how he did his homework, what was going through your mind about it?

IRA: I thought he was cutting corners. He watered down how he did the assignment.

THERAPIST: Did you notice any feeling you were having as you had that thought or after you had it?

IRA: Well, I felt a little uneasy . . . sort of anxious, I guess.

THERAPIST: And perhaps you had some thought in between your assessment that Abdul had not pursued his homework in the way you felt he ought to and your uneasiness.

IRA: Well, I waited to see if anyone else would say something to him about it and no one did. So I felt I should but . . .

AMBER: Come on, Ira!

IRA: I thought it would anger him.

ABDUL: So what's the big deal about that? I get angry a lot.

THERAPIST: So what did you think would happen if you did anger him? What is the risk?

IRA: It would be very uncomfortable being in here because he has an adversarial stance toward me.

HARRIET: You mean he won't like you anymore?

IRA: [laughs] I guess you could put it that way.

THERAPIST: So your belief, Ira, is that if you express anger, you will alienate others, causing them to dislike or reject you. Let's test that out. Abdul, I wonder how you might have responded to Ira had he shared his thoughts?

ABDUL: You know, I probably would have been a little irritated there, too. But I think I would have been less irritated than I was for what he *did* do—I knew he disapproved of something. I just wasn't sure what. It came across as though he disapproved of me in general.

IRA: No, by no means!

ABDUL: But when you don't know what it is, that's how it seems to me—and maybe to others, too.

THERAPIST: So, Ira, it sounds as though we have some evidence against your belief that if you give others negative feedback, they invariably won't like you. So what might be a more accurate, functional thought?

IRA: I'm not sure.

ABDUL: How about: If I hold my opinions back, it could have a negative effect on the relationship.

AMBER: If I'm not forthright, others won't be able to trust me.

[The group continues to identify more functional beliefs for Ira. Later in the session, the group crafts a homework assignment entailing the execution of a behavioral experiment. In this experiment, Ira tries out giving negative feedback to a supervisee and monitoring the individual's response to assess how the communication effects the relationship. Another strategy might have been to work with Ira to recognize what resources he might marshal if the other person did feel alienated because of the constructive feedback he offered.]

Comment on the Session

This brief example illustrates only some of the techniques of group CBT, such as agenda setting, homework, Socratic questioning, and role-playing. For a more extended example of an inpatient group, the reader is referred to Brabender and Fallon (1993, see Chapter 7). The attempt in this vignette was to illustrate the potential for tapping the resources of the group in pursuing therapeutic goals. All of the benefits of using the here-and-now, for example, its capacity to engage members and to offer a behavioral sample that all can witness, were seen in this example. Moreover, the reader could see that the feedback in the here-and-now is immediate. When Ira performs his experiment on the outside, it may take him some time to determine the response of others. In the group, the norm of openness fostered by the therapist enables him to obtain direct responses on the effects of his behaviors.

In this vignette, a cotherapy team led the group. Cotherapy is an extremely useful leadership structure in group CBT given that the tasks the therapists must pursue are great in number. In our vignette, while one therapist wrote on the board, the other pursued the member's automatic thoughts. Moreover, there are particular tasks that are more easily performed by two therapists, such as role plays and demonstrations (Hollon & Evans, 1983; Lang & Craske, 2000). Through their constructive interactions with one another the cotherapy team can model the collaborative style that is the hallmark of the leadership style of the CBT therapist.

Research Support

The support for the effectiveness of group CBT with a wide range of psychological problems is considerable. At the beginning of this chapter, it was noted that a major influence of the behavioral component of CBT is the strong empiricist tradition. Therefore, the study of outcomes has gone hand-in-hand with conceptual and technical developments of this approach. A particular strength of some of the studies is the effort of the investigators not only to examine change as a function of treatment but also to study the effect of possible mediating variables. The greatest concentration of studies on group CBT focuses on depressive symptoms, and these studies will be reviewed first, followed by a description of findings in studies concerning a wide range of other symptoms and psychological problems.

The Use of Group CBT Treating Depression

Meta-analytic studies have resoundingly shown that individual CBT is helpful in the treatment of depression (Kanas, 2000). While far fewer studies look at group CBT, a sufficient number support the efficacy of group CBT for depressive symptomotology across the developmental span. Clarke, Rohde, Lewinsohn, Hops, and Seeley (1999) randomly assigned adolescents with major depression or dysthymia to a CBT group or a wait-list control. They found that 67 percent of the group members and 48 percent of the wait-list individuals exhibited recovery. Adolescents whose parents were simultaneously treated did not show greater improvement. The investigators found that booster sessions did not reduce the rate of reoccurrence but hastened recovery in individuals who still had depressive symptoms at the end of the group. Rohde, Clarke, Lewinsohn, Seeley, and Kaufman (2001) found that comorbidity in adolescents did not limit the effectiveness of a cognitive behavioral group. However, lifetime substance abuse/dependence was associated with slower recovery.

Bright, Baker, and Neimeyer (1999) compared adult depressed patients (bipolar patients were excluded) participating in a psychoeducationally orient CBT group to an interpersonal mutual support group. Outcome measures included scores from the Beck Depression Inventory, Hamilton Rating Scale for Depression, the Hopkins Symptom Checklist-58, and the Automatic Thoughts Questionnaire. Whereas some CBT and support groups were run by professionals, others were run by paraprofessionals. For both groups, depressive symptoms significantly declined during treatment and one type of treatment was not superior to another. However, following treatment, in the professionally led CBT groups, more members were classified as nondepressed than in the paraprofessionally led groups. In the support group, it did not make a difference. Furthermore, those members who exhibited a greater degree of cognitive restructuring showed greater improvement. In the CBT group, neither members' acquired skill in self-disclosure nor time spent on practice in between sessions were related to outcome. Hellerstein, et al. (2001) found that individuals who were receiving antidepressant medication for dysthymia received added benefit from participation in a 16-session cognitive-interpersonal group as reflected in measures of interpersonal and psychosocial functioning.

Steuer et al. (1984) compared cognitive-behavior and psychodynamic group therapy meeting over a nine-month period in the treatment of depressed geriatric patients. While several depression measures were used, only one measure, the Beck Depression Inventory, showed a significant difference between the two groups: It favored the cognitive-behavioral group.

CBT groups have also been found to be helpful to individuals who are depressed because of medical problems. For example, Foley, Bedell, LaRocca, Scheinberg, and Reznikoff (1987) assigned patients with multiple sclerosis to a six-session cognitive-behavioral group or the standard medical care. They found that the cognitive-behavioral group showed greater improvement on measures of depression, state anxiety, and problem-focused coping. These differences could not be attributed to differences in MS symptoms between the two groups. Toner et al. (1998) found that cognitive-behavioral group therapy effected a greater decrease in depression in persons with irritable bowel syndrome than individuals receiving therapy in a psychoeducational group or standard medical treatment.

Depression at times presents alongside other symptoms such as anxiety. In a pilot project, Kush and Fleming (2000) studied the effectiveness of group CBT in treating individuals with comorbid depressive and anxiety disorders. Adult outpatients, most of whom had been using psychotropic medication, participated in a 12-session group in which the symptoms of anxiety and depression were differentially targeted. For example, therapists assisted members in identifying automatic thoughts related to personal inadequacy to address depressive symptoms and thoughts related to danger to treat the anxiety. Participants evidenced lower levels of anxiety, depression, and dysfunctional attitudes upon completion of the group. Given these promising results, this program bears further investigation in the context of a controlled study.

Kush and Fleming suggested that one implication of their findings is the possibility of successfully treating symptomatically heterogeneous individuals in CBT groups. In many clinical settings, there may not be a sufficient number of patients in any one diagnostic category to warrant the establishment of a homogeneous group based on symptoms. There may also be clinical reasons why certain types of compositional heterogensity may be desirable. For example, Bowers (2000) argues that blending anorexic and bulimic patients in one CBT group is helpful because members with differing points of view are better able to challenge one another's irrational thoughts about body size (see Chapter 8 for further discussion). Clearly, the use of CBT groups to treat heterogeneous symptoms, whether they are present within or between members, is an important area of continuing investigation.

Symptoms Other Than Depression

Group CBT has been found to be effective in reducing binge/purge episodes in bulimic patients (e.g., Gray & Hoage, 1990) relative to no treatment and at least as effective as nondirective supportive group therapy (Gordon & Ahmed, 1988). Successful treatment of panic disorder (Telch et al., 1993) and social phobia (Heimberg et al., 1990; Hope & Heimberg, 1993) has been demonstrated. In the treatment of obsessive-compulsive disorder, Group CBT was superior to the control condition in symptom reduction but less effective than traditional behavior therapy (McLean et al., 2001).

Group CBT has also been shown to be effective in treating negative social behaviors. Inpatient male adolescents receiving group CBT were compared to a waiting-list control group and within-ward control group. The members of the CBT group showed a lower level of hostile verbalization, greater self-control, increased reflectiveness, and fewer restrictions on the unit (Feindler, Ecton, Kingsley, & Dubey, 1986). In an outpatient setting, children who had been selected by their teachers for their aggressive behavior in class were randomly assigned to a 10-week group using cognitive-behavioral techniques and a placebo control group that watched films that had no aggressive content. Experimental group members were perceived as being less aggressive and hostile that those in the control group (Omizo, Herschberger, & Omizo, 1988).

In a study involving somewhat older participants, college students (modal age = 19) were randomly assigned to four conditions: one cognitive-relaxation coping skills, two types of social skills training groups, and a no-treatment control condition (Deffenbacher, Thwaites, Wallace, & Oetting, 1994). All participants had provided evidence of having difficulties in anger management. The investigators found that all treatment groups lowered anger control relative to the control group and did so comparably. Only the cognitive-relaxation group, which emphasized developing skills for emotional control, showed a significant diminishment in the outward expression of anger. A similar study showed that anger and anxiety reduction could be maintained over at least a 15-month period (Deffenbacher, Story, Brandon, Hogg, & Hazelus, 1988). Taken together, these studies provide support for the effectiveness of group CBT in the treatment of anger.

The effectiveness of cognitive-behavioral group therapy in helping individuals cope with physical illnesses is an emerging area of investigation. For example, individuals with irritable bowel syndrome were randomly assigned to a cognitive-behavioral group, a psychoeducational group, or conventional medical treatment (Toner et al., 1998). In the cognitive-behavioral group, significant improvement was seen in the following symptoms: diarrhea, constipation, pain, and tenderness. No significant changes were seen in the other two groups.

One of the newest applications of group CBT is in the treatment of individuals with personality disorders. One modification that is typically made with this population is that the length of treatment is extended considerably. Linehan[2] developed a cognitive behavioral approach referred to as dialectical behavior therapy. This approach for persons with borderline personality disorder combines behavioral individual therapy with group therapy. The latter seeks to teach self-regulation skills and self and other acceptance skills (e.g., "The way you are is fine"). While this approach

---

[2] A full explanation of Linehan's approach is beyond the scope of this chapter. The reader is referred to Linehan's 1989 article for a further exposition of her interesting approach.

involves many traditional cognitive-behavioral elements, it also incorporates other therapeutic components such as validation and acceptance treatment strategies.

To test the effectiveness of this approach, Linehan, Tutek, Heard, and Armstrong (1994) randomly assigned female participants to either dialectical behavior therapy or treatment as usual. The latter was a naturalistic treatment condition in which the participants were permitted to participate in any therapy available to them in the community. All research participants were chronically suicidal with varying degrees of severity. After a year of treatment, individuals who had participated in dialectical behavior therapy had better scores on self-reported anger, interview-rated global social adjustment, and the Global Assessment Scale.

Summary

Cognitive-behavioral therapy in groups is based on a cognitive model of personality and psychopathology. According to this model, feelings and behaviors are a consequence of the cognitions people develop in situations. Dysfunctional cognitions are likely to lead to disturbing affects and maladaptive behaviors. By learning how to alter dysfunctional cognitions that are at odds with reality (as most people see it), the individual is likely to have a greater sense of well-being and to behave in adaptive ways and less likely to develop symptoms of many types. The goal of group CBT is to help the person acquire the skills to monitor and alter cognitions in favorable ways. Concomitant with skill acquisition is a decrease in symptomotology.

Group CBT is a structured form of group treatment that is generally short term. During a course of treatment the members learn how to monitor, test, and alter cognitions. This learning occurs through the members' entrance into a special relationship with the therapist and other group members described as collaborative empiricism. The group experience is augmented by the use of the factors unique to group such as group cohesion, interpersonal learning, and the developmental stages. As in the interpersonal and psychodynamic approaches, members' progress in the group requires a rich affective experience organized by an adaptive system of meaning. Group CBT is a technique-abundant approach enabling the therapist to flexibly deploy an array of methods such as role plays, cognitive rehearsal,

Socratic questioning, bibliotherapy, homework assignments, booster sessions, and so on.

Group CBT has been found to be effective with a wide age range. It is helpful in treating persons with various symptoms, especially depression and anxiety but also eating disorders, obsessive disorders, and social phobia. In recent years group CBT approaches have been developed to treat personality disorders. Work with this latter group shows that group CBT is also effective in enhancing interpersonal functioning.

Interpersonal Problem Solving

Emily is an overweight, White, 14-year-old girl of average intelligence. She is currently repeating the eighth grade. Her disruptive behaviors in the classroom have not only tried the patience of her teacher but limited her capacity to learn. She was in detention twice over the past year because of cheating. In one case she paid an older neighbor boy to write a paper for her. In another she cheated on a test by copying the responses of another child. Despite such objectionable behaviors, Emily's teachers describe her as having positive qualities, such as a caring attitude toward her peers.

She is the youngest of three children. Two older brothers are more academically successful, and one is well known for his academic prowess. Emily attempts to affiliate with Patrick, who is 18 months older. However, he rebuffs her efforts to establish a friendship. When he rejects her, she teases him and acts silly in an effort to get him to notice her. He has many friends, all of whom she tries to cultivate when they are visiting her home. Sometimes a friend will respond in an accepting way by conversing with her briefly, but the brother shows disdain and embarrassment on such occasions.

Recently, Emily has taken to calling male classmates on whom she has crushes. One family became upset by her incessant attempts. When Emily continued to call despite a parent's direct request to her to stop, the parent asked the school counselor to intervene. This request led to a referral for an assessment.

Emily was evaluated by both a psychologist and pediatrician for ADHD or some other neuropsychologically based disorder, but no evidence supported such a diagnosis. However, there were manifestations of organizational difficulties, mild depression, and low self-esteem.

Based on all of the evidence, the school counselor felt that in social situations Emily was prone to acting on her impulses, a problem rooted in deficient problem-solving skills. She was referred to a group in which problem solving would be the major focus, especially problem solving in interpersonal situations.

13

chapter

Social or interpersonal problem solving concerns the ways in which individuals think about and respond to those problems that crop up in everyone's daily life (Nezu, Nezu, & Perri, 1989). A problem is a disparity between how one would want a situation to be and how it actually is. For example, Emily has a problem in relation to her brother. Whereas she wishes to be accepted by him and derive companionship from the relationship, his behaviors toward her are rejecting. A solution is a coping response that influences the problem, one's response to the problem, or both. Emily attempts to get attention from Patrick by teasing him. What makes this solution ineffective is that while she may obtain momentary notice, she does not elicit the more positive responses she desires. From a long-term perspective, such behaviors may make it less rather than more likely that Patrick will see her and behave toward her as a friend. In contrast, an effective solution is one that meets the problem solver's goal while minimizing negative consequences, short term and long term (D'Zurilla & Nezu, 1999). The problem-solving model will focus on how Emily arrives at her formulation and how she generates her solutions.

D'Zurilla and Nezu (1999) emphasize the importance of distinguishing between problem solving and solution implementation. Whereas the former encompasses the steps necessary to arrive at a solution, the latter is the process of executing a solution. Both sets of social skills are necessary for social competence, and both require their own focus in treatment because the presence of one does not necessitate the presence of the other. Frequently, the techniques for training in problem solving are combined with modules for those skills necessary to implement a solution. For example, a group designed to help socially phobic persons to solve problems more effectively may also incorporate a unit on assertiveness training. For this population, difficulties in self-assertion may hinder the implementation of solutions.

The problem-solving model is similar to and different from all of the preceding approaches. Like the cognitive-behavioral approach, it places heavy emphasis upon the quality of cognition as a crucial determinant of the well-being of the person. The problem-solving approach also relies upon the development of highly specific goals pursued in a very structured session. These features make it highly suitable for short-term time frames. Many of the cognitive-behavioral techniques such as agenda setting and role-playing are also found in the problem-solving approach. Also, like the cognitive-behavioral approach, this approach has developed in the empiricist tradition, so that there is a relatively large fund of research supporting its application. Like the interpersonal and object-relations approaches, its focus is on activity within the here-and-now of the group. While the content of the problems members solve in the group may refer to external difficulties, the real object of the group is the process of problem solving itself, which is displayed in the group sessions. Also like both of these models, the problem-solving model sees difficulties in negotiating interpersonal situations as the root of psychological symptoms. Finally, the problem-solving approach has in common with the object-relations approach, at least in certain of the latter's applications, the notion that unconscious conflict may underlie difficulties in basic cognitive processes.

Distinguishing the problem-solving approach from the three contrasting approaches is that much of the work on this approach has occurred specifically with children and adolescents. Its easy application to younger age groups in both inpatient and outpatient settings was a primary factor in its selection as our final model. Another factor is that it is a short-term approach compatible with a number of theoretical orientations, as is described in the next section. Finally, the problem-solving approach relative to the other three approaches does not have to be employed solely in relation to psychopathology. The problem-solving approach can be used to promote social competence in the absence of any identified psychological problem in the group members.

Goals and Conceptual Foundation

The premise on which the interpersonal problem-solving approach is based is that the ability to solve problems effectively is critical to psychological health and adaptation to the environment. Skill in problem solving leads to many positive outcomes, such as the capacity to work productively and to enjoy stable relationships. Conversely, poor coping strategies or deficiencies in problem solving can lead to a host of psychological difficulties (Dobson, Backs-Dermott, & Dozois, 2000), with the particular nature of the difficulty being determined by the nature of the problem-solving deficit.

Supporting this premise are many examples within the literature over the past 30 years of how different types of psychopathology are connected to problem-solving difficulties across various populations. For example, suicidal individuals have been shown to exhibit rigidity in their manner of thinking about the problems in their lives. Frequently, they generate fewer possible solutions than do their nonsuicidal counterparts (Cohen-Sandler, 1982). In a sample of reformatory inmates, those who were categorized by prison officials and peers as having disciplinary problems were relatively deficient in problem-solving skills (Higgins & Thies, 1982). The link between depression and problem-solving difficulties is well established in children (Goodman, Gravitt, & Kaslow, 1995), college students (Cheng, 2001; Priester & Clum, 1993), and adults (Nezu, Nezu, & Perri, 1989). Depressed individuals were shown to have a deficit in being able to devise multiple alternatives to a problem (Nezu, 1986). Difficulties in problem solving were associated with depression but also anxiety in a group of middle-aged and elderly community residents (Kant, D'Zurilla, & Maydeu-Olivares, 1997).

Just as psychopathology has been associated with problem-solving deficits, psychological health has been associated with problem-solving skill. For example, healthy individuals are more likely to proceed through the step of introspection before taking action on a problem (Platt & Spivack, 1974). Higher levels of skill in problem solving are associated with lower levels of anxiety and higher assertiveness (Neal & Heppner, 1982, described in Nezu, Nezu, & Perri, 1989) and a more positive self-concept (Heppner, Reeder, & Larson, 1983).

How can the relationship between problem-solving and psychological difficulties be conceptualized? There is no single account because the activity of problem solving can be seen through different theoretical lenses. From the standpoint of cognitive theory, problem solving relates to a set of cognitive processes that affect the types of cognitions an individual generates that in turn influence affects and behaviors. A behavioral perspective defines problem solving as a sequence of covert and overt behaviors. A behavioral perspective sees the description of the problem in operational terms and the implementation of the solution yielded by problem solving as important in the therapeutic process.

From a psychodynamic perspective, a critical aspect is how the individual defines the problem at hand. Through a psychodynamic inquiry that may uncover hidden impulses and affects, the individual is able to define the problem with greater accuracy and thereby develop solutions appropriate to what the problem actually is rather than what the person might deem it to be. Poor problem-solving skills lead to adaptive failures. For example, over time Emily's solution to her problem of wanting a closer, more amiable relationship with Patrick has led to a negatively toned relationship with him. Hence, her characteristic solution has led to an adaptive failure. Adaptive failures in turn beget low self-esteem. Emily is likely to feel negatively about herself in response to being spurned by her much-admired brother. A low level of self-esteem creates a vulnerability to the manifestation or intensification of symptoms (although other elements may predispose the individual to developing symptoms). This sequence is outlined in Table 13.1.

The fact that different theoretical systems are compatible with problem-solving therapy highlights a key aspect of this approach: It does not offer a unidimensional explanation for psychopathology or well-being (Nezu, Nezu, & Perri, 1989). It is an approach that admits of complexity, allowing for the contribution of many types of factors to the problems that people have. For example, the approach is not

Table 13.1 The Problem-Solving Conceptualization of Psychopathology and Its Treatment

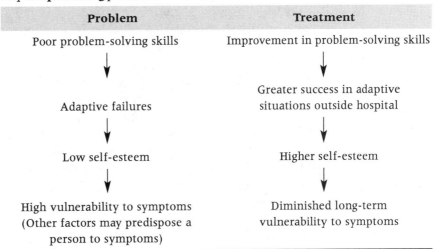

Problem	Treatment
Poor problem-solving skills	Improvement in problem-solving skills
↓	↓
Adaptive failures	Greater success in adaptive situations outside hospital
↓	↓
Low self-esteem	Higher self-esteem
↓	↓
High vulnerability to symptoms (Other factors may predispose a person to symptoms)	Diminished long-term vulnerability to symptoms

at odds with the notion that individuals by virtue of their biochemical make-ups are vulnerable to certain symptom patterns. Within this approach an individual's biochemical status determines whether one reacts to stress with a certain symptomatic pattern. By learning coping responses to stressful circumstances, the individual can circumvent the biochemical reaction associated with a particular set of symptoms. The openness of this approach makes it especially useful in circumstances in which individuals are being treated with a variety of interventions. Rather than creating dissonance, the problem-solving approach offers an overarching perspective that enables the person to see the role of each intervention in enhancing his or her overall adjustment.

Although different theoretical perspectives may provide varying accounts, research is under way to further elucidate the connection between problem solving and symptoms. For example, Kant, D'Zurilla, and Mayden-Olivares (1997) looked at different elements of problem solving in a middle-age and elderly sample to see if any of the elements mediated the relationship between everyday problems and the symptoms of depression and anxiety. They found that one particular dimension, *negative problem orientation*, was most significantly implicated. This orientation entails seeing everyday problems as threats and as having negative significance for the person. This negative problem orientation produces distress and adversely affects the person's ability to use problem-solving techniques. This research, which has also been supported by other studies (e.g., D'Zurilla & Nezu, 1990), suggests the importance of distinguishing between problem orientation[1] and problem-solving skills. Kant, D'Zurilla, and Mayden-Olivares suggest that whereas problem orientation may be more critical to well-being in a "normal" population, problem-solving skills may be more critical in the development of symptoms in clinical groups.

The goal of problem-solving therapy is quite simply to help individuals solve problems more effectively. Movement toward this goal would entail acquiring a positive problem orientation, an ability to identify a problem, a capacity to generate a set of solutions, and a skill in selecting among them. Effective problem solving also involves following through on a chosen solution, removing obstacles to its

---

[1] A study by Chang and D'Zurilla (1996) shows that while negative problem orientation is associated with pessimism and negative trait affectivity, it is not redundant with these constructs.

implementation along the way. While the problem-solving model is a skill-acquisition approach, success in problem solving would be expected to produce adaptive successes, higher self-esteem, and a lessened degree of psychological distress.

Why Group Therapy?

Problem-solving therapy can be conducted on an individual basis. However, groups have resources that make them an especially salubrious environment for learning how to solve problems, resources now quite familiar to the reader. As members present problems of various sorts, they come to realize that there are commonalities among their difficulties (White, 2000a). This factor of universality can help members develop a more positive problem orientation.

Problem solving, as we have noted, entails the generation of multiple alternatives to solving the problem. Group efforts may generate a greater array of alternatives than would be possible by an individual (Perri, Nezu, & Viegener, 1992), although in some groups the opposite trend has been obtained due perhaps to members' concern about others' evaluation (Coskun, Paulus, Brown, & Sherwood, 2000). As members work together to solve a problem, cohesion develops, a therapeutic factor that catalyzes the group's work.

The group allows members to solve problems interpersonally in a way that is experiential. As members form relationships, conflicts emerge. These conflicts can be formulated as problems for the group to solve collaboratively. In inpatient, day hospital, and residential treatment settings in which members spend much of their days together, interpersonal problems are especially common. All of the benefits that accrue from interpersonal learning can be obtained when the problems the group solves are truly its own. D'Zurilla (1986) points out the benefits of the group in providing modeling opportunities and in providing members with social reinforcement as they make strides in mastering problem-solving skills.

Like the cognitive-behavioral approach, the interpersonal problem-solving approach could benefit from further development of techniques that use the resources of the group fully. For example, problem solving group therapists generally pay little attention to stages of group development. The emphasis on group process in this chapter does not characterize group problem-solving literature as a whole.

Change Processes

This section presents the mechanics of conducting interpersonal problem-solving group treatment. The reader will see that as in the cognitive-behavioral approach, the therapist is highly active, the session, extremely structured, and procedures are introduced (such as homework) to ensure that learning in the group is applied to the outside social environment. All of these features are characteristic of approaches that establish skill acquisition as a major goal of the treatment.

The Role of the Leader

In Chapter 5, we explored the four sets of leader activities: executive functions, caring, meaning attribution, and emotional stimulation (Lieberman, Yalom, & Miles, 1973). We learn about how the problem-solving therapist effectively conducts a group by considering activities associated with each of these functions.

The executive function is prominent in the problem-solving approach. It calls for a therapist who is active and directive. At the beginning of treatment the therapist functions at various points as a teacher presenting a clear rationale for the model and the therapeutic processes by which the group members acquire skill in using it. The therapist creates and implements the format of a highly structured session. He or she makes sure that the group does not get bogged down or off track. At various points, the therapist provides reinforcement, model aspects of the problem-solving process, record solutions on the board, and assign and check homework. In fact, there are so many activities in the executive domain that a cotherapy team is often necessary to accomplish them all.

With all the executive activities required, it might be easy for the therapist to become preoccupied with them to the neglect of caring, which is also critical to the effective application of this model. The problem-solving approach should never be applied mechanistically (D'Zurilla & Nezu, 2001). In the early stage of treatment when members may feel doubt about the pertinence of problem solving to their symptoms and other psychological difficulties, it is frequently the therapist's empathy for the patient that fosters the patient's openness to this approach before having had an opportunity to experience its benefits (Nezu, Nezu, & Perri, 1989). The problem-solving approach also entails establishing a collaborative relationship with group members. One aspect of this collaboration is the therapist's respect for what each member can contribute to the treatment process.

Meaning attribution is a conspicuous function in this system. In labeling members' difficulties as problems in need of solutions, the therapist is providing a meaning system to members. On a more individual level, the therapist's assisting members in clarifying their problems serves a meaning-attribution function. For example, in the problem-definition phase Emily may come to recognize that her behavior of teasing Patrick is on a surface level an attempt to secure his attention but more deeply an expression of a wish for his love. In general, the therapist who uses problem solving from a psychodynamic vantage point will work to enhance the psychological mindedness of members during the problem-formulation step.

Emotional stimulation is a function less emphasized than others. Within this approach, confrontation, a tool commonly used to stimulate affect, is employed relatively sparingly. Judicious therapist self-disclosures can occur, not to stimulate emotion, but rather to show that the approach the therapist endorses is one the therapist uses. However, two types of interventions can increase the members' level of emotional engagement. The first is when the therapist identifies conflicts among the group members as problems in need of solution. Interpersonal learning opportunities stimulate members and increase their engagement because the problem is immediate and shared rather than distant and personal. Emotional stimulation is also effected by the brainstorming process—an essential element of the approach. Frequently, pleasurable excitement occurs when members are able to offer solutions with abandon. The pleasure in working together in this fashion can help members develop a more positive problem orientation.

The Structure of Treatment

As in the cognitive-behavioral approach, we examine the group treatment in three phases: the initial sessions in which members are learning about problem solving and its importance for their well-being, the middle sessions in which members practice problem-solving techniques, and the termination steps in which members consolidate learning and prepare for their departure from the group. Generally, problem-solving therapy groups are short term, ranging most typically from 8 to 16 sessions, and close ended, with all members beginning and ending at the same time.

The Initial Session: In the initial session the therapists present a rationale for problem-solving training and an outline of how the group is going to proceed. Members are told that the goal of the group is to help them cope with everyday stressors by mastering a particular problem-solving system. At this time the relationship between interpersonal problem solving and symptoms can also be discussed. Because many members will be entering the group with symptoms, establishing the link between problem solving and symptoms increases their motivation to participate; at the same time the therapist should not suggest that immediate symptomatic relief will occur.

Right from the beginning of the group, the therapist should work to establish group cohesion. A means to foster cohesion is to have members introduce themselves and to have each member describe what brought him or her into the group (Nezu, Nezu, & Perri, 1989).

A major task during the early sessions, particularly the first and second session, is to develop a *positive problem orientation*. The importance of a positive problem orientation is that it motivates individuals to use their resources to both recognize problems and to work constructively to solve them. This orientation requires members to see problems as a natural part of life. This orientation is cultivated in the introduction, when members hear about those difficulties that led the person to join the group. Moreover, some difficulties will overlap. For example, Emily, from our original vignette, may hear that other group members were rejected by peers. Members' awareness of the shared aspect of this problem is especially useful in helping them to see that problems in general and their problems in particular are normal. As members talk about their difficulties, the therapist can identify certain self-statements or beliefs that might lead to a negative problem orientation. Examples of such statements might be:

"If I ignore this situation, it will go away."

"There's just nothing I can do about it."

"Recognizing the problem will make it worse."

"I'll just fly by the seat of my pants."

"This is a catastrophe—it will destroy my life."

Several themes are likely to emerge during the introductions. One is that denial is a frequent strategy in handling problems. Helplessness in the face of a problem is also a common theme. Another theme is that each problem has great destructive potential for the person. Still another is that impulsive solutions work best because they rid the person of the problem quickly.

As these beliefs are identified, they can be refuted. Members can be asked to suggest counters to these beliefs. For example, in response to the notion that a problem is a catastrophe, the person could say, "This is an opportunity for me to experience some growth." This counter would reflect the individual's *problem appraisal,* which is how the individual views the problem in relation to his or her own well-being. Tendencies toward minimization (underestimating an event's significance) or magnification (overestimating its importance) may lead to difficulties in problem perception, difficulties that should be identified and corrected at this time and as they arise in later sessions. At this time, it may be helpful to share with members a worksheet developed by Nezu, Nezu, and Perri (1989) that lists potential statements supporting a positive problem orientation (see Figure 13.1).

Another aspect of problem orientation is being able to recognize a problem when it occurs, a capacity referred to as *problem perception.* As the negative statements identified earlier suggest, one common strategy of individuals who have low social competence is the denial of problems that arise. Group members are helped to see how they can use their own feelings as a guide to realizing when a problem may have surfaced:

THERAPIST: So you say that when you got home from school, you began to have a fight with Patrick. Did it happen when you walked in the door?

EMILY: No, it took about fifteen minutes . . . that's all it usually takes for him to get annoyed with me.

THERAPIST: But let's look at that little bit of time before that . . . right when you walked through the door . . . what happened?

EMILY: I put my book down. I got a snack. I ate it. And then, I was bored.

THERAPIST: Can you talk about that boredom a little more? What was it like?

EMILY: Well, I had nothing to do . . . I had no one to call . . . I felt, just for a moment lonely . . . and . . .

Name: _____   Date: _____

_____

Briefly describe the problem situation.

_____

Briefly describe your initial reaction to this problem.

_____

How does this compare with a POSITIVE ORIENTATIN as described below?

_____

Positive problem orientation:

Problems are a common part of life; many people have similar kinds of problems.

It is better to face or confront a problem when it occurs, rather than avoid it.

I can solve this problem effectively!

I should use my feelings as a *cue* that a problem exists.

I should "STOP and THINK" before I act impulsively!

Figure 13.1

Problem Orientation Worksheet.
Reprinted with permission of John Wiley & Sons, Inc., from Nezu, Nezu, and Perri's (1989) *Problem-Solving Therapy for Depression: Theory, Research, and Clinical Guidelines.* New York, p. 146.

THERAPIST: Maybe sad?

EMILY: Yes because I didn't know what to do with myself. I tried to get Patrick to let me listen to his CD and the next thing I knew we were fighting.

In this brief exchange the therapist has helped Emily recognize her affective state, which could serve as a clue to the presence of a problem. By homing in on her boredom and sadness, Emily could move toward the identification of a problem and its solution. Instead, what Emily did was to short-circuit the process by taking flight into an activity that led to the greater frustration of her needs. This recognition of feelings as cues often is a shift for the group member, who at the outset of treatment may see feelings as the problems themselves (D'Zurilla, 1986).

Another aspect of a member's problem orientation that may be evident early in the group is *problem attribution,* or how the problem came about. Let's suppose Emily continued to describe the exchange between her brother and her:

EMILY: He just got mad at me because I kept asking him for the CD. But that's not unusual. There's just something about me that people hate. My brother treats me the same way the kids at school do. They don't want to have anything to do with me because I'm a big zero.

Here we find Emily attributing her difficulty with Patrick to some global defectiveness. We can imagine that such an attributional style would make it very difficult for Emily to commit herself to pursuing her problems in a systematic way. Helping Emily to recognize her problem-solving set and to appreciate other possible explanations is likely to increase her investment in problem-solving activity. Other group members may have other attributional biases. For example, some members may see external forces as entirely responsible for their difficulties. While these biases probably will not be eliminated by identifying them and discussing other possible sets, they may be relaxed sufficiently to enable the member to be receptive to the next phase of the therapy.

During the first session, the therapist also outlines for members the stages of problem solving. These are as follows:

- Preliminary description of the problem
- Clarification of the problem
- Generation of alternatives
- Evaluation of the alternatives
- Role play
- Implementation of the decision and verification of its correctness

Although in the first session these stages are described and perhaps illustrated, most of the time ensuing sessions will provide members with practice in problem solving. These steps are described in some detail in the next section in terms of how members practice them within the group.

Typically, at the end of the first session members are given homework to complete. Group members may not yet be ready to practice the problem-solving steps outside of group. However, they can begin to prepare for doing so in the group by identifying problems. The therapist may provide various categories in which problems may occur, such as "Home," "School," "Relationship with Friends," "Relationships with Parents," and so on to stimulate the members' thinking.

Sessions Following the First Session: A problem can be established in a variety of ways. The therapist may simply ask members to volunteer problems. Alternately, the therapist may suggest an area of potential problem solving based on his or her knowledge of the areas of difficulty for a given patient population. For example, members might be encouraged to problem solve in relation to self-destructive impulses (Linehan & Wagner, 1990). Rather than simply providing members a topic area, the therapist may develop a composite problem based upon the issues members presented in the opening sessions. A third alternative is for the therapist to identify problems concerning their relationships with one another or, in the case of inpatients, with persons in the broader treatment environment (Coche, 1987). While some therapists may pick a consistent way of choosing problems, others may use different means from session to session in order to strengthen members' skill levels across different situations.

CLARIFICATION OF THE PROBLEM: The member's clear grasp and accurate identification of the problem are of paramount importance in successful problem solving. Often, the initial rendering of the problem is vague. For example, remember that when we last left Emily, she described herself as "a big zero." A vague and global self-condemnatory statement such as this one cannot but beget negative feelings. These negative feelings then hamper her problem-solving efforts. In fact, a recent study shows that group members are more receptive to problem-solving training when they are having a positive mood state (Joiner et al., 2001). Therefore, the effort will be to help Emily to specify the problem in terms as concrete as possible because operationally defined problems are both more solvable and more emotionally manageable.

In the quest for precision in the definition of the problem, group members assist the member by getting as much information about that problem as possible. Members may say to Emily, "Was it your brother's favorite CD you wanted to borrow?" or "How did you make your request?" or "Have there been other times when you've borrowed his stuff?" The other members and the therapist ask whatever questions may help to clarify the problem and through this process may illuminate dimensions of the problem that may not have been originally evident to the problem solver. Often the feel of the group as an investigative team is engaging and enjoyable for members, an affective state that further spurs the process. In some cases a homework assignment will emerge, directing the members to procure some important piece of information the member lacks.

During this step, another aspect of problem clarification is distinguishing the real problem from a possible camouflage problem. Consider the case of Ian:

> *Ian, a 16-year-old boy, came into the group after having made a suicide attempt. His parents had been divorced three years ago and his mother had sole custody of him. Ian, the eldest child of three, had taken on a tremendous amount of responsibility for his younger siblings. After a brief courtship, his mother had recently remarried, and Ian had formed an amiable but distant relationship with his stepfather. Ian complained that the reason he was driven to engage in self-destructive activity was that his mother has become so absorbed in her new relationship that she relied upon him excessively for the care of his siblings and he no longer had time to engage in activities that might bring him pleasure.*
>
> *During the information-gathering step, it became evident that Ian could not substantiate his claim that he was spending more time in providing child care. If anything, it seemed as though his siblings were becoming more self-sufficient. As the group discussion unfolded, what became evident to all was that the real source of pain for Ian was the lessening of the admiring attention paid to him by his mother, attention that he enjoyed prior to the blossoming of her romantic relationship. The problem, then, was clarified as being able to let his mother know that he continued to need her recognition. The redefinition of the problem was facilitated by two other adolescents in the group attesting to how difficult it was for them to accept the*

change in the relationship with the custodial parent when that parent re-married. These members made it less necessary for Ian to erect a defense against his feelings of disappointment in his mother.

The therapist sensed that lurking below that surface was another aspect of Ian's problem: the conflict between competitiveness with his stepfather and his judgment that such competitive strivings in relation to his mother are forbidden. However, the therapist perceived that uncovering this facet of the problem would unduly raise Ian's anxiety and sense of vulnerability, so the therapist refrained from probing in this area. The therapist's exercise of clinical sensitivity is all-important in this problem-clarification process.

The problem-clarification process should yield a goal whose fulfillment will enable the member to know when the problem has been solved. For example, a goal for Emily might be to make a friend with whom she can socialize once a week.

GENERATE ALTERNATIVE SOLUTIONS: Once the group has clarified a problem, the next step is to develop as many solutions to that problem as members working together can muster. The technique guiding this step is Osborn's (1963) *brainstorming* method. The three features of this method are quantity of solutions, deferment of judgment or criticism, and variety of solutions (D'Zurilla & Nezu, 1999). Members might be encouraged not to be fettered by habit or convention through the use of exercises. For example, D'Zurilla and Nezu describe an exercise in which members are asked to think of ways to improve upon a common object.

The therapist guides the process of solution generation by pointing out to members when they are lapsing into a more evaluative stance that hinders creativity. Even solutions that have moral or legal implications should not be rejected. Any critical input at this time is likely to decrease the quantity of all types of solutions. Ultimately, the problem-solving process makes it less rather than more likely that an individual behaves in antisocial ways (Coche & Douglass, 1977). At the same time, the therapist keeps members on track so that the solutions offered are relevant to the problem at hand. Relevance is the only requirement placed on solutions.

To encourage members to offer as many ideas as possible, the therapist should provide verbal encouragement and record all suggestions in a log with the contributor's initials next to the solution. This log is a resource to group members who at some time may want to refer back to the array of solutions for their problems. The therapist also helps the member to keep in mind all of the principles guiding the solution-generation stage with posters on the walls of the room with such tips as "Solutions: the more the better."

To encourage variety, the therapist might have the members categorize potential solutions according to the strategy they suggest. For example, Emily might be given solutions to her brother's rejection that involve obtaining other sources of companionship. There may be few or no solution alternatives concerning how she might engage him in a way that would be likely to be more successful or how she might be less affected by occasions when he is not receptive. The group could then be encouraged to develop alternatives consistent with these newly emerging strategies.

This solution-generating step may be revisited later in the problem-solving sequence. When the group initially provides solutions, they usually have a more general, strategic character. After the member chooses a solution, it may be necessary to return to this step so that more specific tactics for implementing a strategy can be devised. Also, in the next step, if it is revealed that all solutions are unsatisfactory, then, the group must return to this step.

Table 13.2 summarizes tips for successful solution generation.

EVALUATION AND DECISION MAKING: This step entails members' examination of all of the solutions for a given problem so that eventually one can be selected. Potential solutions should be evaluated from several standpoints. The group should consider whether a particular solution would lead to the accomplishment of an established goal: Has the problem, in fact, been solved? The group must also determine whether an alternative solution is feasible, that is, can the solution be implemented given the resources at hand (Nezu, Nezu, & Perri, 1989). The group can quickly scan the list of alternatives

Table 13.2　　**Tips for Successful Solutions Generation**

1. Emphasize quantity.
2. Encourage acceptance of solutions.
3. Reward effort.
4. Use posters with prompts.
5. Record all solutions and note contributors.

and eliminate those that either present unacceptable risks or cannot be implemented (D'Zurilla & Nezu, 1999).

The *value* of a possible solution must be assessed by a system suggested by D'Zurilla and Nezu (1999) in which a solution is evaluated according to the following categories: positive and negative short-term consequences, long-term consequences, personal consequences, and social consequences. D'Zurilla and Nezu point out that included in the category of personal consequences are ethical considerations or affective reactions that the proposed solution might generate. Some writers have suggested that a numerical approach might enhance the costs/benefits analysis. For example, Hussian (1987) suggested a scale from −2 to +2 by which short- and long-term advantages to self and others could be rated. The winning solution would be that which received the highest score. However, such an approach could be cumbersome and also simplistic in its failure to allow for the weighting of factors.

Some members may have difficulties anticipating the likely consequence of implementing a given solution alternative. The demand of this step may be especially great for children and younger adolescents (such as some of the members we will meet in the vignette), who are still developing the imaginal abilities to anticipate consequences. Moreover, some individuals have personality styles in which trial-and-error problem-solving activities are emphasized over a playing out of possibilities in fantasy. D'Zurilla and Nezu (1999) suggest that the therapist initiate a role play in which two or more group members enact a solution so that consequences can be recognized. This use of role play is different from its application once a solution has been chosen in that the latter application occurs so that emerging obstacles can be identified and then overcome.

The careful consideration of each proposed solution and the focus on not only short-term but long-term effects are of particular benefit to impulse-ridden individuals or those with antisocial tendencies who are inclined to emphasize short-term gratification. It is also helpful to persons prone to rumination because through this step, idle worry is changed into purposive thought.

ROLE-PLAYING: The behavioral rehearsal of an interaction can be very useful in a variety of ways. When anxiety impairs the person's ability to engage in a type of interaction outside the group, the role play can provide a mastery experience that strengthens confidence.

The role play provides information. For example, suppose Emily were given an opportunity to role play an interaction in which she invited, in an amiable fashion, her brother to spend time with her. By carefully monitoring her feelings as she proceeded through the role play, Emily might learn that interacting with her brother without resorting to teasing made her feel vulnerable. She would realize that teasing was her armament. The therapist would play an important role in achieving such insight by encouraging Emily to examine her experience before, during, and after the role play. Hence, role-playing can activate the therapeutic factor of self-understanding.

Interpersonal learning may also occur during the role play. Consider how the therapist might orchestrate the group discussion after Emily had the opportunity to role play asking her brother to spend time with her:

THERAPIST: Thanks, Emily. Thanks for playing the brother, Ian. While all of you were watching Emily make a request of her brother, did any of you notice anything in her behavior that might have helped or hindered her cause?

BOBBI: Well, I thought her eye contact was really good.

EMILY: Yeah, I was trying to pay attention to that—I really felt like turning my eyes away because I felt nervous.

THERAPIST: How did you experience Emily's eye contact, Ian?

IAN: I couldn't just slough her off—I had to deal with what she was asking.

In orchestrating the feedback process, it would be important for the therapist to keep in mind the various findings concerning feedback discussed in Chapter 4. For example, positive feedback should generally precede negative feedback, and the former should be abundant so that the latter can be tolerable.

Role play can also increase empathy for other critical figures involved in the problematic situation. As Blatner (1996) wrote, "for a true understanding of a problem, it is necessary for the parties to consider the viewpoints and feelings of the other people involved" (p. 156). In the role play, Emily might play the role of Patrick so she could obtain greater sensitivity to his emotional reactions to the situation. This is the psychodramatic technique of role reversal. Many other psychodramatic techniques might be useful during this step.

SOLUTION IMPLEMENTATION AND VERIFICATION: The problem solver finally carries out the solution and discovers whether the solution was in fact feasible. While good information gathering helps the solver to anticipate most obstacles, it may be impossible to anticipate all of them. Some new circumstances may emerge between the time the solver formulates a solution and implements it. At times, it may be necessary to reinitiate the problem-solving process or to recast the original problem to include the subgoal of overcoming an obstacle (Nezu, Nezu, & Perri, 1989).

Many consequences may occur from the implementation of a solution. We can imagine that if Emily changes how she relates to Patrick, it might have consequences, too, for her relationships with the other three members of her family and her relationship with herself. These effects and any others would be important for Emily to monitor in order to evaluate the success of a part of the chosen solution. This evaluation should be part of the group's work. If a solution is deemed not to have been entirely satisfactory, then the group should consider various possibilities. Was the solution adequately implemented? Are there ways the solution could be modified to be more effective? Is a new solution needed?

After solving as many problems as possible within the available time of the session, the therapist summarizes homework assignments generated in the course of the session. For any members who have not yet received assignments, they are developed at this time. Homework assignments encourage practice, and practice is crucial for the acquisition of problem-solving skills (D'Zurilla & Nezu, 2001).

As the sessions progress, the focus transfers from acquisition of skills to maintenance and generalization training. The endeavor is to enhance members' flexibility in applying the problem-solving steps across a wide variety of situations. Here groups offer some advantages in that a group of members can bring up a greater array of problems than any one member can generate. Moreover, as members come to know one another better, they can become more astute in providing feedback on aspects of each other's interpersonal styles that might interfere with the accomplishment of goals. Role plays can then provide opportunities to alter negative aspects of these styles.

Termination Sessions: In the final sessions, the focus should be anticipating those problems that might emerge following treatment that are associated with the individual's departure from the group.

Such concerns as dealing with loss and self-doubt become new problems to be solved like all of the problems that have proceeded them. The members should be reminded to use whatever handouts were distributed over the course of the groups. Handouts serve not only as informational tools but also, as object-relational thinkers might note, as transitional objects that can cull up the emotional atmosphere of the group, an atmosphere in which problems were greeted with equanimity rather than terror or hopelessness.

Like the cognitive-behavioral approach, the problem-solving approach sometimes uses booster sessions as a way of helping members retain the gains made from participation in the group. Some research (e.g., Lochman, 1992) suggests that these sessions are effective.

Clinical Vignette

The outpatient group met for 16 sessions on a weekly basis. Members could renew for another 16 sessions at the end of the current session. Each session lasts 75 minutes. The group was coled by a male and female therapist. The group was composed of boys and girls in their early adolescence. They ranged in age from 13 to 16.

There were six group members. The reader has already met Emily and Ian, who were on their first 16-week stints in the group. The other members were as follows:

- Billy: This 14-year-old boy was argumentative in school with both teachers and peers. The referral to group was precipitated by his pushing a teacher against the wall. Billy expressed remorse after such episodes that appeared sincere. This is Billy's second stint in the group.

- Veronica: 15-year-old Veronica's parents worried about her involvement in a string of relationships with boys who would become sexually involved with her and after several months leave her. Veronica would show signs of depression until she established another relationship. Investment in school was minimal. She frequently failed to show up for school.

- Martin: This 15-year-old boy was referred to the group after his parents discovered that he was attempting to hack into his high school's computer system in order to change a low grade. His father was a member of the school board and a reverend, who, as he described it, said his son lacked a "work ethic." Martin spent most of his time playing video games and skateboarding. His mother felt Martin failed to study and engaged in rebellious behavior to humiliate his father.

- Bobbi: This 15-year-old girl was a model student at school and got very high grades. However, in the home setting she was intolerant of younger siblings when they intruded upon her privacy. When she baby-sat (which she did quite often because of her parents' work schedules), she used physical means of disciplining her siblings. One sibling reported this practice to a neighbor, who had been disturbed by shrieks coming from the home. The neighbor in turn called Child Protective Services. While an investigation did not support an abuse claim, Bobbi's parents were sufficiently alarmed to place her into treatment.

This session was the group's ninth. All of the members were very well acquainted with the steps of problem solving. The group had completed reviewing members' homework. Typically, in this group three or four problems would be pursued within a session. The group had identified three problems, the first of which had been suggested by an obstacle Bobbi encountered in doing her homework assignment. From the group's earlier sessions, it had become clear that Bobbi greatly resented having to spend so much time taking care of her younger siblings. This past week she was going to go home and talk to her parents about getting a baby-sitter for one night during the week so that she could go out with her friends. Bobbi reported during the beginning of the current session that it was impossible to make this request of her parents at this time. Her father had just been notified by his company that he was going to take a pay cut. The company was facing massive lay-offs. Her father had been fortunate to have retained his job. He was told that he might be able to get some overtime to make up for his lost income. For Bobbi, it would mean providing child care for more rather than fewer hours. Her mood state while reporting this circumstance to the group had been one of dejection, a factor leading the therapist to begin with her problem:

THERAPIST: Okay, let's begin with you, Bobbi. You said you weren't able to ask your parents for some relief so that you could begin to develop a social life.

BOBBI: It's impossible now.

VERONICA: But you still have the same needs. For me, not being able to go out . . . it would just be no life.

EMILY: I never go out.

BOBBI: My parents work so incredibly hard. I just couldn't possibly be so insensitive to their situation as to say I'm not going to help them right now.

VERONICA: Your sisters and brothers are their responsibility, not yours.

[Veronica is rushing in to solve the problem before it has become established. Her solution is for Bobbi to ignore her parent's needs.]

MARTIN: In a family, everyone is responsible for everyone else. If there was one thing my father impressed in me, it was that. But you also have a responsibility to take care of them the right way and if you're so bitter that you can't be a normal teenager with friends and everything, how can you do that?

THERAPIST: Good point. So let's see if we can work this up into a problem. We've already established that Bobbi needs a social life. The solution we developed was based upon different information than we have now. Therefore, what we need to do is go back and look at the problem again and see what solutions are possible. What we're doing is not all that unusual in problem solving. Frequently we have to go back and problem solve again because either the situation is changed or there was something we just didn't know the first time we solved the problem. So the problem is: How can Bobbi reduce her child-care responsibilities without compromising her family's financial situation? Is that right, Bobbi?

BOBBI: Yeah, I think that says it.

THERAPIST: Okay. [writes the problem on the board] Now let's see if we have all of the information we need to solve this problem. Are there any questions?

IAN: Is this a short-term situation for him?

BOBBI: No, I guess this is how it will be until the economy changes or something. . . .

VERONICA: Well, I have a question I'm sort of hesitant to ask because I don't want to make Bobbi angry at me.

BOBBI: Why do you think I'll get angry?

VERONICA: Because in a way, I would be calling you a liar if I say what I'd like to say.

BOBBI: You mean you don't think my father really took a pay cut?

VERONICA: Of course I believe you there. I don't think you're lying to *us*. . . . I think you're lying to *yourself,* maybe.

BOBBI: I won't get mad . . . I really want to hear this . . . c'mon.

VERONICA: Well, it sounds to me like you've never had much of a social life . . . you've never had a serious relationship. All you have are these friends of yours and your idea of a cool time is going to the library on Saturday night. [members laugh]

BOBBI: That's not true!

VERONICA: Okay, so I'm exaggerating. But what I think is that you're just scared. I have a feeling that you are using your parents' money problem so you don't have to go out and try to meet some guys.

THERAPIST: You have a sense that fear is a big factor for Bobbi. I'm wondering . . . does it just have to do with what you've heard about her social life outside the group. Does it have anything to do with how Bobbi is in here?

VERONICA: Something about how she looks only at the two of you [pointing to the therapists] and avoids looking at us.

EMILY: Yeah! I noticed that, too!

BOBBI: Listen—you're right . . . you are . . . about me being scared . . . especially about the guy part. I'll admit it. But I also want to try. I'm in this group and it would be a good time for me to try so I could talk about my problems meeting guys. I have only seven more sessions.

COTHERAPIST: So you feel that this money problem is legit?

BOBBI: I do. But I also think that I'm going to need help with the other.

THERAPIST: And that you can realize it is great. [The therapist attempts to nurture Bobbi's positive problem orientation.] So we have two problems: The one is how you can start a social life even while your family is having these financial struggles and the other is how you can deal with your fear of meeting guys. We haven't even scratched the surface on the second one, so let's come back to it later. Thanks, Veronica, for pursuing that line. You came up with something important. But, Bobbi, you can't deal with your fears unless you have the opportunity to be in social situations, especially social situations with guys present. You can't be with guys the way you're scheduling your time now. So let's go back to the original problem and brainstorm about some possible solutions.

BILLY: Okay, I've got it! You can just give them cough syrup so they'll sleep and then go out.

[The therapist does not challenge this antisocial alternative.]

EMILY: You could have parties in your home.

MARTIN: I find I can't get any girls to come to my home for parties. [Billy laughs.]

THERAPIST: Martin, in sharing your experiences, you are in effect evaluating Emily's suggestion. We'll have plenty of time to evaluate later. Right now we just want to get as many ideas down as we can.

EMILY: How about if she trades off with a friend . . . like, the friend brings her younger brothers and sisters over and Bobbi watches all of them so she can go out. But she does the same for Bobbi.

BOBBI: But where would they sleep?

THERAPIST: Let's wait to think of the practicalities later.

BOBBI: Oh yeah, I forgot.

MARTIN: Maybe she could have relationships over the Internet. After the kids go to sleep, she could go into a chat room.

VERONICA: She could get a job . . . my friend works at a movie store and meets lots of other kids . . . in fact, she met her boyfriend there. Then she could hire the baby-sitter.

EMILY: She could join a club at school where she could meet friends.

[Alternative solutions continue to be generated. The group then moves toward the evaluation stage. Bobbi is asked to pick which solution seems most feasible. She decides that getting a job might work. She could socialize and make money at the same time. She reasons that a baby-sitter might be more patient with her siblings than she is. Her homework is to have a discussion with her parents about this possibility.]

COTHERAPIST: Okay, the next problem was one you brought up, Martin. You feel your parents don't trust you and are keeping you on . . . what did you say . . . "a short leash"? Maybe it would help if we could be a bit more specific. Can you describe what you mean?

MARTIN: Yeah, ever since I got caught trying to break into the school's computer system—which was really dumb—[Billy injects "I think it was cool."] my parents are suspicious of me. They are constantly coming into my room and checking on me. They won't let me leave the house unless they know exactly where I'm going and I've caught them spying on me. I can't stand it!

BOBBI: Martin, you have to realize that of course they're going to worry.

MARTIN: But I feel I've learned my lesson. I've been punished for my crime and it's time to move on.

BOBBI: So you feel they can trust you now?

MARTIN: Yeah, I do. I'm not going to screw up again.

THERAPIST: So the problem is: How can Martin convince his parents that he is trustworthy and won't be tempted to engage in conduct that will be objectionable to them?

MARTIN: That's exactly right. I can't seem to convince them.

[The therapist writes the problem on the board.]

THERAPIST: Okay, so maybe the group can help. But let me ask one thing: How will you know when they trust you?

MARTIN: When they let me leave the house for a few hours and don't check on me all the time. [affects a radio announcer voice] And if any of you can help me with this, I'll offer a cash reward. You can either get it in a lump sum or . . . [Veronica laughs.]

THERAPIST: We have the problem. Next we need to clarify the problem and see what information we need before we suggest possible solutions.

BOBBI: Are there things you're doing that bothers them . . . I don't mean the big things . . . I mean minor things that would just worry them a little?

MARTIN: Well, I get Cs in school. They worry about whether I'll get into a college. I'm lazy and they know it.

IAN: Anything else?

MARTIN: Well, my room's a mess. That's definitely my mom's pet peeve. And when friends come over, I spend all of my time playing computer games . . . that's a big thing . . . they hate that. My mother says, "Did you ever hear of having a conversation?"

VERONICA: Would they rather you were out on dates? My parents would be so happy if I would hang with my friends in my room.

MARTIN: Mine say I'm obsessed.

[The conversation continues with group members getting more information on Martin's parents' concerns.]

THERAPIST: Okay, I think we're ready to work on generating some possible solutions. And remember, no judging.

BOBBI: Well, for starters, I think he could work on staying up on his homework assignments.

[The cotherapist is recording each suggestion.]

VERONICA: What if you have some friends over and did something else? Like listen to music.

BILLY: Next time when you hack into the computer system at school, do it right.

EMILY: Keep your room clean. They'll notice that right away.

THERAPIST: Martin, do you have any ideas?

MARTIN: Just spend less time playing computer games.

IAN: And don't have such an attitude all the time.

THERAPIST: Can you explain that a little more?

IAN: Yeah, you see how he is in here. Always has a joke or a smart comment.

BILLY: And you smirk a lot. People tell me I smirk a lot.

MARTIN: What does that have to do with my parents?

IAN: If you're the same way with them, they probably feel that when you say something, you don't mean it.

THERAPIST: So you're saying that he should talk to his parents in a different way?

IAN: Yeah, that's what I'm saying.

THERAPIST: How so?

IAN: Just try not to make a joke when they say something serious. Answer them in a serious way.

THERAPIST: I'm just wondering: Are there some solutions that we can put together?

[The therapist can help the member to chunk solutions, an especially helpful intervention when the problem is multipronged.]

MARTIN: Well, how about the cleaning up my room with studying and getting better grades. They are both things my parents want me to do.

The group moves on to evaluate the solutions. Group members validate Ian's observations about how Martin acts in the group and agree that even if he were to act responsibly, this fact might be lost on his parents if he did not have a sincere and respectful demeanor. Martin then is given an opportunity to practice responding in a less sarcastic and dismissive way in the group. The solution that was eventually formulated was for Martin to try to adopt a more respectful demeanor when his parents communicate their wishes to him and to keep up with his homework and to maintain a tidy bedroom. His homework assignment for the week was to have two conversations with his parents in which he listened to their input without making jokes that demeaned what they said.

Comment on the Session

Members of this group were variable from one another on many dimensions. For example, we can see a great range of interpersonal styles and behaviors. In general, such diversity is helpful in groups with children and adolescents. Writing on this point, Shechtman (2001) notes that groups treating aggressive children who lack social skills greatly benefit from the presence of children with stronger prosocial tendencies. This variation is useful in the problem-solving approach because it creates a greater range in the ways problems can be formulated, the types of strategies that are proposed, and the possibilities that are recognized for overcoming obstacles in implementing solutions. Moreover, each member will have relative strengths and weaknesses in each step of the problem-solving process. For example, Veronica has a strength in seeing an emotional issue underlying a practical problem. Other members can model her ability to look deeper than the concrete presentation of the problem.

At the same time, this vignette highlights the strength of having members be relatively homogeneous in terms of age. We can see that the problems members presented, although having some uniqueness, were ones to which other members could relate. Veronica had a grasp of the importance of social life for Bobbi because she in a different way longs for greater relational fulfillment. Most of these members can identify with problems in dealing with parents and other authority figures, as could be seen in Billy's identification with Martin's problems with his parents. A number of members had sibling problems of various sorts. Because within this approach each member's problem may not be addressed within a given session, the capacity to identify and the opportunity for vicarious learning to operate are all-important.

This vignette featured two steps of problem solving: clarification of the problem and generation of alternatives. At each of these steps, we can see how the therapist can use the here-and-now of the group to deepen the opportunities for learning. D'Zurilla and Nezu (2001) exhort the therapist to help problem solvers avoid defining their problems in superficial ways. Through the use of the here-and-now, the therapist can accomplish this goal. When the group was working on the clarification of Bobbi's problem, the therapist directed members to see the problem in concrete, practical terms. By the therapist's elicitation of feedback on Bobbi's behavior within the group, a problem was identified that was deeper than the financial problem Bobbi recognized. Admittedly, the therapist did allow Bobbi to go on and work on the practical, financial problem. Focusing on the easier, external problem first could bolster Bobbi's confidence, enabling her to take on the more challenging problem of her fearfulness of entering the social arena. However, it would be extremely important for Bobbi's growth for her to learn how to apply her problem-solving skills to the difficult emotional problems likely to surface in daily life.

A second example of the use of the here-and-now occurred when the group was helping Martin to generate solution alternatives in relation to his parents' lack of trust of him. For many group members, the solutions that may occur to them spontaneously are those lying outside of them. By encouraging members to use their observations of one another in generating solution alternatives, the therapist helps members increase their levels of psychological mindedness and assume greater responsibility for their difficulties.

At each of the steps of problem solving, similar opportunities for tapping the here-and-now could be found. To the extent that the therapist seizes upon these opportunities, the group is likely to be a powerful workplace.

Research Support

As we did for the interpersonal approach, we first examine the support for the major assumption of the problem-solving approach and then proceed to consider the evidence that it fosters various types of positive change.

Theoretical Postulate of the Problem-Solving Approach

A postulate of the problem-solving approach is that underlying symptoms and other psychological problems are often deficits in problem solving, deficits that limit an individual's overall social competence. Earlier in this chapter, evidence was reviewed for this supposition. As noted, the evidence for the link between interpersonal problem-solving skills and emotional adjustment is well established (Spivack, Platt, & Shure, 1976). Research has shown that degree of psychopathology is positive associated with difficulties in problem solving, although the relationship is somewhat stronger in men than women (Gilbride & Hebert, 1980; Platt & Siegel, 1976). Problem-solving deficits are associated not only with psychopathology but with indicators of interpersonal success. For example, interpersonal problem-solving ability is directly associated with number of close friendships (Hansen, St. Lawrence, & Christoff, 1985).

What is more difficult than establishing a relationship between problem solving and adjustment is demonstrating that the former causes the latter. The several investigations that have looked at problem solving as a mediator between life stresses and depression and anxiety have provided support for the role of problem solving as a mediator (Kant, D'Zurilla, & Maydeu-Olivares, 1997; Nezu & Ronan, 1985). Pragmatically, however, if training in problem solving enhances the individual's self-esteem, resistance to developing symptoms, or other indicators of health, then causality need not be established to defend the usefulness of the approach. In the next section, the outcomes associated with the application of this model are reviewed. The studies reviewed are those that entail the overall effectiveness of problem-solving groups. The reader should know, however, that there is a good deal of research on specific components of the approach. This type of research enables continual improvements to be made to this approach.

Effectiveness of the Problem-Solving Approach

Over the past 25 years, research has provided substantial support for the efficacy of the problem-solving approach. This review highlights only a small sample of the studies available and considers three types of effects of application of the model: (a) problem solving itself, (b) interpersonal effectiveness, and (c) symptoms. This sequence follows the theoretical model in which changes in problem solving lead to more effective interpersonal behaviors, which lead to symptom reduction. For a more extensive review of the outcome literature for both individual and group applications of the problem-solving approach, the reader is referred to D'Zurilla and Nezu (1999, 2001).

Changes in Interpersonal Problem-Solving Ability: Problem-solving training is an effort to alter positively how a person solves problems. Does it achieve this goal? In an early investigation Coche and Flick (1975) assigned inpatients to an eight-session problem-solving group, a play-reading group, or a control condition. Before and after group participation the patients' skill in problem solving was measured through paper-and-pencil procedures. The researchers found that the problem-solving group improved more than the other two groups. Especially noted was the capacity of problem-solving members to generate multiple solutions to problems. Jones (1981) assigned inpatients to problem-solving (six-session), recreational, or no-treatment groups. Participants in the problem-solving group showed a higher level of *means-end thinking*, which is the capacity to see the intermediate steps to be taken toward a goal (as reflected in paper-and-pencil measures). On the other hand, an improvement in problem-solving thinking has not been shown in all studies. In a study very similar to the one by Coche and Flick (1975), Coche and Douglas (1977) were unable to show an improvement in problem-solving relative to a play-reading group. McLatchie (1982) found that people with chronic schizophrenia in group problem-solving training and relaxation training performed comparably on measures of problem solving. Arean et al. (1993) found with a sample of research participants age 55 and older that in contrast to a reminiscence group (a group in which members could reflect upon experiences earlier in life) and wait-list control group, a 12-session problem-solving group produced positive change in three of five problem-solving skills: (a) problem definition and formulation, (b) generation of alternatives, and (c) decision making. Problem orientation and solution verification were unimproved.

Changes in Interpersonal Styles or Behaviors: Studies exploring interpersonal behaviors have shown that the problem-solving approach can have a favorable effect on an individual's social adjustment. For example, Coche and Douglas (1977) assigned subjects to problem solving, play-reading, or control groups. They found the problem-solving group showed a greater decline in impulsiveness as reflected through Scale 4 scores on the Minnesota Multiphasic Personality Inventory. They indicate that staff members also observed this change. Members also manifested an increase in self-esteem, an outcome also predicted by the model.

Gendron, Poitras, Dastoor, and Perodeau (1996) investigated the effects of a group combining problem-solving training, assertiveness training, and cognitive restructuring on spousal caregivers of patients with dementia on their ability to be assertive with members of the extended family network. The comparison group was a support group. The findings favored the problem-solving treatment. Changes in interpersonal behavior were also seen in a study of socially phobic persons randomly assigned to a problem-solving group, a wait-list control group, or three cognitively oriented groups. Each treatment group met for 10 sessions, 90 minutes a session. All treatment groups relative to the wait-list group showed less social avoidance and fewer behavioral manifestations of anxiety.

For children and adolescents, managing aggression can create major interpersonal difficulties. Several of the members of our vignette were referred because of difficulties with aggression. Lochman, Burch, Curry, and Lampron (1984) did a study on aggressive boys who had or had not been treated in an anger-control program. The anger-control treatment involved the use of groups that met for 12 to 18 sessions. Members learned the steps of problem solving and had discussions about anger arousal. The investigators found that at a one-month follow-up, the members had decreased their disruptive and aggressive behaviors in the classroom and home relative to the untreated boys. In a three-year follow-up, Lochman (1992) found that the treated boys had lower levels of drug and alcohol use, higher levels of self-esteem, and more effective interpersonal problem solving. However, no differences were found in classroom behavior except for those boys who received booster sessions. Boys receiving the booster sessions had low levels of passive off-task behavior in the classroom.

Symptom Changes: Research has demonstrated the effectiveness of the problem-solving approach in the treatment of symptoms, in both symptom homogeneous and heterogeneous groups. Group problem-solving therapy is helpful in the treatment of depression and suicidality. Nezu and Perri (1989) assigned individuals who were diagnosed as having a major depressive disorder based on Research Diagnostic Criteria (RDC, Spitzer, Indicott, & Robbins, 1978) to a problem-solving group, an abbreviated problem-solving group (problem solving without training in problem orientation), and a wait-list control group. Both problem-solving groups lasted 10 sessions. Using the Beck Depression Inventory to measure depression, the investigators found that over 85 percent in the members of the problem-solving group, 50 percent of the members in the abbreviated problem-solving group, and 9 percent of the members in the wait-list control group manifested a substantial diminishment in depressive symptoms. Therapeutic benefits continued to be observed at the six-month follow-up.

Arean et al. (1993) tested an older population relative to the Nezu and Perri (1989) study. In the Arean et al. investigation described previously, research participants were 55 and older and all met the criteria for the Research Diagnostic Criteria for major depression. Participants were assigned to problem-solving groups, reminiscence groups, or wait-list groups. The investigators found that (a) both treatment groups showed significantly less depression than the control group at the time of posttreatment, (b) these changes held at the three-month follow-up, and (c) the problem solving showed less depression than the reminiscence group on two of the three measures of depression.

Joiner, Voelz, and Rudd (2001) examined the usefulness of group problem-solving therapy with suicidal young adults with comorbid depressive and anxiety disorders. Patients were randomly assigned to a problem-solving group or treatment as usual. Treatment as usual consisted of a combination of inpatient and outpatient treatment. Problem-solving treatment entailed group participation, psychoeducational issues, and discussions concerning the interrelationship between symptoms. Comorbid participants responded similarly across treatment, with both treatment groups showing a drop in suicidal ideation. Participants in the problem-solving treatment did better than treatment-as-usual subjects, who continued to show considerable suicidal ideation at follow-up.

The effectiveness of problem-solving groups has been investigated in the treatment of addictions. In one study problem-solving group participation led to a decrease in duration and severity of relapsed episodes relative to a discussion group or standard hospital treatment (Chaney, O'Leary, & Marlatt, 1978). In another study a problem-solving group was superior in its ability to solve problems relative to a discussion group, but at the one-year follow-up the groups were indistinguishable. With a group of members with opioid-related disorders, participants in a problem-solving group had a significant increase in employment at posttreatment and at the six-month follow-up (Platt, Husband, Hermalin, Cater, & Metzger, 1993). At the 12-month follow-up, however, the problem-solving group showed a decline in employment.

While these studies have explored diagnostically homogeneous groups, there have also been attempts to assess the efficacy of the problem-solving approach in heterogeneous groups. For example, Flowers and Booraem (1990b) evaluated a psychoeducational format involving problem-solving training against a less structured, experiential approach as described by Yalom (1985). All groups met for 16 sessions. The psychoeducational groups improved more on a scale of severity of psychopathology than the experiential groups. For methodological reasons, Flowers and Booraem did not see this study as suggesting the superiority of the psychoeducational format but rather its viability with heterogeneous groups.

In examining the pattern of results across the three areas, we can see that the support for the efficacy of the problem-solving approach in producing positive changes in how a person solves problems is strong. The usefulness of the approach for effecting desired changes in interpersonal behavior is somewhat less firm, although some support does exist. The degree of support for the usefulness approach with different diagnostic groups varies from symptom pattern to symptom pattern. Support is strongest for the helpfulness of the group problem-solving approach in the treatment of depression.

As D'Zurilla and Nezu (1999) note, future research should take into account the specific kind of problem-solving format being used. For example, while some formats involve training on problem orientation, others do not. Given that research (Nezu & Perri, 1989) has shown the importance of training in problem orientation, it is crucial that the presence or absence of this factor be specified in the description of the treatment.

Summary

The interpersonal problem-solving approach is a model for group therapy that is useful for a wide variety of populations from the standpoint of age, psychological problems, and settings. This approach is based upon the supposition that many symptom patterns are rooted in problem-solving deficits. Difficulties in problem solving often lead to adaptive failures. Such failures lower self-esteem and in turn create a vulnerability to developing symptoms under stress. In fact, the link between problem-solving difficulties and symptoms has received considerable empirical support. By learning a system of problem solving that compensates for these deficiencies, the person's overall social competence can be enhanced. The improvement in the person's ability to negotiate interpersonal situations leads to enhanced self-esteem and diminished symptom vulnerability. While the primary target of change is skill acquisition, the anticipated long-term effects are many including a lessening of many types of symptoms and improved relationships.

In this short-term approach, members are assisted in developing a more positive problem orientation, which entails the ability to recognize a problem, the acceptance of problems as inherent in living, the expectation that one's problem-solving efforts will be successful, and the capacity to summon the necessary creativity to respond to each problem's uniqueness. Members then are trained in a sequence of problem-solving steps, which include (a) problem identification, (b) problem clarification, (c) alternative generation, (d) evaluation and decision making, (e) role playing, and (f) implementation of the solution and verification. Problem-solving groups are action oriented in that they foster change by encouraging members to do something differently in the group than they did prior to group participation. Research demonstrates that problem-solving groups can be effective in enhancing a person's ability to solve problems, improving interpersonal behaviors, and diminishing a wide range of symptoms, and that these changes may be long term.

GROUP THERAPY WITH OTHER MODALITIES

The Use of Multiple Modalities

14

Chapter

Group therapy is a unique modality. While it can accomplish many goals, it is especially suited to certain goals— goals that are not as easily pursued in other ways. Furthermore, processes such as interpersonal learning that can be deployed to help members achieve their goals are particular to this modality. Because of the uniqueness of group therapy, it can be used with other modalities without the concern that one may duplicate the other. Rather, many group therapists have found that the use of one or more alternate modalities strengthens the contribution of groups. Reciprocally, group participation can enhance members' use of other types of intervention. Yet the decision to use multiple modalities must be made with great care. A group member's participation in another therapeutic situation adds complexity to the group participation and alters it throughout its course (Gans, 1990). Also, there are ethical considerations associated with participation in two or more modalities. To help the practitioner make effective decisions about multiple modality treatment, this chapter focuses on the most common combinations of group therapy and another modality. However, many of the considerations raised are applicable to combinations of treatments not explicitly discussed in this chapter.

Group Therapy and Individual Therapy

Members of therapy groups are often also in individual therapy, at least for some period during the group experience. The reason for their simultaneous occurrence is that group therapy and individual therapy each can make a distinctive contribution to furthering an individual's well-being. The following situations illustrate how a referral from a group to individual treatment might come about:

> *Fred is seeing an individual therapist who cannot understand what difficulties Fred is having with his co-workers. Fred makes a compelling case for it being their problem and not his, but the therapist remains doubtful. He feels that in group therapy, the problems would both be manifest and more amenable to treatment.*

This example highlights a strength of group therapy that has been emphasized throughout this text. Group therapy provides a venue in which interpersonal difficulties can manifest themselves in a variety of types of relationships. We can also imagine that individual therapy might be enhanced if Fred received feedback from the group members on his relational style. We return later to Fred to see how he fares once he enters the group. Group therapy might also be suggested when the patient in individual therapy does not produce enough information for exploration. As Rutan and Alonso (1982) wrote, "the rich stimuli of the group setting often stimulates many associations, memories, and feelings that can then be explored in both the individual and the group sessions" (p. 270).

The following situation is one that may lead to a referral to individual therapy:

> *Kai had been in group therapy for two years to work on relational difficulties. She came into group one week and reported that several of her immediate co-workers had been killed in a terrorist attack. She had not happened to be at work that day because she decided to take a "mental health day." The group spent that session and the next focusing on Kai's feelings of grief. However, the therapist recognized that other issues would surface in the group that would command its attention. She knew that Kai needed continuing assistance during her crisis. She decided to refer her for individual treatment.*

Goodman and Weiss (2000) write, "Individual therapy is indicated when a detailed examination of the trauma is necessary, and when retrieval of lost memories needs to be conducted in the safest arena possible in the context of a trusted relationship" (p. 48). However, in and of itself trauma does not necessarily suggest the need for individual therapy. Group approaches have been developed for many different types of trauma (Klein & Schermer, 2000). In fact, a traumatized individual who has been in individual therapy might appropriately be referred to group therapy to obtain relief from a sense of social isolation or to enable the individual therapist to continue to address the issues that preceded the trauma (Goodman & Weiss, 2000).

Individual therapy may be indicated when a group member hits on an issue that needs further individual exploration. Rutan and Stone (2001) give the example of a group member who hears other members talk about incidents of sexual abuse in their childhoods and recalls such events in his or her life. Individual therapy may be seen as a safer place to pursue the details of these early experiences. In general, individual therapy is a more optimal place for the in-depth exploration of genetic (or historical) experiences as they link to those in the present (Porter, 1993). In fact, when such investigations protractedly occur in the group, much that is unique about group is lost. Therefore, when such explorations are important, individual therapy is indicated.

When an individual participates in both individual and group therapy, it is referred to as *concurrent* therapy. There are different types of concurrent therapy, the most common subdivisions of which are conjoint and combined therapy. In conjoint therapy, the therapists in the group and individual modalities are different. In combined therapy the therapist is the same individual for both.

Conjoint Therapy

In outpatient settings group therapy will often begin after the individual therapist has recognized a need for the addition of the group modality. In some cases the individual therapist may not conduct therapy groups. In inpatient settings (including day hospital and residential treatment centers) the structure of the treatment program for an individual often involves a variety of modalities, with different therapists for each.

Conjoint therapy has a number of strengths in terms of what it offers both the therapist and the patient. The therapist has the advantage of participation on a treatment team. Rather than operating in isolation, the group therapist can take advantage of the perspective and data offered by the individual therapist. Conjoint therapy "offers the option of binocular vision on the patient" (Rutan & Alonso, 1982, p. 275). This resource can be a crucial one in working with certain types of difficult patients who test to the limit the therapist's ability to maintain a therapeutic stance (Yalom, 1995).

For the patient, having different therapists for each modality creates a richness of therapeutic opportunity that cannot be achieved with a single therapist serving in both roles. Some of these opportunities are created through the therapist as stimulus for patient reactions. To the extent that the stimuli vary, so does the range of potential reactions. Porter (1993) gives the example of how the individual therapist of a male patient had a warm, maternal style while the group therapist had a more confrontational style. These stylistic differences were one factor that led the patient to do different pieces of work in each modality. Expanded therapeutic opportunities may be created when one therapist is male and the other female (Rutan & Alonso, 1982).

For some patients the dilution of transference is a positive aspect of the treatment package. In the object-relations chapter the reader met Arabella, who would find intolerable the emergence of strong feelings of dependency upon the therapist. Having both an individual and group therapist enables an individual such as Arabella to split her dependency, making those impulses more acceptable and thereby available for exploration. As Alonso and Rutan note (1990), some patients may find sharing the individual therapist with the entire group an extreme narcissistic injury. Another benefit of conjoint therapy is that it provides for greater continuity of treatment. Inevitably in the therapist's life, there will be planned and unplanned absences, some of which may be protracted. These interruptions may pose a special hardship for patients who struggle intensively with abandonment issues. They may also pose a hardship for the absent therapist, who may be required to perform case management duties from afar. The availability of the alternate modality helps the patient to bridge these periods.

Conjoint therapy has significant disadvantages. Like cotherapy, conjoint therapy places a great demand upon both therapists to communicate regularly. Potential impediments exist to such communication. The therapist may feel that the patient's sense of safety in the treatment may be undermined by the knowledge that the material is being exported, even if only to the other therapist. The individual therapist is more likely to feel this concern, given that in the group, the member self-discloses to multiple parties. Another factor is the therapist's unwillingness or lack of discipline to take the time and expend the effort to have regular communication. Without payment for such consultations, the therapist may resent spending more time on this patient than that necessary for others.

Another potential impediment is the failure of both therapists to see the alternate therapy as being of value. Ultimately, conjoint therapy works best when all parties see each modality as complementing the other and intensifying the contribution of the other. Yet such a mutual endorsement does not always occur. In some instances the patient rather than the therapist initiates involvement in the second modality, such as an individual therapy patient deciding on his or her own that group might be beneficial. (For example, students in the mental health disciplines who want to become group therapists often recognize that an important part of the training is their own experience as members of therapy groups.) While some individual therapists might recognize the benefit of group participation, others might see it in negative terms. Even if, in the latter case, the individual therapist did not actively oppose the group involvement, there are likely to be covert communications from therapist to patient about the worth of the investment in the group. Genuine theoretical differences may exist between the two therapists, such as a different attitude toward the usefulness of medication (Alonso & Rutan, 1990). Countertransference issues may also arise related to the demand on the therapist to share the patient with another therapist and to have his or her work monitored by another professional.

Another problem in conjoint therapy arises when the group member uses his or her individual sessions to dilute the intensity of his or her reactions to the group:

> Courtney had completed a year of group participation. During this time, members relied upon her for compassion, humor, and support. However, a new member, Jasmine, seemed to be aware of how Courtney was unchallenged by the group. "All you do is coast" was Jasmine's refrain when addressing Courtney. Courtney was incensed, accustomed as she was to being appreciated, if not celebrated, by group members. She revealed to her

individual therapist what had occurred in group. The therapist said, "She must be envious of your skill in finessing social situations." In fact, the individual therapist was correct. Nonetheless, Courtney used this as a mantra to inoculate herself against any of Jasmine's accurate observations.

As Yalom (1995) wrote, "The patient may interact like a sponge in the group, taking in feedback and carrying it away to gnaw on like a bone in the safe respite of the individual therapy hour" (p. 407). Any reservations on the part of the individual therapist about the value of a patient's participation in group may be played out by allowing the individual to externalize any difficulty experienced in the group. Likewise, any feeling of loss on the part of the individual therapist for having to share the patient may be diminished by the individual therapy team providing meta-exploration for the group experience. The individual therapist's offering formulations on the group experience may say to the individual, "This is your real or primary treatment."

Effective conjoint therapy requires that both therapists speak candidly to one another prior to the commencement of the conjoint arrangement about such topics as (a) the importance of both modalities for this particular person, (b) the goals and processes of each modality, (c) how communication will proceed between the therapists, and (d) what information will be shared between therapists.

Combined Therapy

Combined therapy occurs when the same therapist sees the patient in group and individual therapy. Relative to conjoint therapy, this format has a number of strengths (many of which are the converse of the weaknesses of conjoint therapy). One strength is that the therapist gains tremendously from the opportunity to see the individual in both contexts. Most likely, all therapists who practice combined therapy are at some point surprised at the individual's behavior in one of the contexts, particularly if one therapy began before the other. Let us return now to Fred:

Fred had lost two jobs because of difficulties with his colleagues at work. Fred's own analysis of the situation was that these colleagues were back-biters. He felt that his supervisors at work tended to perceive him in a bad light because his coworkers went out of their way to point out his mistakes.

He believed that they alighted on him because his mild-mannered make-up made him vulnerable to others looking for an outlet for their aggression.

Initially, Fred came across in the group as a self-effacing individual, eager to defer to others. However, as time went on it became evident that he was greatly attentive to what each member was receiving from the therapist and the group as a whole. At first his sensitivity to this aspect appeared as a concern about whether particular members were being neglected. For his advocacy, he received favorable attention. Over time his vigilance in this area revealed itself as a worry about his own emotional income. For example, he would become irritated if members had failed to tune into his mood state on a given evening but had done so for another member. Members appeared put off by this quality and showed increasing irritation with him. When he would assume the role of advocate for another member, they responded with cynicism. Like his coworkers, intentionally or inadvertently, they began to reveal his foibles.

The therapist could see from Fred's behavior in the group the contribution he makes to others' negative responses toward him and the dynamic underpinnings of this behavior. With this greater awareness the individual therapist might be more sensitive to material containing issues pertaining to sibling rivalry. At the same time, it would be important for the therapist to refrain from imposing interpretations on the material emerging in Fred's individual sessions. What combined therapy does is to provide the therapist with a great fund of information about an individual being treated in both modalities so that the therapist can intervene optimally in each. Of course, some of the knowledge could be had in a conjoint therapy situation marked by excellent communication between the two therapists. However, the information obtained from the therapist working in the alternate modality would not be experiential and, hence, would be less comprehensive.

A second advantage of combined therapy is that it encourages the patient to avoid premature termination of either individual or group therapy. Consider the following situation, which provides an example of this benefit:

Katie had been in therapy only a few months when she entered a session in which two very intellectualized members exchanged analyses about the group. Katie appeared mystified by the exchange and at several points had asked clarifying questions. Very late in the session, when she tried to expand on one of the member's points, both members began to chuckle in a patronizing way, conveying that she had not grasped their ideas. Other members rallied to her defense and labeled the intellectualization for what it was—an avoidance of more genuine affective contact with one another and the other members.

Despite the support she received, Katie remained upset. She came to her individual therapy session and revealed that she contemplated leaving the group. The therapist explored with her her reaction to the members' laughter. Over the course of the session Katie realized that it reminded her of her family situation. Throughout her adolescence she had been the object of ridicule by her family members for her behavior as a "space cadet." Katie always imagined that the covert message was that she was less intelligent than other family members and perhaps was even an embarrassment to them. Katie had much evidence from her life that her intellectual resources were ample. The recognition then occurred that the laughter was a stimulant to Katie's self-doubt. With this information, Katie could realize that much could be learned from remaining in the group and working on her response to such provocations.

In conjoint therapy, the individual therapist might still have helped Katie remain in the group. However, the individual therapist might not have been able to put together all of the necessary pieces to realize that the two group members were tapping into an area of vulnerability for Katie. Also, the therapist operating in combined therapy may be able to interpret with more conviction and have more credibility in Katie's eyes given that he had directly experienced the group events.

Results from a study (Scheuble, Dixon, Levy, & Kagan-Moore, 1987) of eating disorder patients provide support for the argument that combined therapy assists patients in remaining in treatment. Thirty-eight women with a diagnosis of bulimia or anorexia nervosa completed either combined or conjoint therapy. The members in combined therapy showed a lower frequency of premature termination than those in conjoint treatment.

In combined therapy, the patient is less likely to use the individual sessions as opportunities to defuse remaining tensions from the group work. In some cases members may introduce material from the group in order to be more able to pursue the matter in the group and in other cases, to escape from having to do so. The therapist participating in both modalities is more likely to make this discrimination and thereby recognize how the patient might be supported in the direction of growth.

Combined therapy allows the placement of individuals in group therapy who would never permit themselves a group experience otherwise. Gans (1990) writes, "Reluctance to consider group is often a barometer of shame" (p. 126). With some patients, the strong expectation that they will experience intolerable shame makes it impossible for them to contemplate being in a group. However, a patient who has established a firm relationship with an individual therapist may be more willing to consider group therapy if that therapist is leading the group. Ultimately, there must be other sources of safety for the member in order to benefit from group involvement. Initially, however, the sense on the part of the patient that the individual therapist will have a protective role (and in fact, most of the members of the group will share in this expectation) can be instrumental in enabling the individual's entrance into the group.

Finally, combined therapy may offer an opportunity to make a better placement of the patient. When a person has been in individual therapy for some duration, the individual therapist has an opportunity to know that person well. This knowledge provides the therapist with the material to make a very grounded anticipation of how that member is likely to blend with the other members of the group.

Combined therapy poses certain complications largely but not wholly absent in conjoint therapy. Countertransference issues may affect the therapist's contemplation of combined therapy for a patient. Also, recommendations of combined therapy can serve the therapist's self-interest. As Gans (1990) has noted, "Group therapists stand to benefit when they can fill their groups from their individual practice. They do not have to depend exclusively on referral sources to fill their groups" (p. 132). Typically, an individual therapy patient who enters that therapist's group will pay a higher weekly fee. Therefore, combined therapy has the benefit of being more profitable (Lakin, 1994). How the therapist's self-interest operates depends on the personality of the therapist. Gans (1990) has identified a variety of potential therapist responses. Some therapists may give inadequate scrutiny to the influence of this factor and refer patients to combined therapy who are unsuitable for it. Other therapists may react with undue guilt if a patient out of his or her own dynamic concerns accuses the therapist of acting solely out of self-interest. Similarly, the therapist may fail to

interpret the resistance that an individual therapy patient has to joining a group and take at face value obstacles that the patient presents.
As always, by being aware of countertransference responses, the therapist is likely to respond to them in a productive way. When the therapist reacts to countertransference with a heightened awareness of his
or her own dynamics and those of the patient, this potential disadvantage becomes an advantage.

Another complication occurs when the therapist recommends
combined therapy to the patient. All of the elements of informed consent described in Chapter 9 must be provided at this juncture. Part of
an adequate informed consent entails apprising the patient of other
treatment alternatives. One obvious alternative is conjoint therapy.
This and other possibilities should be identified, along with the potential risks and benefits of each. The therapist should be sensitive to an
inhibition the patient might have in giving serious consideration to
these other possibilities, given that pursuing them would be at odds
with the therapist's recommendation. The patient might fear that failing to pursue combined therapy may be construed as a rejection of the
therapist. To enhance the patient's capacity to give a consent that is
free of coercion, the therapist could provide names of independent
practitioners who might assist in exploring the options.

Perhaps one of the most significant complications of combined
therapy concerns confidentiality. The therapist is interacting with
the patient in two venues and obtaining information about the patient from each. Circumstances may arise when the patient offers
information in individual therapy that he or she does not share or
does not wish to have shared in group therapy. Should the therapist
share this information with the group? Writers on this topic express
various opinions. Some (e.g., Rutan & Stone, 2001) argue that if
the patient is permitted to have, in essence, secrets with the therapist, a ready mechanism of resistance has been offered to the patient to his or her and possibly the group's detriment. Therefore,
before entering the group the patient is told as part of the informed-
consent process that the boundary of confidentiality surrounds
both the individual therapy and the group. Combined therapy, according to this perspective, is a unitary but multifaceted treatment.
Events in individual treatment are viewed on a continuum with
events in the group, with one end of the continuum representing
the intrapsychic and the other end the interpersonal (Schlachet,

1990). The initial agreement provides the therapist with the freedom to introduce the hidden material in the group setting in ways ranging from the extremely subtle (such as a quick glance at a member) to the direct. Writers holding this position generally underscore the importance of the therapist's attending to the vulnerability of the individual. The first route is to work in individual therapy to enable the patient to reveal the information to the group.

Others (e.g., Yalom, 1995) hold that ultimately the therapist should allow the patient to take responsibility to sharing information in the group. Such writers point out that the therapist's conveying information that the member chose to withhold can damage trust. Moreover, if the patient refused to offer material in the group because it evokes shame, then the therapist's volunteering such information could be quite traumatic. Still another factor is that the member may have a legitimate reason for withholding certain information. Alonso and Rutan (1990) provide the example of the potential communication involving a family member or friend who may be known to group members. In other words, the possible disclosure could violate the privacy of an external party. Of particular concern is information shared in the individual setting that has implications for present or possible legal proceedings. As noted in Chapter 9, a group can provide "a pool of legal witnesses" (Foster, 1975, p. 50) in a legal proceeding such as a deposition or trial, given that privilege is not assured. Were the therapist to volunteer information in the group against the member's objection, the therapist could be held liable for any consequences of such disclosures, legal or otherwise. This possibility suggests that despite the member's agreement, the therapist should always use discretion in sharing information.

Most writers on group therapy seem to agree on two points. The first is that the therapist's position on confidentiality should be part of the written informed consent. If the therapist agrees not to voluntarily share specific information that the members disclose in individual therapy, the therapist must nonetheless help the member appreciate that the work in the two modalities cannot but inform the therapist's understanding and that this understanding will affect the therapist's interactions with the patient in both settings. The point is important because otherwise the patient may feel the therapist is violating his or her trust when the member can see a connection between individual work and the therapist's interventions in the group.

The second point is that the therapist in individual work should help the member not to have secrets from the group. Here a secret is regarded as material withheld from the group not for some of the practical reasons described earlier but because the sharing of the information would lead to some psychological discomfort with the group. Secrets lead to a compartmentalization of parts of the self and thereby hinder the individual from movement toward a more integrated, mature personality.

Especially crucial is the member's divulging the secret if it pertains to the integrity of the group. For example, one of my group members mentioned in an individual therapy session that she had violated the rule of no socialization with another member by having coffee with the member on two occasions after the group. She indicated that she had begun to see the merit of this rule and was planning on stopping. When I mentioned the importance of talking about these extragroup contracts, the woman initially resisted. She did not wish to incur the anger of the other member, who was less willing to come forward. For this member, facing others' anger was a major problem in her life outside the group. Frequently, she made major compromises of her own wishes, needs, and standards to appease others. When she finally summoned the courage to address the violation in the group, the work she was able to do in relation to her anger-related conflicts was of enormous benefit. The approbation she received from members for reckoning with the violation served only to enhance her self-esteem.

Two additional concerns have appeared in the literature with respect to combined therapy. One concern is that the therapist will unwittingly disclose material from the individual sessions in the group session (Clay, 2000). Of course, this concern would apply only when the agreement was that the therapist would maintain confidentiality of material in individual therapy. This worry is probably greater among those who are not group therapists. What this apprehension fails to take into account is that therapists work in different ways in the two modalities. For group therapists who use heavily the here-and-now, material that the member has offered in individual sessions outside the group rarely has a high level of relevance. Hence, the therapist may be less at risk for making unauthorized disclosures than it would seem.

A second concern is that the therapist seeing the patient in group and individual therapy is in a powerful position vis-à-vis that patient (Taylor & Gazda, 1991). The question has been raised as to whether the therapist through this arrangement acquires excessive influence over the patient and fosters dependency. Again this argument lacks relevance to group therapy in contemporary practice. In those groups that provide attention to process, the group moves from a leader-centered to peer-centered mode of operation. Through this process members address their authority-related conflicts in a way that makes extreme dependency less rather than more likely. In my own practice I have observed patients who took a rather compliant stance in individual therapy show a movement toward a more mature way of relating after participating in a therapy group in which strides were made by the group as a whole on authority issues. Of course, for group therapists who rely on a charismatic leader-focused style in the group setting, such a concern about the dependency pull of combined therapy may be warranted.

The area of concurrent therapy is one that would benefit from a thoroughgoing research effort. Controlled studies in which participants were randomly assigned to conjoint versus combined conditions would yield results helping us to better understand why a given format is likely to benefit an individual patient.

Group Therapy and Psychopharmacology

The group therapist is likely to be faced with issues pertaining to medication regardless of whether that therapist has prescription privileges. The first reason is that the group therapist is likely to have patients taking psychopharmacologic agents in his or her group. Stone, Rodenhauser, and Markert (1991) did a survey concerning the inclusion of medicated patients in therapy groups. Psychologists, social workers, and psychiatrists were the largest professional groups represented, and among these, 70 percent, 60 percent, and 83 percent included in their groups individuals receiving medication. Most of these practitioners did not see including medicated and nonmedicated members in group together as an impediment. This study suggests that with or without prescription privileges, in the course of their career group therapists are likely to encounter many members for whom psychoactive agents are a component of their treatment packages.

An implication of this reality of group practice is that group therapists need to be knowledgeable about medication issues. No therapist should operate beyond the scope of his or her license to practice, but having an understanding of likely side effects of different medications and being attentive to member complaints about medication increase one's capacity to work effectively with professionals who are responsible for medication. In some cases, the prescribing professional may see the group member after long intervals. A group therapist seeing a group member weekly would have the opportunity to garner current impressions and data on behavioral changes that could be of great benefit to the prescribing professional. What is key is that the prescriber and therapist be close collaborators (Thase, 2000) with an articulated understanding of their respective responsibilities.

A second reason why the group therapist must be ready to grapple with medication issues is that medication has symbolic significance to members. If group members are taking medication, or even if they are not, the topic of medication can readily enter the group conversation because it has some meaning concerning the dynamic issues at hand. El-Mallakh and Hair (1993) provide a beautiful example of how medication can figure into the group process. They reported on an anxiety group in which all members were treated with medication prescribed by the cotherapists. The group session was conducted with a psychodynamic orientation. Members were permitted to raise medication concerns during the first 10 minutes of the session. After that period, members were permitted to introduce any topics with the exception of medication. Because the therapists were in residency training and were about to complete their year, they went through a termination with members. They found that the group dealt with termination by becoming preoccupied with medication. All members who wanted to remain in the group became focused on the medication Buspirone. Those members who were not currently on it asked to be switched to it. The therapists noted that the members seemed to be using the medication focus to avoid their reactions to the loss of the therapists. In fact, members ignored therapists' attempts to get them to explore themes of abandonment. At the same time, the members used the medication as a means of establishing a cohesion that was necessary to withstand the departure of the therapists. However, by emphasizing a commonality that involved members' adoption of a passive-receptive position characteristic of early group development, members showed that the medication preoccupation was part of a regressive process.

Members do not need to take medication to be concerned about medication. At various points the topic of medication will surface, and its meaning will vary. Talk of medication is especially common early in the life of a group. Members may be heard saying, in effect "If only I could find the right pill, I'd be a happy person." Here, the medication interest seems to be an extension of members' perception of the therapist, who is expected—like the medication—to take away all the pain. Technical questions about medication may be an effort to induce the therapist to display expertise. In cultures in which having a physical illness is more acceptable than having a psychological problem, the focus on medication is likely to be more frequent and protracted. In groups in which none of the members take medication, medication may be used as a way to establish a sense of superiority to those outside the group. The notion is "They are out there resorting to medication whereas we are here working on our problems." This is one way among many that the group establishes its external boundaries.

In the authority phase of the group, members may bring up medication as a better alternative to what they are currently doing. Now the expression of longing for the right medication is a way of underscoring the inadequacies of the therapist. Later in the group, the appeal of medication is often evident to members when they tacitly recognize the need to do a difficult piece of psychological work.

Other Multiple Treatments

In settings such as inpatient units, residential treatment facilities, and day hospitals, it is not unusual for group therapists to have other roles with the group member. For example, the group therapist outside of the group sessions may perform a psychological assessment on the person, carry out a behavioral program targeting a particular symptom, give instructions during a fire drill, or all of the preceding. In some cases the behaviors associated with the role may be at odds. That is, the therapist may be directive in one context and exploratory in another. Such role variation, while usually necessary, can create anxiety for the group member, who is given the task of discerning which rules apply to which context and which relationship. There may be other more specific reactions. For example, a member who has gone through a psychological assessment and has received a great deal of individual attention may mourn the loss of the exclusive tie with the therapist and assessor.

What is helpful to the group member is the therapist's sensitivity to possible anxiety over this role variation. Clarity during the preparation concerning how this role differs from other roles the therapist may have is also likely to be beneficial. Finally, the role conflicts can be used to strengthen the microcosmic aspect of the group. In life outside of therapy, relationships are complex. How to negotiate role variability in a relationship is a skill that is likely to enhance the individual's overall interpersonal functioning. By being aware of when a member may be responding to a role conflict, the therapist can use it as an opportunity for development and thereby remove it as an obstacle in the member's group work.

Summary

Group therapy often occurs alongside other interventions. This chapter focused on several common treatment formats in which group therapy was not the sole modality. Frequently, an individual may be in both group therapy and individual therapy, a format referred to as concurrent therapy. Because individual and group therapies each have different focuses and resources, participation in each can enhance involvement in the other. When a different therapist sees the patient in group therapy and individual therapy, it is referred to as conjoint therapy. When the same therapist sees the patient in each modality, it is referred to as combined therapy. Whether conjoint or combined therapy is appropriate depends upon the needs of the individual patient. Each format brings up a distinctive set of informed consent and confidentiality issues, which must be clearly established between patient and therapist.

Attention was given to medication issues, which often enter group therapy. When the prescribing professional is not the group therapist, good communication must be established between the two. The group therapist must also be aware of the symbolic significance of discussions about psychopharmacologic agents in the group.

When group therapy takes place in a larger treatment context (such as an inpatient unit), the group therapist may have many other roles in relation to the members outside of the group. To reduce anxiety-arousing ambiguity, the therapist should clarify the different roles in the preparatory stage of treatment and explore reactions to the multiplicity of roles in the group.

CONCLUSIONS

Effective Group Therapy

15
Chapter

This final chapter echoes a number of themes from the text, all of which suggest how group therapy should be conducted so that the members of groups might derive benefit from participation. As noted in Chapter 1, the evidence that group therapy is effective is overwhelming. However, as also noted, group therapy is most likely to compare favorably to other possible types of interventions only if groups are run according to certain principles. Fortunately, the group therapy literature has been sufficiently ample to permit conclusions about what an effective group This chapter also serves as a vehicle for comparing and contrasting the four theoretical approaches described in this text.

The effective group is one in which the therapeutic processes unique to group therapy are given abundant opportunity to emerge. In the presentation of the four models, it was described how factors such as cohesion, universality, and interpersonal learning can be activated regardless of what other factors are tapped by a particular approach or whether the group is structured or unstructured, time limited or time unlimited. Admittedly, for certain approaches, their activation is more straightforward and easier than for others. The interpersonal approach was developed specifically to focus upon the processes inherent in a group. The therapist's interventions are designed to create a cohesive group that will serve as a fertile environment for members' engagement in interpersonal learning. The psychodynamic approaches use the here-and-now of the group to explore transferences toward the leader and one another. The psychodynamic approaches differ from the interpersonal approach not so much on the extent to which group processes are used but on the group processes that are tapped for exploration and how these processes are employed. For example, although the interpersonal approach acknowledges group-level forces, they are the warp and woof of the group's work and often given center stage.

For those approaches that have their origins in an individual-therapy-in-a-group format the therapist will need to use more ingenuity in finding ways for those unique factors to be tapped. In regard to the cognitive-behavioral approach, we discussed how the therapist's treating the agenda in a flexible way provides the therapist with the latitude to respond to affective issues that arise in the group, especially those pertaining to relational issues among members. In the problem-solving approach, group phenomena such as universality can be tapped in the problem definition stage of treatment. In the selection of problems, priority can be given to those problems emerging in the here-and-now so that during the problem-solving steps, interpersonal learning can take place as fully as possible.

The effective group is one in which the therapist is clear about the target areas of change and goals within the target area that are being pursued in a given group. We have seen that the kinds of positive changes that can be produced through participation in a therapy group are manifold. Because of this fact, therapists may be tempted to pursue an array of ill-defined goals, some of that may not be wholly compatible. Outcome studies in the 1960s and 1970s that were not as supportive of the usefulness of group therapy targeted groups in which treatment goals were less clear than those studies conducted today. In short-term group work, the need for delimitation of goals is especially important. By renouncing the wish to accomplish everything for members, the therapist can achieve something substantial even if the period available is very brief. We saw this scaling down of goals in the application of the interpersonal approach to the inpatient situation. Here, the typical duration of group participation is extremely brief. Usually, the goal of the interpersonal approach is to enable the individual to modify maladaptive interpersonal patterns. However, the interactional agenda model's goal is to have members have a positive group experience so that they will be more receptive to other modalities during their inpatient stays and have a positive association with group therapy, leading them to pursue it after hospitalization (Yalom, 1983).

The effective group is one in which the mechanisms that will lead the group toward change and the interventions that support those mechanisms are clear. Clarity in relation to goals leads directly to a choice of methods to pursue those goals. Whether the therapist uses clarifications, interpretations, confrontations, role-playing, homework, or other types of interventions and activities is crucially dependent upon what types of goals the therapist is pursuing. This point is illustrated through a comparison of all four approaches. The psychodynamic object-relations therapist working toward intrapsychic change in members relies heavily upon reflective comments and interpretations. The problem-solving and cognitive-behavioral therapists helping members to increase their levels of social competence through skill training have a very different intervention style, using structuring, directive interventions such as agenda setting, role-playing, and homework assignments. The interpersonal therapist fosters a spontaneous group process using a variety of verbal interventions ranging from clarifications to interpretations.

Given the introductory nature of this text, the featured theoretical approaches were described in their pure form. However, within the field there is a trend toward integration. For example, formats integrating cognitive-behavioral and psychodynamic orientations are emerging (e.g., Sorensen, 2001). What is crucial is that the melding of different theoretical approaches be thoughtful: Goals and methods should be conceptualized just as explicitly as when a single orientation is employed.

The effective group is one in which the therapist is competent both to do group therapy and to implement a given approach with a particular population. Group therapy is unique in relation to other modalities, and, consequently, competency requires that the person endeavoring to conduct therapy groups have both the knowledge base and skills pertinent to the modality. Training in individual therapy or any other modality will not suffice to prepare a professional for group work. Historically, training in group therapy in academic programs has been limited, and today the number of courses on group therapy in curricula varies greatly from discipline to discipline (Fuhriman & Burlingame, 2001). In general, group therapy is given relatively short shrift in favor of individual treatment. Many mental health professionals seeking to practice group therapy will benefit from taking advantage of the didactic and experiential training opportunities available through such organizations as the American Group Psychotherapy Association, the American Society for Group Psychotherapy and Psychodrama, and the Association for Specialists in Group Work. The offerings of these organizations will be especially useful to the seasoned group therapist who wishes to employ theoretical orientations or techniques with which he or she has little experience or to conduct groups with new populations or settings. Supervision is useful not only to assist the therapist making forays into new areas but also to ensure the competent delivery of services ongoingly.

For any given group, the structure of the leadership should be a very carefully considered dimension of the group design; if the structure is a cotherapy team, the members of that team should allocate considerable time and attention to addressing their relationship as cotherapists. For some theoretical approaches, cotherapy is highly desirable. For example, in the cognitive-behavioral approach, a cotherapy team is extremely helpful because of the multiplicity of tasks to be performed by the therapist in each session and because certain techniques (e.g., role-playing) are optimally used when they can be performed by two therapists. For other approaches, there may be no clear advantage to having one format over another across contexts. However, within a given treatment context there may be an advantage to one arrangement. For example, Kibel (1992) notes that cotherapy is helpful when the object-relations approach is being applied on an inpatient unit because each member of the cotherapy team helps the other tolerate and understand members' primitive projective identifications.

If cotherapy is the leadership format for a given group, it is crucial that the team give adequate time prior to the selection of members to collaborating on the group design sufficiently to achieve an agreement on goals, processes, and interventions. Ongoingly, cotherapists must allocate time and attention to exploring their reactions to the sessions as well as their relationship as it develops within the group.

The effective group is one in which the various diversities of the patient population are considered in all aspects of the treatment. Group therapy is a modality in which diversities can be celebrated because effective group work requires that members be diverse; without a multiplicity of perspectives, interpersonal learning is very limited. However, learning how to work with differences effectively is an essential task. Although the focus on diversity may be more significant in the curricula of advanced degree programs than was once the case, graduates will nonetheless be required to supplement their academic training through continuing education. All that defines the group members—their ethnic/racial status, sexual preference, mode of spirituality, abilities and disabilities—may be relevant to their therapeutic needs, their receptivity to different types of group processes and therapist interventions, and the resources they bring to the group.

An important area for future investigation is the exploration of how different theoretical approaches accommodate (or fail to do so) different types of diversity. For example, the psychodynamic object relations approach in lessening the tenacity of certain primitive defenses such as projection and projective identification at least in principle should contribute to fostering members' tolerance of other human beings. Schoenholtz-Read (1996) writing from a feminist perspective notes that historically, cognitive-behavioral approaches (like many other theoretical approaches) with its emphasis upon the correction of faulty thinking has not taken into account the more relational and less linear modes of cognition of some women. She suggests that the recent influence of constructivist thinking (Mahoney, 1995) on cognitive-behavioral theory with the former's emphasis on the individual's development of unique narrative as it is affected by his or her context, broadens cognitive behavioral theory such that gender differences in thinking styles can be accommodated. Efforts such as Schoenholtz-Read's will enable us to use theory to expand rather than limit our view of the individual group member.

The therapist should also be aware of all that defines him or her in relation to both how the therapist experiences the group and each of the members, and how the group experiences the therapist. The therapist should be aware of his or her beliefs and values, especially in regard to how they may differ from those of the group members (Sue & Sue, 1999).

The effective group is one in which the members are adequately prepared for the group. A considerable body of research suggests that preparation is useful from a variety of standpoints (Yalom, 1995). Preparation as part of the informed consent process is consistent with the ethical principle of autonomy (see Chapter 9). Preparation by adding structure to a member's early group experience reduces the likelihood of unproductively high levels of anxiety (Kaul & Bednar, 1994). It appears to help members to get off to a very strong beginning in the group by leading them to participate actively. Some studies have shown a positive relationship between preparation and outcome. Group therapists use many preparation formats, and such variables as theoretical orientation, time frame, and member characteristics should determine what type of preparation is most important. For example, preparation for an interpersonal group entailing some small-group processing of members' interactions can help members form a very reasonable anticipation of what the group is likely to be. Preparation for the psychodynamic group might involve exercises designed to enhance a member's level of psychological mindedness.

The effective group is one in which the therapist keeps in mind developmental stage principles. Regardless of the type of group, every group is likely to show developmental aspects. Members tend to behave very differently toward one another in the beginning, middle, and end of the group not simply because of any particular set of therapist interventions but because the group has matured. By having a cognizance of the level of maturity of the group, the therapist can ascertain what tasks the group is capable of undertaking and what resources can be brought to bear in accomplishing these tasks. Some approaches, such as the object-relations orientation, are designed to use the group's developmental aspects as the centerpiece of the treatment. Other approaches (e.g., problem solving and cognitive-behavioral) are not explicitly oriented to take development of the group into account, but the effectiveness of the approach could be enhanced by the therapist's doing so. For example, within both cognitive-behavioral and problem-solving approaches, the group-wide neglect of homework may reflect a disappointment with the failure of the group to magically remove members' difficulties. The therapist's awareness of this possibility will enhance the therapist's skill in identifying automatic thoughts or helping members to formulate here-and-now problems.

The effective group is designed with a consideration of the context in which the group will take place. The group design should always take into account the characteristics of the setting in which the group will be held. For example, in an inpatient setting the group therapist should take into account the other components of the treatment package. By not duplicating the work of other modalities, the therapist is likely to make a greater contribution to increasing the patient's fund of resources upon leaving the hospital. The therapist is likely also to secure the critical cooperation of other staff members, who will see the role of the group as unique but also supportive of other therapeutic activities.

The effective group is one in which the therapist keeps in mind that group therapy has its own ethical and legal aspects and responds to these aspects with a high level of knowledge and a systematic way of engaging in ethical/legal decision making. Issues pertaining to confidential and privileged communication, informed consent, the use of multiple modalities, and so on that are particular to group therapy. The therapist is best equipped by a familiarity with these issues and the relevant ethical codes and laws. Therapists must always be prepared to encounter situations that are unique in his or her their group therapy practices. The therapist is best able to handle them in an ethically and legally sound way by knowing broad ethical principles and having a system by which to reconcile them.

The effective group is one in which the therapist carefully monitors progress of members and recognizes when progress is or is not being made toward goals. For the therapist to have clear treatment goals is insufficient to ensure the usefulness of group work. The therapist must also have a concrete conception of the indicators that an individual member is thriving in the group over its course. Such monitoring enables the therapist to know when treatment in a particular group is not working. When treatment is working, feedback from such monitoring may invigorate a group member whose motivation is flagging. We have seen that member progress can be defined in tangible ways regardless of whether the group's theoretical orientation is cognitive-behavioral, psychodynamic, interpersonal, or problem solving. Many other theoretical approaches are currently used, and to the extent that the theoretical framework has been elucidated in sufficient detail, it should be possible to find ways of measuring members' progress.

Another purpose of an investigative attitude toward group work is to help us to improve our group work continually by leading us to link therapeutic goals with the processes that move the group toward these goals. For example, in the last chapter we saw how outcome research on the problem-solving approach reveals the importance of cultivating members' positive problem orientation. This discovery strengthened an already efficacious approach. The investigator's ability to link process to outcome is abetted by the development of process measures that capture the complex interactional patterns that occur in a therapy group (A. P. Beck & Lewis, 2000). These measures will help us to address in a more thoroughgoing way than was ever possible before the seminal issue of why groups work.

Through the application of an investigative attitude, we will also be able to address such practical questions as, "How long of a tenure in the group is necessary for a member to fulfill the goals of the group?" Given that the cost-containment pressures on therapists of all modalities to render the most efficient treatment will most likely increase (MacKenzie, 2001), such information would be invaluable in the therapist's advocacy for patients with third-party payers.

Regardless of the theory he or she employs, the group therapist adhering to these guidelines, is likely to create an environment that nurtures members' development and furthers their well-being. The therapist is also likely to realize the enormous personal and professional fulfillment to be had from the experience of conducting groups.

References

Abramowitz, S. I., & Abramowitz, C. V. (1974). Psychological—mindedness and benefit from insight—oriented group therapy. *Archives of General Psychiatry, 30*(5), 610–615.

Abramowitz, S. I., & Jackson, C. (1974). Comparative effectiveness of there-and-then versus here-and-now therapist interpretations in group psychotherapy. *Journal of Counseling Psychology, 21,* 288–293.

Addis, M. E., Wade, W. A., & Hatgis, C. (1999). Barriers to dissemination of evidence-based practices: Addressing practitioners' concerns about manual-based psychotherapies. *Clinical Psychology: Science and Practice, 1999, 6*(4), 430–441.

Agazarian, Y. (1997). *Systems-centered therapy for groups.* New York: Guilford Press.

Agazarian, Y. (1999). Phases of development in the systems-centered psychotherapy group. *Small Group Research, 30*(1), 82–107.

Agazarian, Y., & Peters, R. (1981). *The visible and invisible group: Perspectives on group psychotherapy and group process.* London: Routledge & Kegan Paul.

Albrecht, E., & Brabender, V. (1983). Alcoholics in inpatient, short-term interactional group psychotherapy: An outcome study. *Group, 7,* 50–54.

Allen, J. G. (1973). Implications of research in self-disclosure for group psychotherapy. *International Journal of Group Psychotherapy, 23,* 306–321.

Alonso, A., & Rutan, J. S. (1984). The impact of object relations theory on psychodynamic group therapy. *American Journal of Psychiatry, 141*(11), 1376–1380.

Alonso, A., & Rutan, J. S. (1990). Common dilemmas in combined individual and group treatment. *Group, 14*(1), 5–12.

Alonso, A., & Rutan, J. S. (1993). Character change in group psychotherapy. *International Journal of Group Psychotherapy, 43*(4), 439–451.

Alonso A., & Swiller, H. I. (1993). Introduction: The case for group therapy. In A. Alonso & H. I. Swiller (Eds.), *Group therapy in clinical practice* (pp. xxi–xxv). Washington, DC: American Psychiatric Association.

American Association for Marriage and Family Therapy. (1991). *AAMFT code of ethics.* Washington, DC: Author.

American Counseling Association. (1995). *The code of ethics and standards of practice.* Alexandria, VA: Author.

American Group Psychotherapy Association. (1991). *AGPA Guidelines for ethics.* New York: Author.

American Psychological Association. (1992). Ethical principles of psychologists and code of conduct. *American Psychologist, 47,* 1597–1611.

American Psychological Association. (1997). Services by telephone, teleconferencing, and Internet: A statement by the Ethics Committee of the American Psychological

Association. Washington, DC: Author. [Online.] Available: www.apa.org/ethics/stmnt01.html

Andreason, N. C., & Olsen, S. (1982). Negative v. positive schizophrenia. *Archives of General Psychiatry, 39,* 789–794.

Andrews, H. B. (1995). *Group design and leadership: Strategies for creating successful common-theme groups.* Boston: Allyn & Bacon.

Arean, P. A., Perri, M. G., Nezu, A. M., Schein, R. L., Christopher, F., & Joseph, T. X. (1993). Special populations: Comparative effectiveness of social problem-solving therapy and reminiscence therapy as treatment for depression in older adults. *Journal of Consulting and Clinical Psychology, 61*(6), 1003–1010.

Aries, E. (1976). Interaction patterns and themes of male, female, and mixed groups. *Small Group Behavior, 7*(1), 7–18.

Ashbach, C., & Schermer, V. L. (1987). *Object relations, the self, and the group: A conceptual paradigm.* New York: Routledge & Kegan Paul.

Association for Specialists in Group Work. (1989). *Ethical guidelines for group counselors.* Washington, DC: American Association for Counseling and Development.

Barlow, S. H., Burlingame, G. M., Harding, J. A., & Behrman, J. (1997). Therapeutic focusing in time-limited group psychotherapy. *Group Dynamics: Theory Research, and Practice, 1*(3), 254–266.

Bateman, A., & Fonagy, P. (1999). Effectiveness of partial hospitalization in the treatment of borderline personality disorder: A randomized controlled trial. *American Journal of Psychiatry, 156,* 1563–1569.

Beard, M. T., & Scott, P. Y. (1975). The efficacy of group therapy by nurses for hospitalized patients. *Nursing Research, 24*(2), 120–124.

Beck, A. P. (1974). Phases in the development of structure in therapy and encounter groups. In D. A. Wexler & I. N. Rice (Eds.), *Innovations in client-centered therapy* (pp. 421–463). New York: Wiley.

Beck, A. P., & Lewis, C. L. (2000). *The process of group psychotherapy: Systems for analyzing change.* Washington, DC: American Psychological Association.

Beck, A. T. (1976). *Cognitive therapy and the emotional disorders.* New York: International Universities Press.

Beck, A. T., & Greenberg, R. L. (1974). *Coping with depression.* New York: Institute for Rational Living.

Beck, A. T., Rush, A. J., Shaw, B. F., & Emery, G. (1979). *Cognitive therapy of depression.* New York: Guilford Press.

Beck, J. S. (1995). *Cognitive therapy: Basics and beyond.* New York: Guilford Press.

Bednar, R. L., & Kaul, T. J. (1994). Experiential group research: Can the cannon fire. In A. E. Bergin & S. L. Garfield (Eds.), *Handbook for psychotherapy and behavior change* (4th ed., pp. 631–663). New York: Wiley.

Bellack, A. S., Gold, J. M., & Buchanan, R. W. (1999). Cognitive rehabilitation for schizophrenia: Problems, prospects, and strategies. *Schizophrenia Bulletin, 25*(2), 257–274.

Benjamin, L. R., & Benjamin, R. (1995). A therapy group for mothers with dissociative disorders. *International Journal of Group Psychotherapy, 45*(3), 381–403.

Bennis, W. G., & Shepard, H. A. (1956). A theory of group development. *Human Relations, 9,* 415–437.

Berger, M. M. (1958). Nonverbal communication in group psychotherapy. *International Journal of Group Psychotherapy, 8,* 161–178.

Bernstein, B. E., & Hartsell, T. L. (1998). *The portable lawyer for mental health professionals.* New York: Wiley.

Bersoff, D. N., & Koeppl, D. M. (1995). The relation between ethical codes and moral principles. In D. N. Bersoff (Ed.), *Ethical conflicts in psychology* (pp. 132–134). Washington, DC: American Psychological Association.

Berzon, B., Pious, C., & Farson, R. (1963). The therapeutic event in group psychotherapy: A study of subjective reports of group members. *Journal of Individual Psychology, 19,* 204–212.

Beutler, L. E., Frank, M., Schieber, S., Calvert, S., & Gaines, J. (1984). Comparative effects of group psychotherapies in a short-term inpatient setting: An experience with deterioration effects. *Psychiatry, 47,* 66–76.

Bion, W. (1959). *Experiences in groups.* New York: Basic Books.

Bion, W. (1962). *Learning from experience.* New York: Basic Books.

Blatner, A. (1996). *Acting-in: Practical applications of psychodramatic methods* (3rd ed.). New York: Springer.

Bloch, S., & Crouch, E. (1985). *Therapeutic factors in group psychotherapy.* New York: Oxford University Press.

Block, S., Bond, G., Qualls, B., Yalom., I., & Zimmerman, E. (1976). Patients' expectations of therapeutic improvement and their outcomes. *American Journal of Psychiatry, 133*(12), 1457–1460.

Bolman, L. (1973). Some effects of trainers on their groups: A partial replication. *Journal of Applied Behavioral Sciences, 9,* 534–539.

Bowers, W. A. (2000). Eating disorders. In J. R. White & A. S. Freeman (Eds.), *Cognitive-behavioral group therapy for specific problems and populations* (pp. 127–148). Washington, DC: American Psychological Association.

Bowlby, J. (1963). Pathological mourning and childhood mourning. *Journal of the American Psychoanalytic Association, 11,* 500–541.

Brabender, V. (1985). Time-limited inpatient group therapy: A developmental model. *International Journal of Group Psychotherapy, 35*(3), 373–390.

Brabender, V. (1987). Vicissitudes of countertransference in inpatient group psychotherapy. *International Journal of Group psychotherapy, 37,* 549–567.

Brabender, V. (1988). A closed model of short-term inpatient group psychotherapy. *Hospital and Community Psychiatry, 39*(5), 542–545.

Brabender, V. (2000). Chaos, group psychotherapy, and the future of uncertainty and uniqueness. *Group, 24*(1), 23–32.

Brabender, V. (2001). The future of group psychotherapy: Expanding the conversation. *International Journal of Group Psychotherapy, 51*(2), 181–189.

Brabender, V., & Fallon, A. (1993). *Models of inpatient group psychotherapy.* Washington, DC: American Psychological Association.

Brabender, V., & Fallon, A. (1996). Termination in inpatient groups. *International Journal of Group Psychotherapy, 46*(1), 81–98.

Bricklin, P. (2001). Being ethical: More than obeying the law and avoiding harm. *Journal for Personality Assessment, 77*(2), 195–202.

Brigham, P. M. (1992). Object relations and regression in groups. *International Journal of Group Psychotherapy, 42*(2), 247–266.

Bright, J. I., Baker, K. D., & Neimeyer, R. A. (1999). Professional and paraprofessional group treatments for depression: A comparison of cognitive-behavioral and mutual support interventions. *Journal of Consulting and Clinical Psychology, 67*(4), 491–501.

Brunswik, E. (1956). *Perception and the representative design of psychological experiments* (2nd ed.). Berkeley: University of California Press.

Bryant, M. J., Simons, A. D., & Thase, M. E. (1999). Therapist skill and patient variables in homework compliance: Controlling an uncontrolled variable in cognitive therapy outcome research. *Cognitive Therapy and Research, 23*(4), 381–399.

Budman, S. H., Cooley, S., Demby, A., Koppenaal, G., Koslof, J., & Powers, T. (1996). A model of time-effective group psychotherapy for patients with personality disorders: The clinical model. *International Journal of Group Psychotherapy, 46*(3), 329–355.

Budman, S. H., Demby, A., Soldz, S., & Merry, J. (1996). Time-limited psychotherapy for patients with personality disorders: Outcomes and dropouts. *International Journal of Group Psychotherapy, 46*(3), 357–377.

Budman, S. H., Simione, P. G., Reilly, R., & Demby, A. (1994). Progress in short-term and time-limited group psychotherapy: Evidence and implications. In A. Fuhriman & G. M. Burlingame (Eds.), *Handbook of group psychotherapy: An empirical and clinical synthesis* (pp. 319–339). New York: Wiley.

Budman, S. H., Soldz, S., Demby, A., Feldstein, M., Springer, T., & Davis, M. S. (1989). Cohesion, alliance and outcome in group psychotherapy. *Psychiatry, 52,* 339–350.

Burns, D. D., & Spangler, D. L. (2000). Does psychotherapy homework lead to improvements in depression in cognitive-behavioral therapy or does improvement lead to increased homework compliance? *Journal of Consulting and Clinical Psychology, 68*(1), 46–56.

Byrnes, E. I., Hansen, K. G., Malloy, T. E., Carter, C., & Curry, D. (1999). Reductions in criminality subsequent to group, individual, and family therapy in adolescent residential and day treatment settings. *International Journal of Group Psychotherapy, 49*(3), 307–322.

Caine, T. N., & Wijesingle, B. (1976). Personality, expectancies, and group psychotherapy. *British Journal of Psychiatry, 129,* 384–387.

Carbonell, D. M., & Parteleno-Barehmi, C. (1999). Psychodrama groups for girls coping with trauma. *International Journal of Group Psychotherapy, 49*(3), 285–306.

Carloch, C. H., & Martin, P. Y. (1977). Sex composition and the intensive group experience. *Social Work, 22,* 27–32.

Carter, M. M., Turovsky, J., & Barlow, D. H. (1994). Interpersonal relationships in panic disorder with agoraphobia: A review of empirical evidence. *Clinical Psychology Science and Practice, 1*(1), 25–35.

Cashdan, S. (1988). Object relations therapy: Using the relationship. New York: Norton.

Chaney, E. F., O'Leary, M. R., & Marlatt, G. A. (1978). Skill training with alcoholics. *Journal of Consulting and Clinical Psychology, 46*(5), 1092–1104.

Chang, E. C., & D'Zurilla, T. J. (1996). Relations between problem orientation and optimism, pessimism, and trait affectivity:

A construct validation study. *Behavior, Research and Therapy, 34,* 185–195.

Cheng, S. K. (2001). Life stress, problem solving, perfectionism, and depressive symptoms in chinese. *Cognitive Therapy and Research, 25*(3), 303–310.

Clarke, G. N., Rohde, P., Lewinsohn, P. M., Hops, H., & Seeley, J. R. (1999). Cognitive-behavioral treatment of adolescent depression: Efficacy of acute group treatment and booster sessions. *Journal of the American Academy for Child and Adolescent Psychiatry, 38*(3), 272–279.

Clay, R. (2000). APA task force considers changes to proposed ethics code. *Monitor on Psychology, 31*(7), 86–87.

Cloitre, M., & Koenen, K. C. (2001). The impact of borderline personality disorder on process group outcome among women with posttraumatic stress disorder related to childhood abuse. *International Journal of Group Psychotherapy, 51*(3), 379–398.

Coche, E. (1987). Problem-solving training: A cognitive group therapy modality. In A. Freeman & V. Greenwood (Eds.), *Cognitive therapy: Applications in psychiatric and medical settings* (pp. 83–102). New York: Human Sciences.

Coche, E., Cooper, J. B., & Petermann, K. J. (1984). Differential outcomes of cognitive and interactional group therapies. *Small Group Behavior, 15*(4), 497–509.

Coche, E., & Douglas, A. A. (1977). Therapeutic effects of problem-solving training and play-reading groups. *Journal of Clinical Psychology, 33*(3), 820–827.

Coche, E., & Flick, A. (1975). Problem-solving training groups for hospitalized psychiatric patients. *Journal of Psychology, 91,* 19–29.

Cohen, B. D., & Ettin, M. F. (1999). Self-structure and self-transformation in group psychotherapy. *International Journal of Group Psychotherapy, 49*(1), 71–83.

Cohen, B. D., Ettin, M. F., & Fidler, J. W. (1998). Conceptions of leadership: The "analytic stance" of the group psychotherapist. *Group Dynamics: Theory, Research, and Practice, 2*(2), 118–131.

Cohen-Sandler, R. (1982). Interpersonal problem-solving skills of suicidal and non-suicidal children: Assessment and treatment. *Dissertation Abstracts International, 43*(2), 519-B.

Concannon, C. (1995). The dynamics of the cotherapy relationship: A symposium: The senior-senior team. *Group, 19*(5), 71–78.

Connelly, J. L., & Piper, W. E. (1989). An analysis of pretraining work behavior as a composition variable in group psychotherapy. *International Journal of Group Psychotherapy, 3*(2), 173–189.

Corey, G. (1995). *Theory and practice of group counseling* (4th ed.). Pacific Grove, CA: Brookes/Cole.

Corey, M. S., & Corey, G. (1997). *Groups: Process and practice* (5th ed.). Pacific Grove, CA: Brookes/Cole.

Corsini, R., & Rosenberg, B. (1955). Mechanisms of group psychotherapy: Processes and dynamics. *Journal of Abnormal and Social Psychology, 51,* 406–411.

Coskun, H., Paulus, P. B., Brown, V., & Sherwood, J. J. (2000). Cognitive stimulation and problem presentation in idea-generating groups. *Group Dynamics: Theory, Research, and Practice, 4,* 307–329.

Crouch, E. C., & Bloch, S. B., & Wanless, J. (1994). Therapeutic factors: Interpersonal and intrapersonal mechanisms. In

A. Fuhriman & G. M. Burlingame (Eds.), *Handbook of group psychotherapy: An empirical and clinical synthesis* (pp. 269–315). New York: Wiley.

Cunningham, A. J., Edmonds, C. V. I., Jenkins, G. P., Pollack, H., Lockwood, G. A., & Warr, D. (1998). A randomized controlled trial of the effects of group psychological therapy on survival in women with metastatic breast cancer. *Psycho-Oncology, 7,* 508–517.

Curry, L. A., Snyder, C. R., Cook, D. L., Ruby, B. C., & Rehm, M. (in press). The role of hope in academic and sport performance. *Journal of Personality and Social Psychology, 73*(6), 1257–1267.

Davis, K. (1980). Is confidentiality in group counseling realistic? *Personnel and Guidance Journal, 59,* 197–201.

Deffenbacher, J. L., Story, D. A., Brandon, A. D., Hogg, J. A., & Hazelus, S. L. (1988). Cognitive and cognitive-relaxation treatments of anger. *Cognitive Therapy and Research, 12,* 167–184.

Deffenbacher, J. L., Thwaites, G. A., Wallace, T. L., & Oetting, E. R. (1994). Social skills and cognitive-relaxation approaches to general anger reduction. *Journal of Counseling Psychology, 41,* 386–396.

Dembert, M. L., & Simmer, E. D. (2000). When trauma affects a community: Group interventions and support after a disaster. In R. H. Klein & V. L. Schermer (Eds.), *Group psychotherapy for psychological trauma.* New York: Guilford Press.

Dies, R. R. (1973). Group therapist self-disclosure: An evaluation by clients. *Journal of Counseling Psychology, 20*(4), 344–348.

Dies, R. R. (1977). Group therapist transparency: A critique of theory and research. *International Journal of Group Psychotherapy, 27,* 177–200.

Dies, R. R. (1983). Clinical implications of research on leadership in short-term group psychotherapy. In R. Dies & K. MacKenzie (Eds.), *Advances in group psychotherapy* (pp. 27–79). New York: International Universities Press.

Dies, R. R. (1993). Research in group psychotherapy: Overview and clinical applications. In A. Alonso & H. Swiller (Eds.), *Group therapy in clinical practice* (pp. 473–518). Washington, DC: American Psychiatric Association.

Dies, R. R. (1994). Therapist variables in group psychotherapy research. *Handbook of group psychotherapy: An empirical and clinical synthesis.* New York: Wiley.

Dies, R. R., & Cohen, L. (1976). Content considerations in group therapist self-disclosure. *International Journal of Group Psychotherapy, 26,* 71–88.

Dies, R. R., & Dies, K. R. (1993). The role of evaluation in clinical practice: Overview and group treatment illustration. *International Journal of Group Psychotherapy, 43*(1), 77–105.

District of Columbia Laws 6–2002(b).

Dobson, K. S., Backs-Dermott, B. J., & Dozois, D. J. A. (2000). Cognitive and cognitive-behavioral therapies. In C. R. Snyder & R. E. Ingram (Eds.), *Handbook of psychological change: Psychotherapy processes and practices for the 21st century* (pp. 409–428). New York: Wiley.

Doi, T. (1963). Some thoughts on helplessness and the desire to be loved. *Psychiatry, 26,* 266–272.

Douglas, M. S., & Mueser, K. T. (1990). Teaching conflict resolution skills to the chronically mentally ill. *Behavior Modification, 14*(4), 519–547.

Drob, S., Bernard, H., Lifshutz, H., & Nierenberg, A. (1986). Brief group psychotherapy for herpes patients: A preliminary study. *Behavior Therapy, 17,* 299–338.

Dublin, R. A. (1995). The junior-senior team. *Group, 19*(2), 79–86.

Dugo, J. M., & Beck, A. P. (1984). A therapist's guide to issues of intimacy and hostility viewed as group-level phenomena. *International Journal of Group Psychotherapy, 34,* 25–45.

Dugo, J. M., & Beck, A. P. (1997). Significance and complicity of early phases in the development of the co-therapy relationships. *Group Dynamics: Theory, Research, and Practice, 1*(4), 294–305.

Durkin, H. E. (1981). The technical implication of general systems theory for group psychotherapy. In J. E. Durkin (Ed.), *Living groups: Group psychotherapy and general system theory* (pp. 171–198). New York: Brunner/Mazel.

Durst-Palmer, K., Baker, R. C., & McGee, T. F. (1997). The effects of pretraining on group psychotherapy for incest-related issues. *International Journal of Group Psychotherapy, 47*(1), 71–89.

D'Zurilla, T. J. (1986). *Problem-solving therapy: A social competence approach to clinical intervention.* New York: Springer.

D'Zurilla, T. J., & Nezu, A. M. (1982). Social problem solving in adults. In P. C. Kendall (Ed.), *Advances in cognitive-behavioral research and therapy* (Vol. 1, pp. 201–274). New York: Academic Press.

D'Zurilla, T. J., & Nezu, A. M. (1990). Development and preliminary evaluation of the social problem-solving inventory. *Psychological Assessment, 2,* 156–163.

D'Zurilla, T. J., & Nezu, A. M. (1999). *Problem-solving therapy: A social competence approach to clinical intervention* (2nd ed.). New York: Springer.

D'Zurilla, T. J., & Nezu, A. M. (2001). Problem-solving therapies. In K. S. Dobson (Ed.), *Handbook of cognitive-behavioral therapies* (2nd ed., pp. 145–211). New York: Guilford Press.

Ehly, S. W., & Garcia-Vazquez, E. (1998). Groups in the school context. In K. C. Stoiber & T. R. Kratochwill (Eds.), *Handbook of group intervention for children and families* (pp. 9–28). Boston: Allyn & Bacon.

Eisenberg, N., Liew, J., & Pidada, S. U. (2001). The relations of parental emotional expressivity with quality of Indonesian children's social functioning. *Emotion, 1*(2), 116–136.

Elfant, A. B. (1997). Submergence of the personal and unique in developmental models of psychotherapy groups and their leaders. *Group Dynamics: Theory, Research, and Practice, 1*(4), 311–315.

Ellis, A. (1962). *Reason and emotion in psychotherapy.* New York: Lyle Stuart Press.

Ellis, A. (1992). Group rational-emotive and cognitive-behavioral therapy. *International Journal of Group Psychotherapy, 42,* 63–80.

Ellsworth, J., & Hoag, M. (2000, Fall). Inpatient group psychotherapy: Improvement through group skills training and outcomes tracking. *Group Solution, 3,* 7.

El-Mallakh, R. S., & Hair, C. S. (1993). Medication dynamics in group psychotherapy. *Group, 17*(2), 101–106.

Ends, E. J., & Page, C. W. (1957). A study of three types of group psychotherapy with hospitalized male inebriates. *Quarterly Journal of Studies on Alcohol, 18,* 263–277.

Eriksen, L., Bjornstad, S., & Grotestam, G. (1986). Social skills training in groups for alcoholics: One-year treatment outcome for groups and individuals. *Addictive Behaviors, 11,* 309–329.

Ettin, M. (1994). Symbolic representation and the components of a group-as-a-whole model. *International Journal of Group Psychotherapy, 44*(2), 209–231.

Ettin, M. (2000). Group psychotherapy and group psychology in the 21st century: From future shock to a shocking future. *Group, 24*(1), 1–12.

Evans, N. J., & Jarvis, P. A. (1980). Group cohesion: A review and re-evaluation. *Small Group Behavior, 11,* 359–370.

Exner, J. (1993). *The Rorschach: A comprehensive system: Basic foundations* (3rd ed., Vol. 1). New York: Wiley.

Fallon, A., & Brabender, V. (2002). *Awaiting the therapist's baby: A guide for expectant therapists.* Mahwah, NJ: Erlbaum.

Fallon, A., Brabender, V., Anderson, N., & Maier, L. (1998, November). Therapists' perceptions of differences in the responses of group and individual psychotherapy patients to the therapists' pregnancy. *Focus,* 3–5.

Falloon, I. R. H. (1981). Interpersonal insights in behavioral group therapy. *British Journal of Medical Psychology, 54,* 133–141.

Falloon, I. R. H., Lindley, P., McDonald, R., & Marks, I. M. (1977). Social skills training of out-patient groups. *British Journal of Psychiatry, 131,* 599–609.

Fals-Stewart, W., Marks, A., & Schafer, J. (1993). A comparison of behavioral group therapy and individual behavior therapy in treating obsessive-compulsive disorder. *Journal of Nervous and Mental Diseases, 181,* 189–193.

Farrell, L. v. Superior Court, 203 Cal. App. 3d 521 (1988).

Fawzy, F. I., & Fawzy, N. W. (1994). A structured psychoeducational intervention with metastatic cancer. *Archives of General Psychiatry, 16,* 149–192.

Fawzy, F. I., Fawzy, N. W., Arndt, L. A., & Pasnau, R. O. (1995). Critical review of psychosocial intervention in cancer care. *Archives of General Psychiatry, 52,* 100–113.

Feindler, E. L., Ecton, R. B., Kingsley, D., & Dubey, D. R. (1986). Group anger-control training for institutionalized psychiatric male adolescents. *Behavior Therapy, 17*(2), 109–123.

Fenichel, O. (1945). *The psychoanalytic theory of neurosis.* New York: Norton.

Ferber, S., DeMartino, R. A., & Prout, H. T. (1989). Ethical and legal issues in psychological interventions with children and adolescents. In D. T. Brown & H. T. Prout (Eds.), *Counseling and psychotherapy with children and adolescents* (2nd ed., pp. 39–67). Brandon, VT: Clinical Psychology.

Fiedler, P. E., Orenstein, H., Chiles, J., Fritz, G., & Breitt, S. (1979). Effects of assertive training on hospitalized adolescents and young adults. *Adolescence, 14*(5), 523–528.

Flowers, J. V. (1979). Behavioral analysis of group therapy and a model for behavioral group therapy. In D. Upper & S. M. Ross (Eds.), *Behavioral group therapy 1979: An annual review* (pp. 5–37). Champaign, IL: Research Press.

Flowers, J. V., & Booraem, C. D. (1990a). The effects of different types of interpretation on outcome in group psychotherapy. *Group, 14*(2), 81–88.

Flowers, J. V., & Booraem, C. D. (1990b). The frequency and effect of different types of interpretation in psychodynamic and cognitive-behavioral group psychotherapy.

International Journal of Group Psychotherapy, 40(2), 203–214.

Flowers, J. V., & Schwartz, B. (1985). Behavioral group therapy with heterogeneous clients. In D. Upper & S. M. Ross (Eds.), *Handbook of behavioral group therapy* (pp. 145–170). New York: Plenum Press.

Foley, F. W., Bedell, J. R., LaRocca, N. G., Scheinberg, L. C., & Reznikoff, M. (1987). Efficacy of stress-inoculation training in coping with multiple sclerosis. *Journal of Consulting and Clinical Psychology, 55*(6), 919–922.

Foster, L. M. (1975). Group psychotherapy: Pool of legal witnesses. *International Journal of Group Psychotherapy, 25,* 50–53.

Foulkes, S. H. (1964). *Therapeutic group analysis.* London: Allen & Unwin.

Foulkes, S. H. (1986). *Group analytic psychotherapy: Method and principles.* London: H. Karnas.

Foxx, R. M., McMorrow, J., Bittle, R. G., & Fenton, S. J. (1985). Teaching skills to psychiatric inpatients. *Behavioral Research Therapy, 23*(5), 531–537.

Frable, D. E. S., Platt, L., & Hoey, S. (1998). Concealable stigmas and positive self-perceptions: Feeling better around similar others. *Journal of Personality and Social Psychology, 74*(4), 909–922.

Frank, J. D., & Frank, J. B. (1991). *Persuasion and healing* (3rd ed.). Baltimore: Johns Hopkins University Press.

Free, M. L., Oei, T. P. S., & Sanders, M. R. (1991). Treatment outcome of a group cognitive therapy program for depression. *International Journal of Group Psychotherapy, 41*(4), 533–547.

Freeman, A. (1983). *Cognitive therapy with couples and groups.* New York: Plenum Press.

Freeman, A., Schrodt, R., Gilson, M., & Ludgate, J. (1993). Group cognitive therapy with inpatients. In J. Wright, M. Thase, A. Beck, & J. Ludgate (Eds.), *Cognitive therapy with inpatients* (pp. 121–153). New York: Guilford Press.

Freud, S. (1953). The future prospects of psycho-analytic therapy. In J. Strachey (Ed.), *The Standard edition of the complete psychological works of Sigmund Freud.* (Vol. 11, pp. 139–151). London: Hogarth Press. (Original work published in 1910)

Freud, S. (1953). Three essays on the theory of sexuality. I: The sexual aberrations. In J. Strachey (Ed.), *The Standard edition of the complete psychological works of Sigmund Freud* (Vol. 7, pp. 135–243). London: Hogarth Press. (Original work published in 1905)

Freud, S. (1955). Group psychology and the analysis of the ego. In J. Strachey (Ed. and Trans.), *The standard edition of the complete psychological works of Sigmund Freud* (Vol. 14, pp. 243–258). London: Hogarth Press. (Original work published 1921)

Freud, S. (1957). Mourning and melancholia. In J. Strachey (Ed.), *The Standard edition of the complete works of Sigmund Freud* (Vol. 14, pp. 243–258). London: Hogarth Press. (Original work published 1917)

Freud, S. (1958). The dynamics of the transference. In J. Strachey (Ed.), *The Standard edition of the complete works of Sigmund Freud* (Vol.12, pp. 97–108). London: Hogarth Press. (Original work published in 1912)

Freud, S. (1977). Five lectures on psychoanalysis. In J. Strachey (Ed.), *The Standard edition of the complete psychological works of Sigmund Freud.* New York: Norton. (Original work published in 1910)

Frieze, I. H., & Schafer, P. C. (1984). Alcohol use and marital violence: Female and male differences in reactions to alcohol. In S. C. Wilsnack & L. J. Beckman (Eds.), *Alcohol problems in women: Antecedents, consequences and intervention* (pp. 260–279). New York: Guilford Press.

Froberg, W., & Slife, B. D. (1987). Overcoming obstacles to the implementation of Yalom's model of inpatient group psychotherapy. *International Journal of Group Psychotherapy, 37*(3), 371–388.

Fromme, D. K., & Smallwood, R. E. (1983). Group modification of affective verbalizations in a psychiatric population. *British Journal of Clinical Psychology, 22,* 251–256.

Frost, J. C., & Alonso, A. (1993). On becoming a group therapist. *Group, 17*(3), 179–184.

Fuhriman, A., & Burlingame, G. M. (1994). Group psychotherapy: Research and practice. In A. Fuhriman & G. M. Burlingame (Eds.), *Handbook of group psychotherapy: An empirical and clinical synthesis* (pp. 3–40). New York: Wiley.

Fuhriman, A., & Burlingame, G. M. (2001). Group psychotherapy training and effectiveness. *Journal of Group Psychotherapy Special issue, 51*(3), 399–416.

Gans, J. S. (1990). Broaching and exploring the question of combined group and individual therapy. *International Journal of Group Psychotherapy, 40*(2), 123–137.

Gans, J. S. (1992). Money and psychodynamic group psychotherapy. *International Journal of Group Psychotherapy, 42*(1), 133–152.

Garland, J. A. (1981). Loneliness in the group: An element of treatment. *Social Work with Groups, 4,* 95–110.

Garrison, J. (1978). Written vs. verbal preparation of patients for group psychotherapy. *Psychotherapy: Theory, Research and Practice, 15,* 130–134.

Geczy, B., & Sultenfuss, J. (1995). Group psychotherapy on state hospital admission wards. *International Journal of Group Psychotherapy, 45*(1), 1–15.

Gendron, C., Poitras, L., Dastoor, D. P., & Perodeau, G. (1996). Cognitive-behavioral group intervention for spousal caregivers: Findings and clinical considerations. *Clinical Gerontologist, 17*(1), 3–19.

Gilbride, T. V., & Hebert, J. (1980). Pathological characteristics of good and poor interpersonal problem-solvers among psychiatric outpatients. *Journal of Clinical Psychology, 36,* 121–127.

Gioe, V. J. (1975). *Cognitive modification and positive group experience as a treatment for treatment depression.* (Doctoral dissertation, Temple University, 1975). *Dissertation Abstracts International, 36,* 3039–3040.

Goldberg, D. A., Schuyler, W. R., Bransfield, D., & Savino, P. (1983). Focal group psychotherapy: A dynamic approach. *International Journal of Group Psychotherapy, 33*(4), 413–431.

Goldstein, W. N. (1991). Clarification of projective identification. *International Journal of Psychiatry, 148*(2), 153–161.

Goodman, M., Marks, M., & Rockberger, H. (1964). Resistance in group psychotherapy enhanced by the countertransference reactions of the therapist: A peer group experience. *International Journal of Group Psychotherapy, 14*(3), 332–343.

Goodman, M., & Weiss, D. (2000). Initiating, screening, and maintaining psychotherapy groups for traumatized patients. In R. H. Klein & V. L. Schermer (Eds.), *Group psychotherapy for psychological trauma* (pp. 47–63). New York: Guilford Press.

Goodman, S. H., Gravitt, G. W., & Kaslow, N. J. (1995). Social problem solving: A moderator of the relation between negative life stress and depression symptoms in children. *Journal of Abnormal Child Psychology, 23*(4), 473–485.

Gordon, P. K., & Ahmed, W. (1988). A comparison of two group therapies for bulimia. *British Review of Bulimia and Anorexia Nervosa, 3*(1), 17–31.

Gotleib, I. H., & Schraedley, P. K. (2000). Interpersonal psychotherapy. In C. R. Snyder & R. E. Ingram (Eds.), *Handbook of psychological change: Psychotherapy processes and practices for the 21st century* (pp. 258–279). New York: Wiley.

Graca, J. (1985). Whether informed consent to psychotherapy? *American Psychologist, 40*, 1062–1063.

Gray, J. J., & Hoage, C. M. (1990). Bulimia nervosa: Group behavior therapy with exposure plus response prevention. *Psychological Reports, 66*(2), 667–674.

Greanias, T., & Siegel, S. (2000). Dual Diagnoses. In J. R. White & A. S. Freeman (Eds.), *Cognitive-behavioral group therapy for specific problems and populations* (pp. 149–173). Washington, DC: American Psychological Association.

Greenberg, J. R., & Mitchell, S. A. (1983). *Object relations in psychoanalytic theory.* Cambridge, MA: Harvard University Press.

Greene, L. (1983). Relationships among semantic differential change measures of splitting, self-fragmentation, and object relations in borderline psychopathology. *British Journal of Medical Psychology, 63*, 21–32.

Greene, L. R., & Cole, M. B. (1991). Level and form of psychopathology and the structure of group therapy. *International Journal of Group Psychotherapy, 41*(4), 499–521.

Greene, L. R., Rosenkrantz, J., & Muth, D. (1985). Borderline defenses and countertransference: Research findings and implications. *Psychiatry, 9*(3), 253–264.

Haas, L. J. (1991). Hide and seek or show and tell? Emerging issues of informed consent. *Ethics and Behavior, 1*, 175–189.

Haas, L. J., & Malouf, J. L. (1995). *Keeping up the good work: A practitioner's guide to mental health ethics.* Sarasota, FL: Professional Resource Press.

Haas, L. J., & Malouf, J. L. (2002). *Keeping up the good work: A practitioner's guide to mental health ethics* (2nd ed.). Sarasota, FL: Professional Resource Press.

Halberstadt, A. G., Crisp, V. W., & Eaton, K. L. (1999). Family expressiveness: A retrospective and new directions for research. In P. Philippot, R. S. Feldman, & E. Coats (Eds.), *The social context of nonverbal behavior* (pp. 109–155). New York: Cambridge University Press.

Halligan, F. R. (1995). The challenge: Short-term dynamic psychotherapy for college counseling centers. *Psychotherapy, 32*(1), 113–121.

Hansen, D. J., St. Lawrence, J. S., & Christoff, K. A. (1985). Effects of interpersonal problem-solving training with chronic aftercare patients on problem-solving component skills and effectiveness of solutions. *Journal of Consulting and Clinical Psychology, 53*(2), 167–174.

Hanson, N. D., & Goldberg, S. G. (1999). Navigating the nuances: A matrix of considerations for ethical-legal dilemmas.

Professional Psychology: Research and Practice, 30(5), 495–503.

Hayes, J. A. (1995). Countertransference in group psychotherapy: Waking a sleeping dog. *International Journal of Group Psychotherapy, 45*(4), 521–536.

Heimberg, R. G., Dodge, C., Hope, D., Kennedy, C., Zollo, L., & Bednar, R. (1990). Cognitive-behavioral group treatment for social phobia: Comparison with a credible placebo control. *Cognitive Therapy and Research, 14*, 1–23.

Heitler, J. B. (1973). Preparation of lower-class patients for expressive group psychotherapy. *Journal of Consulting and Clinical Psychology, 41*(2), 251–260.

Hellerstein, D. J., Little, S. A. S., Samstag, L. W., Batchelder, S., Muran, J. C., Fedak, M., et al. (2001). Adding group psychotherapy to medication treatment in dysthymia: A randomized prospective pilot study. *Journal of Psychotherapy Practice and Research, 10*(2), 93–103.

Heppner, P. P., Reeder, B. L., & Larson, L. M. (1983). Cognitive variables associated with personal problem-solving appraisal: Implications for counseling. *Journal of Counseling Psychology, 30*, 537–545.

Hersey, P., & Blanchard, K. (1977). *Management of organizational behavior: Utilizing human resources* (3rd ed.). Englewood Cliffs, NJ: Prentice-Hall.

Higgins, J. P., & Thies, A. P. (1982). Social effectiveness and problem solving thinking of reformatory inmates. *Journal of Offender Counseling, Services and Rehabilitation, 5*(3/4), 93–98.

Hilkey, J., Wilhelm, C., & Horne, A. (1982). Comparative effectiveness of videotape pretraining versus no pretraining as selected process and outcome variables in group therapy. *Psychological Reports, 50,* 1151–1159.

Hill, C. E., Mahalik, J. R., & Thompson, B. J. (1989). Therapist self-disclosure. *Psychotherapy, 26*(3), 290–295.

Hills, H. I., & Strozier, A. A. (1992). Multicultural training in APA approved counseling psychology programs: A survey. *Professional Psychology: Research and Practice, 23,* 43–51.

Hollon, S. D., & Evans, M. D. (1983). Cognitive therapy for depression in a group format. In A. Freeman (Ed.), *Cognitive therapy with couples and groups* (pp. 11–41). New York: Plenum Press.

Hooley, J. M., & Candela, S. F. (1999). Interpersonal functioning in schizophrenia. In T. Millon, P. H. Blaney, & R. D. Davis (Eds.), *Oxford textbook of psychopathology* (pp. 311–338). New York: Oxford University Press.

Hope, D. A., & Heimberg, R. G. (1993). Social phobia and social anxiety. In D. H. Barlow (Ed.), *Clinical handbook of psychological disorders* (2nd ed., pp. 99–136). New York: Guilford Press.

Horwitz, L. (1994). Depth of transference in groups. *International Journal of Group Psychotherapy, 44*(3), 271–290.

Howard, K. I., Moran, K., Brill, P. L., Martinovich, Z., & Lutz, W. (1996). Efficacy, effectiveness, and patient progress. *American psychologist, 51,* 1059–1064.

Humphreys, K., Winzelberg, A., & Klaw, E. (2000). Psychologists' ethical responsibilities in Internet-based groups: Issues, strategies, and a call for dialogue. *Professional Psychology: Research and Practice, 31*(5), 493–496.

Hurley, J. R., & Force, E. J. (1973). T-group gains in acceptance of self and others. *International Journal of Group Psychotherapy, 23,* 166–176.

Hussian, R. A. (1987). Problem-solving training and institutionalized elderly patients. In A. Freeman & V. Greenwood (Eds.), *Cognitive therapy: Applications in psychiatric and medical settings* (pp. 199–212). New York: Human Sciences Press.

Ingram, R. E. (2001). Developing perspectives on the cognitive-developmental origins of depression: Back is the future. *Cognitive Therapy and Research, 25*(4), 497–504.

Ingram, R. E., Scott, W., & Seigle, G. (1999). Depression: Social and cognitive aspects. In T. Millon, P. H. Blaney, & R. D. Davis (Eds.), *Oxford textbook of psychopathology* (pp. 203–226). New York: Oxford University Press.

Intagliata, J. C. (1978). Increasing the interpersonal problem-solving skills of an alcoholic population. *Journal of Consulting and Clinical Psychology, 46*(3), 489–498.

Jackson, D. A. (1999). The team meeting on a rapid turnover psychiatric ward: Clinical illustration of a model for stages of group development. *International Journal of Group Psychotherapy, 49*(1), 41–59.

Jacobs, A. (1974). *The group as agent of change.* New York: Behavioral Publications.

Jacobs, M., Jacobs, A., Gatz, M., & Schaible, T. (1973). The credibility and desirability of positive and negative structural feedback in groups. *Journal of Consulting and Clinical Psychology, 40,* 244–252.

Jacobson, N. S., & Anderson, E. A. (1982). Interpersonal skill and depression in college students: An analysis of the timing of self-disclosures. *Behavior Therapy, 13,* 271–282.

Janoff, D. S., & Schoenholtz-Read, J. (1999). Group supervision meets technology: A model for computer-mediated training at a distance. *International Journal of Group Psychotherapy, 49,* 255–272.

Jerome, L. W., & Zaylor, C. (2000). Cyberspace: Creating a therapeutic environment for telehealth applications. *Professional Psychology: Research and Practice, 31*(5), 478–483.

Jeske, J. O. (1973). Identification and therapeutic effectiveness in group therapy. *Journal of Counseling Psychology, 20*(6), 528–530.

Johnson, D. W., & Johnson, F. P. (2000). *Joining together: Group theory and group skills* (6th ed.). Boston: Allyn & Bacon.

Joiner, T. E., Jr., & Metalsky, G. I. (1995). A prospective test of an integrative interpersonal theory of depression: A naturalistic study of college roommates. *Journal of Personality and Social Psychology, 69,* 778–788.

Joiner, T. E., Jr., Petit, J. W., Perez, M., Burns, A. B., Gencoz, T., Gencoz, F., et al. (2001). Can positive emotion influence problem-solving attitudes among suicidal adults? *Professional Psychology: Research and Practice, 32*(5), 507–512.

Joiner, T. E., Jr., Voelz, Z. R., & Rudd, M. D. (2001). For suicidal young adults with comorbid depressive and anxiety disorders, problem-solving treatment may be better than treatment as usual. *Professional Psychology: Research and Practice, 32*(3), 278–282.

Jones, D. E. (1981). Interpersonal cognitive problem-solving training: A skills approach with hospitalized psychiatric patients. *Dissertation Abstract International, 42*(5-B), 2060–2061.

Jones, E. J., & McCall, M. A. (1991). Development and evaluation of an interactional life skills group for offenders. *Occupational Therapy Journal of Research, 11*(2), 81–92.

Kanas, N. (2000). Cognitive-behavioral group therapy for depression. *International Journal of Group Psychotherapy, 50*(3), 413–416.

Kanas, N., Stewart, P., Deri, J., Ketter, T., & Haney, K. (1989). Group process in short-term out patient therapy groups for schizophrenics. *Group, 13*(2), 67–73.

Kangas, J. A. (1971). Group members' self-disclosure: A function of preceding self-disclosure by leader or other group member. *Comparative Group Studies, 2,* 65–70.

Kant, G. L., D'Zurilla, T. J., & Mayden-Olivares, A. (1997). Social problem solving as a mediator of stress-related depression and anxiety in middle-aged and elderly community residents. *Cognitive Therapy and Research, 21*(1), 73–96.

Kaplan, E. (1997). Telepsychotherapy by telephone, videophone and computer videoconferencing. *Journal of Psychotherapy, Practice and Research, 6,* 27–37.

Karau, S. J., & Williams, K. D. (1997). The effects of group cohesiveness on social loafing and social compensation. *Group Dynamics: Theory, Research, and Practice, 1*(2), 156–168.

Kaul, T. J., & Bednar, R. L. (1986). Experiential group research: Results, questions, and suggestions. In S. L. Garfield & A. E. Birgin (Eds.), *Handbook of psychotherapy and behavior change* (3rd ed., pp. 671–714). New York: Wiley.

Kazantzis, N., & Deane, F. P. (1999). Psychologists' use of homework assignments in clinical practice. *Professional Psychology: Research and Practice, 30*(6), 581–585.

Kearney, M. (1984). Confidentiality in group psychotherapy. *Psychotherapy in Private Practice, 2*(2), 19–20.

Kelly, G. A. (1955). *The psychology of personal constructs.* New York: Norton.

Kelly, J., Murphy, D., Bahr, R., Kalichman, S., Morgan, M., Stevenson, Y., et al. (1993). Outcome of cognitive-behavioral and support group brief therapies for depressed, HIV infected persons. *American Journal of Psychiatry, 150,* 1679–1686.

Kernberg, O. (1976). *Object relations and clinical psychoanalysis.* New York: Aronsen.

Kibel, H. D. (1981). A conceptual model for short-term inpatient group psychotherapy. *American Journal of psychiatry, 181*(1), 74–80.

Kibel, H. D. (1987). Inpatient group psychotherapy: Where treatment philosophies converge. In *Yearbook of psychoanalysis and psychotherapy* (Vol. 2, pp. 94–116). New York: Gardner Press.

Kibel, H. D. (1992). The clinical application of object relations theory. In R. H. Klein, H. S. Bernard, & D. L. Singer (Eds.), *Handbook of contemporary group psychotherapy* (pp. 141–176). Madison, CT: International Universities Press.

Kibel, H. D. (1993). Inpatient group psychotherapy. In A. Alonso & H. I. Swiller (Eds.), *Group therapy in clinical practice* (pp. 93–111). Washington, DC: American Psychiatric Press.

Kilmann, P. R., Laughlin, J. E., Carranza, L. V., Downer, J. T., Major, S., & Parnell, M. M. (1999). Effects of an attachment-focused group preventive intervention on insecure women. *Group Dynamics: Theory, Research, and Practice, 3*(2), 138–147.

Kirman, J. (1995). Working with anger in groups: A modern analytic approach. *International Journal of Group Psychotherapy, 45*(3), 303–329.

Kitchener, K. S. (1984). Intuition, critical evaluation and ethical principles: The foundation for ethical decisions in counseling psychology. *Counseling Psychologist, 12*, 43–55.

Kivlighan, D. M. (1997). Leader behavior and therapeutic gain: An application of situational leadership theory. *Group Dynamics: Theory, Research, and Practice, 1*(1), 32–38.

Kivlighan, D. M., & Jacquet, C. (1990). Quality of group member agendas and group session climate. *Small Group Research, 21,* 205–219.

Kivlighan, D. M., McGovern, T. V., & Corazzini, J. G. (1995). Effects of content and timing of structuring interventions on group therapy process and outcome. *Journal of Counseling Psychology, 31*(3), 363–370.

Kivlighan, D. M., & Tarrant, J. M. (2001). Does group climate mediate the group leadership-group member outcome relationship? A test of Yalom's hypotheses about leadership priorities. *Group Dynamics: Theory, Research, and Practice, 5*(3), 230–234.

Klein, M. (1935). A contribution to the psychogenesis of manic-depressive states. *International Journal of Psycho-Analysis, 16,* 145–174.

Klein, M. (1948). *Contributions to psycho-analysis, 1921–45.* London: Hogarth.

Klein, R. H., & Schermer, V. L. (2000). Introduction and overview: Creating a healing matrix. In R. H. Klein & V. L. Schermer (Eds.), *Group psychotherapy for psychological trauma* (pp. 3–46). New York: Guilford Press.

Koch, H. C. H. (1983). Correlates of changes in personal construing of members of two psychotherapy groups: Changes in affective expression. *British Journal of Medical Psychology, 56,* 323–327.

Kosten, T. R., & Ziedonis, D. M. (1997). Substance abuse and schizophrenia: Editors' introduction. *Schizophrenia Bulletin, 23*(2), 181–186.

Kush, F. R., & Fleming, L. M. (2000). An innovative approach to short-term group cognitive therapy in the combined treatment of anxiety and depression. *Group Dynamics, 4*(2), 176–183.

Lakin, M. (1994). Morality in group and family therapies: Multiperson therapies and the 1992 ethics code. *Professional Psychology: Research and Practice, 25*(4), 344–348.

LaMothe, R. (2001). Vitalizing objects and psychoanalytic psychotherapy. *Psychoanalytic Psychology, 18*(2), 320–339.

Lang, A. J., & Craske, M. G. (2000). Panic and phobia. In J. R. White & A. S. Freeman (Eds.), *Cognitive-behavioral group therapy for specific problems and populations* (pp. 63–97). Washington, DC: American Psychological Association.

Langfred, C. (1998). Is group cohesiveness a double-edged sword: An investigation of the effects of cohesiveness on performance. *Small Group Research, 29*(1), 124–143.

Lasch, C. (1979). *The culture of narcissism.* New York: Norton.

Laurenceau, J., Barrett, L. F., & Pietromonaco, P. R. (1998). Intimacy as an interpersonal process: The importance of self-disclosure, partner disclosure, and perceived partner responsiveness in interpersonal exchanges. *Journal of Personality and Social Psychology, 74*(5), 1238–1251.

Lazarus, A. (1976). *Multimodal behavioral therapy.* New York: Springer.

Lazell, E. W. (1921). The group treatment of dementia praecox. *Psychoanalytic Review, 8,* 168–179.

Leopold, H. (1961). The new member in the group: Some specific aspects of the literature. *International Journal of Group Psychotherapy, 11,* 367–371.

Leopold, H. S. (1977). Selective group approaches with psychotic patients in hospital settings. *Journal of Psychotherapy, 30,* 95–105.

Leszcz, M. (1992). The interpersonal approach to group psychotherapy. *International Journal of Group Psychotherapy, 42*(1), 37–62.

Leszcz, M., Yalom, I. D., & Norden, M. (1985). The value of inpatient group psychotherapy: Patients' perceptions. *International Journal of Group Psychotherapy, 35*(3), 411–433.

Liberman, R. (1970). A behavioral approach to group dynamics: Reinforcement and prompting of cohesiveness in group therapy. *Behavior Therapy, 1,* 141–175.

Lieberman, M. A., Yalom, I., & Miles, M. B. (1973). *Encounter groups: First facts.* New York: Basic Books.

Lindon, J. A. (1988). Psychoanalysis by telephone. *Bulletin of the Menninger Clinic, 52,* 521–528.

Linehan, M. M. (1989). Cognitive and behavior therapy for borderline personality disorder. *Annual Review of Psychiatry, 8,* 84–102.

Linehan, M. M. (1993). *Cognitive-behavioral treatment of borderline personality disorder.* New York: Guilford Press.

Linehan, M. M., Tutek, D. A., Heard, H. L., & Armstrong, H. E. (1994). Interpersonal outcome of cognitive behavioral treatment for chronically suicidal borderline patients. *American Journal of Psychiatry, 151*(12), 1771–1776.

Lochman, J. E. (1992). Cognitive-behavioral intervention with aggressive boys: Three-year follow-up and preventive effects. *Journal of Consulting and Clinical Psychology, 60*(3), 426–432.

Lochman, J. E., Burch, P. R., Curry, J. F., & Lampron, L. B. (1984). Treatment and generalization effects of cognitive-behavioral and goal-setting interventions with aggressive boys. *Journal of Consulting and Clinical Psychology, 52*(5), 915–916.

Lothstein, L. M. (2001). Treatment of non-incarcerated sexually compulsive/addictive offenders in an integrated, multimodal, and psychodynamic group therapy model. *International Journal of Group Psychotherapy, 51*(4), 553–570.

Lubin, D., & Johnson, D. R. (1997). Interactive psychoeducational group therapy for traumatized women. *International Journal of Group Psychotherapy, 47*(3), 271–290.

Lubin, H., Loris, M., Burt, J., & Johnson, D. (1998). Efficacy of psychoeducational group therapy in reducing symptoms of posttraumatic stress disorder among multiply-traumatized women. *International Journal of Group Psychotherapy, 47,* 271–290.

Macaskill, N. D. (1982). Therapeutic factors in group therapy with borderline patients. *International Journal of Group Psychotherapy, 32,* 61–73.

MacKenzie, K. R. (1983). The clinical application of the group climate measure. In R. R. Dies & K. R. MacKenzie (Eds.), *Advances in group psychotherapy: Integrating research and practice* (pp. 159–170). Madison, CT: International Universities Press.

Mackenzie, K. R. (1987). Therapeutic factors in group psychotherapy: A contemporary view. *Group, 11,* 26–34.

MacKenzie, K. R. (1990). *Introduction to time-limited group psychotherapy.* Washington, DC: American Psychiatric Association.

MacKenzie, K. R. (1994). Group development. In A. Fuhriman & G. M. Burlingame (Eds.), *Handbook of group psychotherapy: An empirical and clinical synthesis* (pp. 223–268). New York: Wiley.

MacKenzie, K. R. (1995). Rationale for group psychotherapy in managed care. In K. R. MacKenzie (Ed.), *Effective use of group psychotherapy in managed care* (pp. 1–25). Washington, DC: American Psychiatric Press.

MacKenzie, K. R. (1996). Time-limited group psychotherapy. *International Journal of Group Psychotherapy, 46*(1), 41–60.

MacKenzie, K. R. (2001). An expectation of radical changes in the future of group psychotherapy. *International Journal of Group Psychotherapy, 51*(2), 175–180.

MacKenzie, K. R., & Dies, R. R. (1981). *CORE battery clinical outcome results.* New York: American Group Psychotherapy Association.

MacKenzie, K. R., Dies, R. R., Coche, E., Rutan, J. S., & Stone, W. N. (1987). An analysis of AGPA Institute groups. *International Journal of Group Psychotherapy, 37,* 55–74.

MacKenzie, K. R., & Grabovac, A. D. (2001). Interpersonal psychotherapy group (IPT-G) for depression. *Journal of Psychotherapy Practice and Research, 10*(1), 46–51.

MacLennan, B. W. (1965). Co-therapy. *International Journal of Group Psychotherapy, 15,* 154–166.

Maddi, S. R. (1972). *Personality theories: A comparative analysis* (2nd ed.). Homewood, IL: Dorsey Press.

Mahler, M. S. (1972). On the first three subphases of the separation-individuation process. *International Journal of Psycho-Analysis, 53*(3), 333–338.

Mahoney, M. J. (1995). *Constructive psychotherapy: Principles and ractice.* New York: Guilford Press.

Mann, J. (1981). The core of time-limited psychotherapy: Time and the central issue. In S. H. Budman (Ed.), *Forms of brief psychotherapy* (pp. 25–43). New York: Guilford Press.

Marcowitz, J. S., Weissman, M. M., Ouellette, R., Lish, J. D., & Klerman, G. L. (1989). Quality of life in panic disorder. *Archives of General Psychiatry, 46,* 984–992.

Marcowitz, R., & Smith, J. (1983). Patient perceptions of curative factors in short-term group psychotherapy. *International Journal of Group Psychotherapy, 33,* 21–37.

Marin, P. (1976, October). The new narcissism. *Harpers,* 44–56.

Marsh, L. C. (1935). Group therapy in the psychiatric clinic. *Journal of Nervous and Mental Diseases, 82,* 381–392.

Martin, R. (1971). Videotape self-confrontation in T groups. *Journal of Counseling Psychology, 18,* 341–347.

Massel, H. K., Corrigan, P. W., Liberman, R. P., & Macmillan, M. A. (1991). Conversation skills training of thought-disordered schizophrenic patients through attention focusing. *Psychiatric Research, 38,* 51–61.

Maxmen, J. (1973). Group therapy as viewed by hospitalized patients. *Archives of General Psychiatry, 28,* 404–408.

May, O. P., & Thompson, C. L. (1973). Perceived levels of self-disclosure, mental health, and helpfulness of group leaders. *Journal of Counseling Psychology, 20*(4), 349–352.

McCormick, C. T. (1972). *McCormick's handbook of the law of evidence* (2nd ed.). St. Paul, MN: West.

McCullough, L. B., & Ashton, C. M. (1994). A methodology for teaching ethics in the clinical setting: A clinical handbook for medical ethics. *Theoretical Medicine, 15,* 39–52.

McCutchen, A. J. (2000). Dissociative disorders. In J. R. White & A. S. Freeman (Eds.), *Cognitive-behavioral group therapy for specific problems and populations* (pp. 175–210). Washington, DC: American Psychological Association.

McGuire, J. M., Taylor, D. R., Broome, D. H., Blau, B. I., & Abbott, D. W. (1986). Group structuring techniques and their influence on process involvement in a group counseling training group. *Journal of Counseling Psychology, 33*(3), 270–275.

McLatchie, L. R. (1982). Interpersonal problem-solving group therapy: An evaluation of a potential method of social skills training for the chronic psychiatric patient. *Dissertation Abstracts International, 42*(7), 2995-B.

McLean, P. D., Whittal, M. L., Thordarson, D. S., Taylor, S., Sochting, I., Koch, W. J., et al. (2001). Cognitive versus behavior therapy in the group treatment of obsessive-compulsive disorder. *Journal of Consulting and Clinical Psychology, 69*(2), 205–214.

McMinn, M. R., Buchanan, T., Ellens, B. M., & Ryan, M. K. (1999). Technology, professional practice, and ethics: Survey findings and implications. *Professional Psychology: Research and Practice, 30*(2), 165–172.

McNary, S. W., & Dies, R. R. (1993). Cotherapist modeling in group psychotherapy: Fact or fantasy? *Group, 17*(3), 131–142.

McWilliams, N. (1964). *Psychoanalytic diagnosis: Understanding structure in the clinical process.* New York: Guilford Press.

McWilliams, N. (1994). *Psychoanalytic diagnosis: Understanding personality structure in the clinical process.* New York: Guilford Press.

Meichenbaum, D. (1975). A self-instructional approach to stress management: A proposal for stress inoculation training. In I. Saranson & C. D. Spielberger (Eds.), *Stress and anxiety* (pp. 337–360). New York: Plenum Press.

Meichenbaum, D. (1977). *Cognitive-behavioral modification: An integrative approach.* New York: Plenum Press.

Meichenbaum, D. H., Gilmore, J. B., & Fedoravicius, A. L. (1971). Group insight versus group desensitization in treating speech anxiety. *Journal of Consulting and Clinical Psychology, 36,* 416–421.

Miller, R., & Berman, J. (1983). The efficacy of cognitive behavior therapies. A quantitative review of research evidence. *Psychological Bulletin, 94,* 39–53.

Mishna, F., Muskat, B., & Schamess, G. (2002). Food for thought: The use of food in group therapy with children and adolescents. *International Journal of Group Psychotherapy, 52*(1), 27–47.

Moreno, J. K. (1994). Group treatment for eating disorders. In A. Fuhriman & G. M. Burlingame (Eds.), *Handbook of group psychotherapy: An empirical and clinical synthesis* (pp. 416–457). New York: Wiley.

Morgan, R. D., Ferrell, S. W., & Winterowd, C. L. (1999). Therapist perceptions of important therapeutic factors in psychotherapy groups for male inmates in state correctional facilities. *Small Group Research, 30*(6), 712–729.

Morran, D. K., Robison, F. F., & Stockton, R. (1985). Feedback exchange in counseling groups: An analysis of message content and receiver acceptance as a function of leader versus member delivery, session, and valence. *Journal of Counseling Psychology, 32*(1), 57–67.

Morran, D. K., Stockton, R., Cline, R. J., & Teed, C. (1998). Facilitating feedback exchange in groups: Leader interventions. *Journal for Specialists in Group Work, 23*(3), 257–268.

Morran, D. K., Stockton, R., & Harris, M. (1991). Analysis of group leader and member feedback messages. *Journal of Group Psychotherapy, Psychodrama, and Sociometry, 44*, 126–135.

Moss, E. (1995). Group supervision: Focus on countertransference. *International Journal of Group Psychotherapy, 45*(4), 537–548.

Motherwell, L. (2002). Women, money, and psychodynamic group psychotherapy. *International Group Psychotherapy, 52*(1), 49–66.

Mueser, K. T., Bellack, A. S., Douglas, M. S., & Wade, J. H. (1991). Prediction of social skill acquisition in schizophrenic and major affective disorder patients from memory and symptomatology. *Psychiatry Research, 37*, 281–296.

Mullan, H. (1987). The ethical foundations of group psychotherapy. *International Journal of Group Psychotherapy, 37*(3), 403–416.

Murphy, L., Leszcz, M., Collings, A. K., & Salvendy, J. (1996). Some subjective experience of neophyte group therapy trainers. *International Journal of Group Psychotherapy, 46*(4), 543–552.

Mussell, M. P., Mitchell, J. E., Crosby, R. D., Fulkerson, J. A., Hoberman, H. M., & Romano, J. L. (2000). Commitment to treatment goals in prediction of group cognitive-behavioral therapy treatment outcome for women with bulimia nervosa. *Journal of Consulting and Clinical Psychology, 68*(3), 432–437.

National Association of Social Workers. (1999). *NASW Code of ethics.* Washington, DC: Author.

National Board for Certified Counselors. (2001). *Standards for the ethical practice of webcounseling.* Retrieved February 12, 2002 from www.nbcc.org/ethics/webethics.htm

Neimeyer, R. A., & Feixas, G. (1990). The role of homework and skill acquisition in the outcome of group cognitive therapy for depression. *Behavior Therapy, 21*, 281–282.

Nezu, A. M. (1986). Efficacy of a social problem-solving therapy approach for unipolar depression. *Journal of Consulting and Clinical Psychology, 54*, 196–202.

Nezu, A. M., Nezu, C. M., & Perri, M. G. (1989). *Problem-solving therapy for depression: Theory, research, and clinical guidelines.* New York: Wiley.

Nezu, A. M., & Perri, M. G. (1989). Social problem solving therapy for unipolar depression: An initial dismantling investigation. *Journal of Consulting and Clinical Psychology, 57*, 408–413.

Nezu, A. M., & Ronan, G. F. (1985). Life stress, current problems, problem solving, and depressive symptomatology: An integrative model. *Journal of Consulting and Clinical Psychology, 53,* 693–697.

Nickelson, D. W. (1998). Telehealth and the evolving health care system: Strategic opportunities for professional psychology. *Professional Psychology: Research and Practice, 29*(6), 527–533.

Nitsun, M. (1996). *The anti-group: Destructive forces in the group and their creative potential.* London: Routledge.

Oei, T. P. S., & Kazmierczak, T. (1997). Factors associated with dropout in a group cognitive behaviour therapy for mood disorders. *Behavior Research and Therapy, 35*(11), 1025–1030.

Ogden, T. (1979). On projective identification. *International Journal of Psychoanalysis, 60,* 357–373.

Omizo, M. M., Herschberger, J. M., & Omizo, S. A. (1988). Teaching children to cope with anger. *Elementary School Guidance and Counseling, 22*(3), 241–245.

Organista, K. C. (2000). Latinos. In J. R. White & A. S. Freeman (Eds.), *Cognitive-behavioral group therapy for specific problems and populations* (pp. 281–303). Washington, DC: American Psychological Association.

Ormont, L. (1991). Use of the group in resolving the subjective countertransference. *International Journal of Group Psychotherapy, 41*(4), 433–447.

Osborn, A. (1963). *Applied imagination: Principles and procedures of creative problem solving* (3rd ed.). New York: Charles Scribner's Sons.

Pastushak, R. J. (1978). The effects of videotaped pretherapy training on interpersonal openness, self-disclosure and group psychotherapy outcome (Doctoral dissertation, Temple University). *Dissertation Abstract International, 39*(2-B) 993.

Pattison, E. M., Brissenden, A., & Wohl, T. (1967). Assessing specific effects of inpatient group psychotherapy. *International Journal of Group Psychotherapy, 17,* 283–297.

Pauli, P., Wiedemann, G., Dengler, W., Blaumann-Benninghoff, F., & Kuehlkamp, V. (1999). Anxiety in patients with an automatic implantable cardioverter defibrillator: What differentiates them from panic patients? *Psychosomatic-Medicine, 61*(1), 69–76.

Pearson, M. J., & Girling, A. J. (1990). The value of the Claberry Selection Battery in predicting benefit from group psychotherapy. *British Journal of Psychiatry, 157,* 384–388.

Perri, M. G., Nezu, A. M., McKelvey, W. F., Shermer, R. L., Renjilian, D. A., & Viegener, B. J. (2001). Relapse prevention training and problem-solving therapy in the long-term management of obesity. *Journal of Consulting and Clinical Psychology, 69*(4), 722–726.

Perri, M. G., Nezu, A. M., & Viegener, B. J. (1992). *Improving the long-term management of obesity: Theory, research, and clinical guidelines.* New York: Wiley.

Persons, J. B., Davidson, J., & Tompkins, M. A. (2001). *Essential components of cognitive-behavior therapy for depression.* Washington, DC: American Psychological Association.

Peterson, R. L., Peterson, D. R., Abrams, J. C., & Stricker, G. (1997). The national council of schools and programs of professional psychology education model. *Professional*

Psychology: Research and Practice, 28(4), 373–386.

Pierce, C. V. M. (1980). Interpersonal problem-solving training for psychiatric patients. *Dissertation Abstracts International, 41*(10), 4339-A.

Pine, C., & Jacobs, A. (1991). The acceptability of behavioral and emotional feedback on reception in personal growth groups. *Journal of Clinical Psychology, 47,* 115–122.

Pino, C. J., & Cohen, H. (1971). Trainer style and trainee self-disclosure. *International Journal of Group Psychotherapy, 21,* 202–213.

Piper, W. E. (1994). Client variables. In A. Fuhriman & G. M. Burlingame (Eds.), *Handbook of group psychotherapy: An empirical and clinical synthesis* (pp. 83–113). New York: Wiley.

Piper, W. E., Debbane, E. G., Bienvenu, J. P., & Gerant, J. (1982). A study of group pretraining for group psychotherapy. *International Journal of Group Psychotherapy, 32,* 309–325.

Piper, W. E., Debbane, E. G., Garant, J., & Bienvenu, J. P. (1979). Pretraining for group psychotherapy. *Archives of General Psychiatry, 36,* 1250–1256.

Piper, W. E., Marrache, M., Lacroix, R., Richardsen, A., & Jones, B. (1983). Cohesion as a basic bond in groups. *Human Relations, 36,* 93–108.

Piper, W. E., McCallum, M., & Azim, H. F. A. (1992). *Adaptation to loss through short-term group psychotherapy.* New York: Guilford Press.

Piper, W. E., McCallum, M., Joyce, A. S., Rosie, J. S., & Ogrodniczuk, J. S. (2001). Patient personality and time-limited group psychotherapy for complicated grief. *International Journal of Group Psychotherapy, 51*(4), 525–552.

Piper, W. E., Rosie, J. S., Joyce, A. S., & Azim, H. F. A. (1996). *Time-limited day treatment for personality disorders: Integration of research and practice in a group program.* Washington, DC: American Psychological Association.

Platt, J. J., Husband, S. D., Hermalin, C., Cater, J., & Metzger, D. (1993). A cognitive problem-solving employment readiness intervention for methadone clients. *Journal of Cognitive Psychotherapy: An international Quarterly, 7,* 21–33.

Platt, J. J., Prout, M. F., & Metzger, D. S. (1987). Interpersonal cognitive problem-solving therapy (ICPS). In W. Dryden & W. L. Golden (Eds.), *Cognitive-behavioural approaches to psychotherapy* (pp. 261–289). London: Hemisphere.

Platt, J. J., & Siegel, J. M. (1976). MMPI characteristics of good and poor social problem solvers among psychiatric patients. *Journal of Community Psychology, 94,* 245–251.

Platt, J. J., & Spivack, G. (1974). Means of solving real-life problems: Psychiatric patients vs. controls and cross-cultural comparisons of normal females. *Journal of Community Psychology, 2*(1), 45–48.

Porter, K. (1993). Combined individual and group psychotherapy. In A. Alonso & H. I. Swiller (Eds.), *Group therapy in clinical practice* (pp. 309–341). Washington, DC: American Psychiatric Press

Priester, M. J., & Clum, G. A. (1993). Perceived problem-solving ability as a predictor of depression, hopelessness, and suicide ideation in a college population. *Journal of Counseling Psychology, 40*(1), 79–85.

Query, W. T. (1964). Self-disclosure as a variable in group psychotherapy. *International Journal of Group Psychotherapy, 14,* 107–115.

Rabin, H. M. (1967). How does co-therapy compare with regular therapy? *American Journal of Psychotherapy, 21,* 244–255.

Rachman, A. W. (1990). Judicious self-disclosure in group analysis. *Group, 14*(3), 132–144.

Racker, H. (1972). The meanings and uses of countertransference. *Psychoanalytic Quarterly, 41,* 487–506.

Rae, W. A., & Fournier, C. J. (1999). Ethical and legal issues in the treatment of children and families. In S. W. Russ & T. H. Ollendick (Eds.), *Handbook of psychotherapies with children and families* (pp. 67–83). New York: Kluwer Academic/Plenum Publishers.

Reed, K. G. (1987). *Members' perceptions of therapists' behavior in short-term psychotherapy groups.* (Doctoral dissertation, University of Maryland, 1986). *Dissertation Abstracts International, 47*(08), 3540.

Reisner, R., Slobogin, C., & Rai, A. (1999). *Law and the mental health system: Civil and criminal aspects* (3rd ed.). St. Paul, MN: West.

Rice, C. (1992). Contributions from object relations theory. In R. H. Klein, H. S. Bernard, & D. L. Singer (Eds.), *Handbook of contemporary group psychotherapy* (pp. 27–54). Madison, CT: International Universities Press.

Rice, C. (1995). The junior-junior term. *Group, 19*(2), 87–99.

Rice, C., & Rutan, S. (1981). Boundary maintenance in inpatient therapy groups. *International Journal of Group Psychotherapy, 31*(3), 297–309.

Rieger, E. (1993). *Correlates of adult hope, including high- and low-hope young adults' recollections of parents.* Honor's thesis, University of Kansas, Department of Psychology, Lawrence, Kansas.

Riva, M. T., Lippert, L., & Tackett, M. J. (2000). Selection practices of group leaders: A national survey. *Journal for Specialists in Group Work, 25*(2), 157–169.

Roback, H. B. (1972). Experimental comparison of outcomes in insight and non-insight-oriented therapy groups. *Journal of Consulting and Clinical Psychology, 38,* 411–417.

Roback, H. B. (2000). Adverse outcomes in group psychotherapy: Risk factors, prevention, and research directions. *Journal of Psychotherapy Practice and Research, 9*(3), 113–122.

Roback, H. B., Moore, R. F., Waterhouse, G. J., & Martin, P. R. (1996). Confidentiality dilemmas in group psychotherapy with substance-dependent physicians. *American Journal of Psychiatry, 153*(10), 1483–1484.

Roback, H. B., Ochoa, E., Bloch, F., & Purdon, S. (1992). Guarding confidentiality in clinical groups: The therapist's dilemma. *International Journal of Group Psychotherapy, 42,* 81–103.

Robinson, L., Berman, J., & Neimeyer R. (1990). Psychotherapy for the treatment of depression: A comprehensive review of controlled outcome research. *Psychological Bulletin, 108*(1), 30–49.

Robinson, M., & Jacobs, A. (1970). Focused videotape feedback and behavior change in group psychotherapy. *Psychotherapy: Theory, Research, and Practice, 7,* 169–172.

Roether, H. A., & Peters, J. J. (1972). Cohesiveness and hostility in group psychotherapy.

American Journal of Psychiatry, 128, 1014–1017.

Rohde, P., Clarke, G. N., Lewinsohn, P. M., Seeley, J. R., & Kaufman, N. K. (2001). Impact of comorbidity on a cognitive-behavioral group treatment for adolescent depression. *Journal American Academy of Child and Adolescent Psychiatry, 40*(7), 795–802.

Roller, B. (1997). *The promise of group therapy: How to build a vigorous training and organizational base for group therapy in managed behavioral healthcare.* San Francisco: Jossey-Bass.

Roller, B., & Nelson, V. (1991). *The art of co-therapy.* New York: Guilford Press.

Rose, S. (1990). Putting the group into cognitive-behavioral treatment. *Social Work with Groups, 13,* 71–83.

Rose, S. D. (1999). Group therapy: A cognitive-behavioral approach. In J. R. Price, D. R. Hescheles, & A. R. Price (Eds.), *A guide to starting psychotherapy groups* (pp. 99–113). San Diego, CA: Academic Press.

Rose, S. D., Tolman, R. M., & Tallant, S. (1985). Group process in cognitive-behavioral therapy. *Behavior Therapist, 8*(4), 71–75.

Rosenberg, S. A., & Zimet, C. N. (1995). Brief group treatment and managed mental health care. *International Journal of Group Psychotherapy, 45*(3), 367–379.

Rosenthal, L. (1992). The new member: "infanticide" in group psychotherapy. *International Journal of Group Psychotherapy, 42*(2), 277–286.

Rudd, M. D., Rajab, M. H., Orman, D. T., Stulman, D. A., Joiner, T., & Dixon, W. (1996). Effectiveness of an outpatient intervention targeting suicidal young adults: Peliminary results. *Journal of Consulting and Clinical Psychology, 64*(1), 179–190.

Rutan, J. S., & Alonso, A. (1982). Group therapy, individual therapy, or both? *International Journal of Group Psychotherapy, 32*(3), 267–282.

Rutan, J. S., & Alonso, A. (1994). Some guidelines for group therapists. *Group, 18*(1), 56–63.

Rutan, S., & Stone, W. (1993). *Psychodynamic group psychotherapy* (2nd ed.). New York: Guilford Press.

Rutan, S., & Stone, W. (2001). *Psychodynamic group psychotherapy* (3rd ed.). New York: Guilford Press.

Sabin, J. E. (1981). Short-term group psychotherapy: Historical antecedents. In S. H. Budman (Ed.), *Forms of brief psychotherapy* (pp. 271–282). New York: Guilford Press.

Sacco, W. P., & Dunn, V. K. (1990). Effect of actor depression on observer attributions: Existence and impact of negative attributions toward the depressed. *Journal of Personality and Social Psychology, 59,* 517–524.

Safan-Gerard, D. (1996). Kleinian approach to group psychotherapy. *International Journal of Group Psychotherapy, 46*(2), 177–191.

Salvendy, J. T. (1999). Ethnocultural considerations in group psychotherapy. *International Journal of Group Psychotherapy, 49*(4), 429–464.

Satterfield, J. M. (1994). Integrating group dynamics and cognitive behavioral groups: A hybrid model. *Clinical Psychology: Science and Practice, 1*(2), 185–196.

Scheidlinger, S. (1960). Group process in group psychotherapy: Trends in the integration of individual and group psychotherapy. *American Journal of Psychotherapy, 14,* 104–120.

Scheidlinger, S. (1964). Identification, the sense of belonging and of identity in small groups. *International Journal of Group Psychotherapy, 14,* 291–306.

Scheidlinger, S. (1974). On the concept of the "mother group." *International Journal of Group Psychotherapy, 24,* 417–428.

Scheidlinger, S. (1993). History of group psychotherapy. In H. I. Kaplan & B. J. Sadock (Eds.), *Comprehensive group psychotherapy* (3rd ed., pp. 2–10). Baltimore: Williams & Wilkin.

Scheidlinger, S. (2000). The group psychotherapy movement at the millennium: Some historical perspectives. *International Journal of Group Psychotherapy, 50*(3), 315–339.

Scheuble, K. J., Dixon, K. N., Levy, A. B., & Kagan-Moore, L. (1987). Premature termination: A risk in eating disorder groups. *Group, 11*(2), 85–93.

Schlachet, P. J. (1990). Unity in duality: The synthesis of individual and group psychoanalytic psychotherapy. *Group, 14*(4), 205–217.

Schoener, G. R., & Luepker, E. T. (1996). Boundaries in group therapy: Ethical and practical issues. In B. DeChant (Ed.), *Women and group psychotherapy: Theory and practice* (pp. 373–399). New York: Guilford Press.

Schoenholtz-Read, J. (1994). Selection of group intervention. In H. S. Bernard & K. R. MacKenzie (Eds.), *Basic of group psychotherapy* (pp. 157–188). New York: Guilford Press.

Schoenholtz-Read, J. (1996). The supervisor as gender analyst: Feminist perspectives on group supervision and training. *International Journal of Group Psychotherapy, 46*(4), 479–500.

Schopler, J. H., & Galinsky, M. J. (1990). Can open-ended groups move beyond beginnings? *Small Group Research, 21*(4), 435–449.

Segal, H. (1974). *Introduction to the work of Melanie Klein* (2nd ed.). New York: Basic Books.

Segrin, C., & Abramson, L. Y. (1994). Negative reactions to depressive behaviors: A communication theories analysis. *Journal of Abnormal Psychology, 103*(4), 655–668.

Shapiro, D., & Shapiro, D. (1982). Meta-analysis of comparative therapy outcome studies: A replication and refinement. *Psychological Bulletin, 92,* 581–604.

Shapiro, E. L., & Ginzberg, R. (2001). The persistently neglected sibling relationship and its applicability to group therapy. *International Journal of Group Psychotherapy, 51*(3), 327–341.

Shechtman, Z. (2001). Prevention groups for angry and aggressive children. *Journal for Specialists in Group Work, 26*(3), 228–236.

Shechtman, Z., & Ben-David, M. (1999). Individual and group psychotherapy of childhood aggression: A comparison of outcomes and processes. *Group Dynamics: Theory, Research, and Practice, 3*(4), 263–274.

Shechtman, Z., & Yanov, H. (2001). Interpretives (confrontation, interpretation, and feedback) in preadolescent counseling groups. *Group Dynamics: Theory, Research and Practice, 5*(2), 124–135.

Shields, W. (2000). Hope and the inclination to be troublesome: Winnicott and the treatment of character disorder in group psychotherapy. *International Journal of Group Psychotherapy, 50*(1), 87–103.

Shuman, D. W., & Foote, W. (1999). *Jaffe v. Redmond's* impact: Life after the Supreme Court's recognition of a psychotherapist-patient privilege. *Professional Psychology: Research and Practice, 30*(5), 479–487.

Skolnick, M. (2000). Microcosm-macrocosm. *Group, 24*(2/3), 133–145.

Slavin, R. (1993). The significance of here-and-now disclosure in promoting cohesion in group psychotherapy. *Group, 17*(3), 143–150.

Slocum, Y. S. (1987). A survey of expectations about group therapy among clinical and nonclinical populations. *International Journal of Group Psychotherapy, 37,* 29–54.

Slovak, J. (2000). *The cognitive and emotional impact of the implantable cardioverter defibrillator pre- and post-participation in a time-limited support group.* (Doctoral dissertation, Widener University, 2000). *Dissertation Abstracts International, 61,* 2223. Ann Arbor, MI: Dissertation Information Services.

Slovenko, R. (1998). *Psychotherapy and confidentiality: Testimonial privileged communication, breach of confidentiality, and reporting duties.* Springfield, IL: Charles C Thomas.

Small, R. W., & Schinke, S. P. (1983). Teaching competence in residential group care: Cognitive problem solving and interpersonal skills training with emotionally disturbed preadolescents. *Journal of Social Service Research, 7*(1), 1–16.

Smead, R. (1995). *Skills and techniques for group work with children and adolescents.* Champaign, IL: Research Press.

Smith, M. H., Glass, G. V., & Miller, T. (1980). *The benefits of psychotherapy.* Baltimore: Johns Hopkins University Press.

Snyder, C. R. (1994). *The psychology of hope: You can get there from here.* New York: Free Press.

Snyder, C. R., Cheavens, J., & Sympson, S. C. (1997). Hope: An individual motive for social commerce. *Group Dynamics: Theory, Research, and Practice, 1*(2), 107–118.

Snyder, C. R., & Hackman, A. (1998). *Hope and pain tolerance: A replication.* Unpublished manuscript, University of Kansas, Lawrence.

Snyder, D. R., Ilardi, S., Michael, S. T., & Cheavens, J. (2000). Hope theory: Updating a common process for psychological change. In C. R. Snyder & R. E. Ingram (Eds.), *Handbook of psychological change: Psychotherapy processes and practices for the 21st century* (pp. 128–153). New York: Wiley.

Somberg, D. R., Stone, G. L., & Claiborn, P. C. (1993). Informed consent: Therapists' beliefs and practices. *Professional Psychology: Research and Practice, 24,* 153–159.

Soo, E. S. (1998). Is training and supervision of children and adolescents group therapists necessary? *Journal of Child and Adolescent Group Therapy, 8*(4), 181–196.

Sorenson, M. (2001, Fall). Resting on common ground: Integrating psychodynamic group therapy with other models. *The group solution,* Newsletter of the National Registry of Certified Group Psychotherapists.

Sorrels, J. P., & Myers, B. (1983). Comparison of group and family dynamics. *Human Relations, 35*(5), 477–492.

Spiegel, D., Bloom, J. R., Kraemer, H. C., & Gottheil, E. (1989). Effect of psychosocial treatment on survival of patients with metastatic breast cancer. *Lancet, 2,* 888–891.

Spillius, E. B. (1993). Varieties of envious experiences. *International Journal of Psychoanalysis, 24,* 1199–1212.

Spitz, H. E. (1997). The effect of managed mental health care on group psychotherapy:

Treatment, training and therapy morale issues. *International Journal of Group Psychotherapy, 47*(1), 23–30.

Spitzer, R. L., Indicott, J., & Robbins, E. (1978). Research diagnostic criteria: Rationale and reliability. *Archives of General Psychiatry, 35,* 773–782.

Spivack, G., Platt, J. J., & Shure, M. B. (1976). *The problem-solving approach to adjustment.* San Francisco: Jossey-Bass.

State v. Andring Supreme Court of Minnesota. (1984). 342 N. W.2d 128: In R. Reisner, C. Slobogin, & A. Rai (Eds.), *Law and the mental health system: Civil and criminal aspects* (3rd ed., pp. 358–360). St. Paul, MN: West.

Steenbarger, B. N., & Budman, S. H. (1996). Group psychotherapy and managed behavioral health care: Current trends and future challenges. *International Journal of Group Psychotherapy, 46,* 297–309.

Steinmetz, J. L., Lewinsohn, P. M., & Antonuccio, D. O. (1983). Prediction of individual outcome in a group intervention for depression. *Journal of Consulting and Clinical Psychology, 51*(3), 331–337.

Stern, J. (2000). Parent training. In J. R. White & A. S. Freeman (Eds.), *Cognitive-behavioral group therapy for specific problems and populations* (pp. 331–360). Washington, DC: American Psychological Association.

Steuer, J. L., Mintz, J., Hammen, C. L., Hill, M. A., Jarvik, L. F., McCarley, T., et al. (1984). Cognitive-behavioral and psychodynamic group psychotherapy in treatment of geriatric depression. *Journal of Consulting and Clinical Psychology, 52*(2), 180–189.

Stockton, R., Morran, D. K., & Nitza, A. G. (2000). Processing group events: A conceptual map for leaders, *Journal for Specialists in Group Work, 25*(4), 343–355.

Stockton, R., Rohde, R. I., & Haughey, J. (1992). The effects of structured group exercises on cohesion, engagement, avoidance, and conflict. *Small Group Research, 23*(2), 155–168.

Stone, W. (1995). The dynamics of the cotherapy relationship: A symposium: Discussion. *Group, 19*(2), 117–119.

Stone, W. N., Rodenhauser, P. H., & Markert, R. J. (1991). Combining group psychotherapy and pharmacotherapy: A survey. *International Journal of Group Psychotherapy, 41,* 449–464.

Strassberg, D. S., Roback, H. B., Anchor, K. N., & Abramowitz, S. I. (1975). Self-disclosure in group therapy with schizophrenics. *Archives of General Psychiatry, 32*(10), 1259–1261.

Stravynski, A., Gaudetter, G., Lesage, A., Arbel, N., Petit, P., Clerc, D., et al. (1997). The treatment of sexually dysfunctional men without partners: A controlled study of three behavioral group approaches. *British Journal of psychiatry, 170,* 338–344.

Stricker, G., & Healey, B. (1990). Projective assessment of object relations: A review of the empirical literature. Psychological assessment. *Journal of Consulting and Clinical Psychology, 2,* 219–230.

Subich, L. M., & Coursol, D. H. (1985). Counseling expectations of clients and non-clients for group and individual treatment modes. *Journal of Counseling Psychology, 32,* 245–251.

Sue, D. W., & Sue, D. (1999). *Counseling the culturally different: Theory and practice.* New York: Wiley.

Sullivan, H. S. (1953). *Conceptions of modern psychiatry: The first William Alanson White memorial lectures* (2nd ed.) New York: Norton.

Talbot, N. L., Houghtalen, R. P., Duberstein, P. R., Cox, C., Giles, D. E., & Wynne, L. C. (1999). Effects if group treatment for women with a history of childhood sexual abuse. *Psychiatric Services, 50*(5), 686–692.

Taylor, R. E., & Gazda, G. M. (1991). Concurrent individual and group therapy: The ethical issues. *Journal of Group Psychotherapy Psychodrama and Sociometry, 44*(2), 51–59.

Telch, M. J., Lucas, J. A., Schmidt, N. B., Hanna, H., Haimez, T. L., & Lucas, R. A. (1993). Group cognitive-behavioral treatment of panic disorder. *Behavior Research and Therapy, 31*, 279–287.

Thase, M. E. (2000). Psychopharmacology in conjunction with psychotherapy. In C. R. Snyder & R. E. Ingram (Eds.), *Handbook of psychological change: psychotherapy processes and practices for the 21st century* (pp. 474–497). New York: Wiley.

Thase, M. E., & Beck, A. T. (1993). An overview of cognitive therapy. In J. H. Wright, M. E. Thase, A. T. Beck, & J. W. Ludgate (Eds.), *Cognitive therapy with inpatients: Developing a cognitive milieu* (pp. 3–34). New York: Guilford Press.

Tiller, J. M., Sloane, G., Schmidt, U., Troop, N., Power, M., & Treasure, J. L. (1997). Social support in patients with anorexia nervosa and bulimia nervosa. *International Journal of Eating Disorders, 21*, 31–38.

Tillitski, L. (1990). A meta-analysis of estimated effect sizes for group versus individual versus control treatments. *International Journal of Group Psychotherapy, 40*(2), 215–224.

Tinsely, H. E., Roth, J. A., & Lease, S. H. (1989). Dimensions of leadership and leadership style among group intervention specialists. *Journal of Counseling Psychology, 36*(1), 48–53.

Toner, B. B., Segal, Z. V., Emmott, S., Myran, D., Ali, A., DiGasbarro, I., et al. (1998). Cognitive-behavioral group therapy for patients with irritable bowel syndrome. *International Journal of Group Psychotherapy, 48*(2), 215–243.

Toseland, R., & Siporin, M. (1986). When to recommend group treatment. *International Journal of Group Psychotherapy, 36*, 172–201.

Truax, C. B., & Carkhuff, R. R. (1965). Client and therapist transparency in the psychotherapeutic encounter. *Journal of Counseling Psychology, 12*(1), 3–9.

Truax, C. B., & Carkhuff, R. R. (1967). *Towards effective counseling and psychotherapy.* Chicago: Aldine.

Truax, C. B., Carkhuff, R. R., & Kodman, J. (1965). Relationships between therapist-offered conditions and patient change in group psychotherapy. *Journal of Clinical Psychology, 21*(3), 327–329.

Tschuschke, V., & Dies, R. R. (1994). Intensive analysis of therapeutic factors and outcome in long term inpatient groups. *International Journal of Group Psychotherapy, 44*, 185–208.

Tuttman, S. (1992). The role of the therapist from an object relations perspective. In R. H. Klein, H. S. Bernard, & D. L. Singer (Eds.), *Handbook of contemporary group psychotherapy: Contributions from object relations, self psychology, and social systems theories* (pp. 241–277). Madison, CT: International Universities Press.

Vinogradov, S., & Yalom, I. (1989). *A concise guide to group psychotherapy.* Washington, DC: American Psychiatric Press.

Von Bertalanffy, L. (1950). The theory of open systems in physics and biology. *Science, 3,* 23–29.

Waldinger, R., & Gunderson, J. (1984). Completed psychotherapies with border-line patients. *American Journal of Psychotherapy, 38,* 190–202.

Weigel, R. G., Dinges, N., Dyer, R., & Straumfjord, A. A. (1972). Perceived self-disclosure, mental health, and who is liked in group treatment. *Journal of Counseling Psychology, 19*(1), 47–51.

Weigel, R. G., & Warnath, C. F. (1968). The effects of group therapy on reported self-disclosure. *International Journal of Group Psychotherapy, 18,* 31–41.

Weinberg, H. (2001). Group process and group phenomena on the Internet. *International Journal of Group Psychotherapy, 51*(3), 361–378.

Weiner, M. (1993). Role of the leader in group psychotherapy. In H. I. Kaplan & B. J. Sadock (Eds.), *Comprehensive group psychotherapy* (3rd ed., pp. 84–98). Baltimore: Williams & Wilkins.

Weiner, N. (1948). *Cybernetics or control and communication in the animal and in the machine.* New York: Wiley.

Weishaar, M. E., & Beck, A. T. (1987). Cognitive therapy. In W. Dryden & W. L. Golden (Eds.), *Cognitive-behavioral approaches to psychotherapy* (pp. 61–91). New York: Hemisphere.

Wetcher, C. (2000). *Counseling groups in schools can aid in adolescent identity development.* (Doctoral dissertation, Widener University, 2000). *Dissertation Abstracts International, 61,* 2230. Ann Arbor, MI: Dissertation Information Services.

Wheelan, S. (1997). Group development and the practice of group psychotherapy. *Group Dynamics: Theory, Research, and Practice, 1*(4), 288–293.

White, J. R. (2000a). Introduction. In J. R. White & A. S. Freeman (Eds.), *Cognitive-behavioral group therapy: For specific problems and populations* (pp. 3–25). Washington, DC: American Psychological Association.

White, J. R. (2000b). Depression. In J. R. White & A. S. Freeman (Eds.), *Cognitive-behavioral group therapy: For specific problems and populations* (pp. 29–61). Washington, DC: American Psychological Association.

Widiger, T. A., & Rorer, L. G. (1984). The responsible psychotherapist. *American Psychologist, 39*(5), 503–515.

Wilhite, S. C., & Payne, D. E. (1992). *Learning and memory: The basis of behavior.* Boston: Allyn & Bacon.

Winnicott, D. W. (1945). Primitive emotional development. *International Journal of Psycho-Analysis, 26,* 137–143.

Winnicott, D. W. (1958). *Collected papers: Through paediatrics to psycho-analysis.* New York: Basic Books.

Winnicott, D. W. (1965). *The maturational processes and the facilitating environment: Studies in the theory of emotional development.* New York: International Universities Press.

Winnicott, D. W. (1971). *Playing and reality.* Baltimore, MD: Penguin.

Wong, N. (1980). Combined group and individual treatment of borderline and narcissistic patients: Heterogeneous versus homogeneous groups. *International Journal of Group Psychotherapy, 30*(4), 389–404.

Woolf, H. B. (Ed.). (1981). *Webster's new collegiate dictionary*. Springfield, MA: Merriam.

Wright, F. (2000). The use of the self in group leadership: A relationship perspective. *International Journal of Group Psychotherapy, 50*(2), 181–198.

Wright, J. H., Thase, M. E., Beck, A. T., & Ludgate, J. W. (1993). *Cognitive therapy with inpatients: Developing a cognitive milieu.* New York: Guilford Press.

Yalom, I. (1983). *Inpatient group psychotherapy.* New York: Basic Books.

Yalom, I. (1985). *The theory and practice of group psychotherapy* (3rd ed.). New York: Basic Books.

Yalom, I. (1990). *Understanding group psychotherapy: Process and practice* [Film]. Pacific Grove, CA: Brookes/Cole.

Yalom, I. (1993). *Inpatient group psychotherapy.* New York: Basic Books.

Yalom, I. (1995). *The theory and practice of group psychotherapy* (4th ed.). New York: Basic Books.

Yalom, I. D. (1970). *The theory and practice of group psychotherapy.* New York: Basic Books.

Yalom, I. D. (1975). *The theory and practice of group psychotherapy* (2nd ed.). New York: Basic Books.

Yalom, I., Tinklenberg, J., & Gilula, M. (1968). *Curative factors in group therapy.* Unpublished study, Stanford University, Department of Psychiatry, Stanford, CA.

Zappe, C., & Epstein, D. (1987). Assertive training. *Journal of Psychosocial Nursing and Mental Health Services, 25*(8), 23–26.

Zerhusen, J., Boyle, K., & Wilson, W. (1991). Out of the darkness: Group cognitive therapy for depressed elderly. *Journal of Psychosocial Nursing, 29,* 16–21.

Author Index

Subject Index

A

B

C

H

I